Uncommon Infections
and Special Topics

DEDICATION

To the patients whose lives have been
changed by reproductive tract infections,
and to the doctors who have treated them

* * * * * * * *

"Without life, there is no joy; without
joy there is no life."

After Sophocles

To J.V. from L.K.

Infections in Reproductive Health

VOLUME II

Uncommon Infections and Special Topics

EDITOR

Louis G. Keith, MD, FACOG

Professor
Department of Obstetrics and Gynecology
Northwestern University Medical School, and
Attending Obstetrician-Gynecologist
The Prentice Women's Hospital and Medical Center
of Northwestern Memorial Hospital
Chicago, Illinois, USA

ASSOCIATE EDITOR

Gary S. Berger, MD, MSPH, FACOG

Director, Chapel Hill Fertility Services, and
Adjunct Associate Professor
Department of Maternal and Child Health
University of North Carolina School of Public Health
Chapel Hill, North Carolina, USA

ASSISTANT EDITOR

David A. Edelman, PhD

President
Medical Research Consultants, Inc.
Chapel Hill, North Carolina, USA

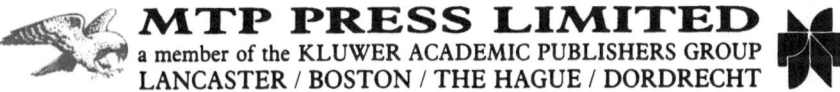

MTP PRESS LIMITED
a member of the KLUWER ACADEMIC PUBLISHERS GROUP
LANCASTER / BOSTON / THE HAGUE / DORDRECHT

Published in the UK and Europe by
MTP Press Limited
Falcon House
Lancaster, England

British Library Cataloguing in Publication Data

Uncommon infections and special topics. — (Infections in
  reproductive health; v. 2)
  1. Generative organs—Diseases
  I. Keith, Louis II. Berger, Gary, S.
  III. Edelman, David A. IV. Series 616.6′5 RC875
  ISBN-13: 978-94-010-8671-4   e-ISBN-13: 978-94-009-4902-7
  DOI: 10.1007/978-94-009-4902-7

Published in the USA by
MTP Press
A division of Kluwer Boston Inc
190 Old Derby Street
Hingham, MA 02043, USA

Library of Congress Cataloging in Publication Data

Main entry under title:

Infections in reproductive health.

  Includes bibliographies and index.
  Contents: v. 2. Uncommon infections and special topics.
  1. Generative organs—Infections—Collected works. 2.
Generative organs—Infections—Complications and
sequelae—Collected works. 3. Human reproduction—
Collected works. 4. Pregnancy, Complications of—
Collected works. I. Keith, Louis G. II. Berger, Gary
S. III. Edelman, David A. IV. Title: Common
infections. [DNLM: 1. Genital Diseases, Female. 2.
Genital Diseases, Male. 3. Infection—in pregnancy. 4.
Urinary Tract Infections. WP 140 I43]
RC877.I54   1984   618   84–26132

Phototypesetting by Titus Wilson, Kendal, Cumbria

Contents

CONTENTS

CONTENTS

vii

Contents

Index

Foreword

Infectious diseases remain a major problem for physicians and other health professionals dealing with problems of the reproductive system. Accordingly, this two-volume comprehensive presentation of infectious diseases involving the male and female reproductive systems promises to be a major contribution in this field and to fill a much-needed vacuum.

During the past three decades, the introduction of antimicrobial therapy has dramatically altered both the clinical presentation and the therapeutic approaches employed in dealing with the traditional infections of the reproductive system. In addition, the changing demographics of infectious problems in the industrial countries and the developing world have been a source of concern. A good deal of important information on this topic is included in this series.

In recent years, considerable attention has been given to the role of *Mycoplasma* and *Chlamydia* in both male and female infertility and the problems related to genital herpes and human papilloma virus infections. Current clinical information is included on these infections as well as on newer aspects of diagnosis, such as the use of laparoscopy in the diagnosis and treatment of pelvic inflammatory disease. Also addressed is new information regarding the role of actinomycosis in pelvic infections; current problems such as toxic shock syndrome and acquired immune deficiency syndrome (AIDS) are reviewed as well.

New concepts are included in these volumes to complement the clinical information. The attachment of microbial organisms to sperm may help to explain access of these and other organisms to the upper female genital tract. Similarly, the role of asymptomatic bacteriospermia and the reproductive effects of other microorganisms in semen are carefully considered. There are also information relating to animal models for the study of human genital infections that may be of value to researchers in this field, important clinical information relating to infections and contraception, detailed discussions of human papilloma virus infections and their oncogenic potential, and separate discussions of sexually transmitted diseases in children of both sexes.

The editors of this two-volume series have undertaken and completed an enormous task assembling and coordinating the contributions to this series made by international experts. The state of the art of diagnosis and therapy of infections in reproductive health has been presented in a comprehensive and readable fashion. These two volumes will be of value to clinicians in the field of family medicine, public health, international health, internal medicine, obstetrics and gynecology, and urology, and indeed, to all health professionals dealing with those infectious diseases that affect the reproductive systems of men and women.

FOREWORD

The editors have aimed for a comprehensive presentation and have accomplished this objective. The publication of this two-volume series should prove to be a highly useful contemporary reference source. The editors and the contributors are to be congratulated on a job well done.

JOHN J. SCIARRA, MD, PhD
Thomas J. Watkins Professor and Chairman,
Department of Obstetrics and Gynecology,
Northwestern University Medical School,
Chicago, Illinois

Acknowledgments

The editors wish to acknowledge the following individuals and organizations without whose support these volumes could not have come into being:

Professor E. S. E. Hafez, for the idea;

Paula Hamilton, for keeping the project going in the face of a multitude of problems of organization and communication;

Vito Maiorano, for meticulous copy editing;

Barbara Carlson, for initial secretarial help;

The Center for the Advancement of Reproductive Health, Chicago and Chapel Hill, for providing funds to edit and coordinate the authors' manuscripts;

The Departments of Obstetrics and Gynecology, Northwestern University Medical School and Chapel Hill Fertility Services, for technical and secretarial support.

Last, but by no means least, it has been a pleasure to work with Mr. David Bloomer, and his successor, Dr. Peter Clarke, their staff at MTP Press – in particular their editor, Mr. Philip Johnstone – who have made this international collaboration a rewarding endeavor.

Louis G. Keith

Preface

It hardly seems necessary to justify the preparation of a book on infections in reproductive health. These afflictions have bothered mankind since antiquity and have accounted for untold numbers of personal tragedies. Unfortunately, until relatively recently, there was little that could be done either to prevent or to treat the spread of these infections. Moreover, the fact that they often afflicted both partners of a conjugal unit was so obvious that it was frequently lost by the practitioners who attempted to treat individual patients, be they male or female.

The advent of antibiotic therapies was supposed to be the dawn of a new era, but in many ways it wasn't. It soon became painfully apparent that the treatment of a specific patient by a specific drug was not enough. As is often the case in medicine, the literature lagged behind clinical practice, and textbooks and monographs spoke about genital infections in males and in females as if there were no connection between them. Clearly, such is not the case, and clinicians who are concerned about appropriately treating genital infections must often deal with their patient's partner(s) or be doomed to failure from the start.

These two volumes were conceived with the idea that clinicians must consider the broader aspects of genital tract infections, even though their primary specialities may be obstetrics and gynecology, or urology, internal medicine, dermatology, or family practice. Perhaps some individuals practicing in clinics treating sexually transmitted diseases might be exempt from this admonition, but certainly not all.

This book had its genesis at the International Conference on Infections in Reproductive Health held in Maui, Hawaii, in 1982 under the aegis of Professor E. S. E. Hafez. Some of the chapters were prepared by speakers at this conference; other authors were invited to contribute. As a result, the authors come from a number of distinguished medical centers and universities throughout the world. In some chapters there will be overlap; in others, there are differences of opinion. Not only are both of these circumstances inevitable in a multiauthored text, but the reader should appreciate that the complexity of the subject contributes to the difficulty of arriving at a consensus. The various chapters contain much information not usually readily accessible to the average practitioner. It is our sincere hope that the readers will have a greater appreciation of the subject of infections in reproductive health after reading this book.

Louis G. Keith
Gary S. Berger
David A. Edelman

POSTSCRIPT

After the manuscripts had gone to the printer, the editor became aware of a series of publications on the incidence of colonization with *Actinomyces* in normal women written by Elizabeth Persson, from the Department of Obstetrics and Gynecology, the Karolinska Institutet, Danderyd Hospital, Danderyd, Sweden, and the Section for Medical Mycology, the National Bacteriological Laboratory, Stockholm, Sweden. Since it was not possible at that late moment to revise the text and reset type on every comment dealing with *Actinomyces*, we encourage interested readers to read the following references:

1. Persson, E., Holmberg, K., Dahlgren, S. and Nilsson, L. (1983). *Actinomyces israelii* in the genital tract of women with and without intra-uterine contraceptive devices. *Acta Obstet. Gynecol. Scand.*, **62,** 563

2. Persson, E. and Holmberg, K. (1984). Genital colonization by *Actinomyces israelii* and serologic immune response to the bacterium after five years use of the same copper intra-uterine device. *Acta Obstet. Gynecol. Scand.*, **63,** 202

3. Persson, E. and Holmberg, K. (1984). A longitudinal study of *Actinomyces israelii* in the female genital tract. *Acta Obstet. Gynecol. Scand.*, **63,** 207

Paper No. 3 reports that *A. israelii* was recovered in 24% of the perineal, 13% of the vaginal, and 6% of the cervical samples, respectively. The occurrence of *A. israelii* was not related to the phase of the menstrual cycle, amount of bleeding or discharge, vaginal pH, the contraceptive method used (including the IUD) or the use of different sanitary products. The authors concluded that *A. israelii* was a part of the indigenous genital flora of healthy women.

Paper No. 2 reports that no significant differences were found in the rate of colonization in a group of 74 women wearing IUDs for 60 ± 6 months compared to 44 women in a control group wearing their IUDs for 36 ± 6 months.

Paper No. 1 reports that immunofluorescent staining and cultures identified *A. israelii* in 4% of 68 IUD users and 3% of 68 women without IUDs. This difference was not significant.

Louis G. Keith

List of Contributors

J. J. AMY
Department of Gynecology and
  Obstetrics
Vrije Universiteit Brussels,
Laarbeeklaan 101,
B-1090 Brussels, Belgium

Department of Gynecology,
  Andrology and Obstetrics,
Academisch Ziekenhuis Vrije
  Universiteit Brussels,
Laarbeeklaan 101,
B-1090 Brussels, Belgium

O. P. ARYA
Department of Genito-Urinary
  Medicine,
Liverpool University Medical School,
Prescot Street,
Liverpool L7 8XP, UK

Department of Genito-Urinary
  Medicine,
Royal Liverpool Hospital,
Prescot Street,
Liverpool L7 8XP, UK

B. F. ATKINSON
Department of Cytopathology,
University of Pennsylvania,
3400 Spruce Street Ground Floor
  Gibson Building,
Philadelphia,
Pennsylvania 19104, USA

Department of Cytopathology,
Hospital of the University of
  Pennsylvania,
3400 Spruce Street Ground Floor
  Gibson Building,
Philadelphia,
Pennsylvania 19104, USA

A. S. BASALAMAH
Department of Obstetrics and
  Gynecology,
King Abdulaziz Medical School,
P.O. Box 6615,
Jeddah,
Saudi Arabia 21452

Department of Obstetrics and
  Gynecology
King Abdulaziz University Hospital,
P.O. Box 6615,
Jeddah,
Saudi Arabia 21452

M. D. BENSON
Department of Obstetrics and
  Gynecology,
The Prentice Women's Hospital and
  Medical Center of Northwestern
  Memorial Hospital,
333 East Superior Street,
Chicago, Illinois 60611, USA

G. S. BERGER
Chapel Hill Fertility Services
109 Conner Drive
Suite 2104,
Chapel Hill,
North Carolina 27514, USA

E. R. BROWN
Department of Microbiology,
Chicago Medical School,
3333 Greenbay Road,
North Chicago, Illinois 60064, USA

American International Hospital,
Zion, Illinois 60099, USA

I. BURZACO
Hospital Clinico y Provincial,
Departamento de Obstetricia y
  Ginecologia,
Casanova, 143
Barcelona 11, Spain

J. E. FOWLER, Jr.
Department of Urology,
University of Virginia School of
  Medicine,
P.O. Box 422,
Charlottesville, Virginia 22908, USA

E. R. CASAS
Department of Obstetrics and
  Gynecology,
The Prentice Women's Hospital and
  Medical Center of Northwestern
  Memorial Hospital,
333 East Superior Street,
Chicago, Illinois 60611, USA

M. GALBRAITH
Department of Medicine,
Uniformed Services University of the
  Health Sciences School of Medicine,
Bethesda, Maryland, USA.

Department of Infectious Diseases,
SGHMMI/Wilford Hall,
USAF Medical Center,
Lackland AFB, Texas 78236, USA

T. A. CHAPEL
Department of Dermatology,
Wayne State University,
Detroit, Michigan 48207, USA

J. GONZALEZ-MERLO
Department of Obstetrics and
  Gynecology,
Barcelona University School of
  Medicine,
Calle Casanova, 143,
08036, Barcelona, Spain

A. W. CHOW
Division of Infectious Diseases,
University of British Columbia,
1119 Gilston Road,
West Vancouver,
British Columbia,
Canada V7S 2E7

Division of Infectious Diseases,
Vancouver General Hospital,
Vancouver, British Columbia,
Canada V7S 2E7

Department of Obstetrics and
  Gynecology,
Hospital Clinico y Provincial,
c/. Casanova 143,
Barcelona 36, Spain

D. H. GREMILLION
Department of Internal Medicine,
University of Texas Health Science
  Center S.A.,
San Antonio, Texas, USA

D. L. COHN
Department of Infectious Diseases,
University of Colorado Health
  Sciences Center,
605 Bannock Street,
Denver, Colorado 80204, USA

Wilford Hall USAF Medical Center,
Infectious Diseases Service,
Lackland AFB,
Texas 78236, USA

Department of Denver Health &
  Hospitals,
Denver Metro Tuberculosis Clinic,
Denver, Colorado 80204, USA

L. IGLESIAS-CORTIT
Department of Obstetrics and
  Gynecology,
Barcelona University,
50 P. San Gervasio,
Barcelona-08022, Spain

W. FOULON
Department of Gynecology,
  Andrology and Obstetrics,
Academisch Ziekenhuis Vrije
  Universiteit Brussels,
Laarbeeklaan, 101,
B-1090 Brussels, Belgium

Department of Family Planning,
Hospital Clinico,
Barcelona-08022, Spain

J. IGLESIAS-GUIU
Department of Obstetrics and
  Gynecology,
Hospital Clinico y Provincial,
c/. Casanova 143,
Barcelona 36, Spain

P. J JEWESSON
Faculty of Pharmaceutical Sciences,
University of British Columbia,
2146 East Mall,
Vancouver, British Columbia,
Canada V6T 1W5

P. JOU
Department of Obstetrics and
  Gynecology,
Hospital Clinico y Provincial,
Casanova 143,
Barcelona 36, Spain

F. N. JUDSON
Department of Medicine,
University of Colorado Health
  Sciences Center,
605 Bannock Street,
Denver, Colorado 80204, USA

Division of Infectious Diseases,
Denver Health and Hospitals,
Denver, Colorado 80204, USA

L. G. KEITH
Department of Obstetrics and
  Gynecology
Northwestern University Medical
  School
333 East Superior Street,
Chicago, Illinois 60611, USA

Department of Obstetrics and
  Gynecology,
The Prentice Women's Hospital and
  Maternity Center of Northwestern
  Memorial Hospital,
333 East Superior Street,
Chicago, Illinois 60611, USA

E. KITA
Department of Bacteriology
Nara Medical College,
840, Shijyocho Kashihara City,
Nara 634, Japan

M. KOCHHAR
Department of Medical Sciences,
University of Delhi,
5-A Kalindi Colony,
Darya Gunj,
New Delhi-110065, India

Department of Obstetrics and
  Gynecology,
Kasturba Hospital,
5-A Kalindi Colony,
Darya Gunj,
New Delhi-110065, India

G. VON KROGH
Karolinska Institute,
School of Medicine,
10064 Stockholm 38,
Sweden

Department of Dermatology,
Södersjukhuset,
10064 Stockholm 38,
Sweden

S. LAUWERS
Department of Microbiology,
Academisch Ziekenhuis Vrije
  Universiteit Brussels,
Laarbeeklaan 101,
B-1090 Brussels, Belgium

V. A. LIVOLSI
Department of Pathology and
  Laboratory Medicine,
University of Pennsylvania School of
  Medicine,
3400 Spruce Street,
Philadelphia, Pennsylvania 19104,
  USA

Surgical Pathology Section,
Hospital of the University of
  Pennsylvania,
3400 Spruce Street,
Ground Floor Gibson Building,
Philadelphia, Pennsylvania 19104,
  USA

M. MARQUEZ
Department of Obstetrics and
  Gynecology,Hospital Clinico y
  Provincial,
Casanova, 143,
Barcelona-11, Spain

M. W. METHOD
Department of Obstetrics and
  Gynecology,
The Prentice Women's Hospital and
  Maternity Center of Northwestern
  Memorial Hospital,
333 East Superior Street,
Chicago, Illinois 60611, USA

A. NAESSENS
Department of Microbiology,
Academische Ziekenhuis Vrije
  Universiteit Brussels,
Laarbeeklaan 101,
1090 Brussels, Belgium

J. RAHMAN
Department of Obstetrics and
  Gynecology,
King Faisal University,
College of Medicine,
P.O. Box 2114, Dammam-31451,
Saudi Arabia

Department of Obstetrics and
  Gynecology,
King Fahd Hospital of the University,
Al-Khobar, Saudi Arabia

M. S. RAHMAN
Department of Obstetrics and
  Gynecology,
King Faisal University,
College of Medicine,
P.O. Box 2114, Dammam-31451,
Saudi Arabia

Department of Obstetrics and
  Gynecology,
King Fahd Hospital of the University,
Al-Khobar, Saudi Arabia

P. J. RETTIG
Department of Pediatrics,
College of Medicine,
University of Oklahoma Health
  Sciences Center,
430 NW 20th Street,
Oklahoma City,
Oklahoma 73103, USA

Pediatric Infectious Diseases,
Oklahoma Children's Memorial
  Hospital,
P.O. Box 26307,
Oklahoma City,
Oklahoma 73125, USA

F. E. SEREBOUR
Department of Immunology,
King Abdulaziz University Hospital,
P.O. Box 6615,
Jeddah 21452, Saudi Arabia

A. F. SINGLETON
Department of Pediatrics,
Charles R. Drew Medical School and
  University of California at Los
  Angeles,
11908 Dorothy Street,
Los Angeles,
California 90049, USA

Department of Ambulatory Pediatrics,
Martin Luther King, Jr. General
  Hospital,
Los Angeles,
California 90059, USA

M. P. SMELTZER
Columbus Health Department,
181 So. Washington Building,
Columbus, Ohio 43215, USA

C. E. SWENSON
Department of Laboratory Medicine,
University of California,
San Francisco, California 94110, USA

The Liposome Co., Inc.,
1 Research Way,
Princeton Forrestal Center,
Princeton, New Jersey 08540, USA

K. J. SYRJÄNEN
Department of Pathology,
University of Kuopio,
P.O. Box 6 Sf-70211,
Kuopio 21, Finland

Department of Pathology,
Kuopio University Central Hospital,
Kuopio, Finland

A. TOTH
Department of Obstetrics and
  Gynecology,
Cornell Medical Center,
525 E 68th Street,
New York, New York 10021, USA

1
Uncommon Infections

1
Tuberculous infections of the female genital tract

J. GONZÁLEZ-MERLO, I. BURZACO, P. JOU and M. MARQUEZ

INTRODUCTION

Since first described by Morgagni in 1779, tuberculosis of the female genital tract has classically presented with a florid group of symptoms and palpable pelvic masses. In the past 40 years, however, with the advent of potent chemotherapeutic agents, the mode of presentation has become milder. Physicians now are able to treat patients with silent genital tuberculosis, the so-called latent forms, which are usually associated with infertility. Indeed, many such patients present without any symptoms and with a normal pelvic examination. Only later are they diagnosed as having genital tuberculosis. Unfortunately, modern antituberculous therapy is followed by serious side-effects, including abortion and ectopic pregnancy. In this regard the spontaneous cure of tuberculous salpingitis may also cause the same type of complications. In recent years the prevalence of genital tuberculosis has declined greatly in Western countries, although some authors have reported a significant rise of tuberculosis in menopausal women (Hutchins, 1977; Falk *et al.*, 1980; Sutherland, 1982).

ETIOPATHOGENESIS

Genital tuberculosis is generally caused by *Mycobacterium tuberculosus hominis*. Only in rare cases are bovine strains of this organism implicated, as occurs in cases of women consuming nonpasteurized milk. In women, genital tuberculosis is nearly always secondary to primary lesions in the lung, although peritoneal and lymph node involvement may precede genital tuberculosis.

Starting from a primary focus, the tubercle bacilli may reach the genital tract by hematogenous, lymphatic, or direct spread. Hematogenous spread is the most common mechanism and represents 80–90% of cases. The well-vascularized ampullary portions of the tubes are particularly susceptible to infection,

3

which is usually bilateral. Fluid, exudate, and pus then either descend from the tubes to the lower genital tract or reach the ovary and peritoneal cavity. The infection may spread to lower sites of the genital tract, including the endometrium, cervix, vagina, and vulva. Rarely are any of these lower sites directly infected via hematogenous dissemination or direct contact with infected secretions from a male sexual partner.

When the primary focus is abdominal, dissemination to the genital tract may take place by lymphatic spread, although this type of occurrence is rare. Also very uncommon is direct spread to the genital organs from the neighboring viscera, such as the bladder or gut. However, the tubes can be infected from the serosa or through the abdominal ostium via canalicular spread. Ascending primary infection is rarely a result of sexual transmission by a male partner with genital tuberculosis. This is somewhat surprising, since tuberculous bacilli are commonly found in the urine, semen, and epididymal aspirates of infected males.

Primary infection commonly occurs during puberty or in the early teens; it may remain latent for years before symptoms become evident or before any clinical investigation is made. Often, no evidence of the primary focus remains when genital tuberculosis is finally diagnosed. This was the case in 10–40% of the patients in the review by Magnin *et al.* (1981).

PATHOLOGY

Gross appearance

The tubes may appear normal or present with slight edema, and erythema in the presence of filmy adhesions to neighboring organs; in about one-third of the cases the tubes remain patent (Nogales *et al.*, 1979). Gross thickening and dilatation due to occlusion, particularly evident in clubbing of the ampullae, and multiple adhesions occur in the remaining two-thirds of cases (Fig. 1). Serosal involvement with greyish-yellow granules occurs in 20% of cases (Nogales *et al.*, 1979).

On section the tubal wall appears normal, but a greyish-yellow rim of fibrosis surrounds the lumen. Ulceration of the mucosa and caseation occur occasionally. A blood-stained exudate or pus is often due to secondary infection.

The uterus remains small in 30% of cases. The cavity is generally normal, although ulcers may be noted in the cornual regions or there may even be extensive areas of caseation. While the cervix is rarely affected, copious exudate and caseum may be seen. The canal may have a fungoid or polipoid granulomatous appearance that resembles carcinoma. Ulcers are rare.

The ovary is seldom affected, but perioophoritis is charactererized by miliary seedings, which are usually associated with perisalpingitis or peritoneal tuberculosis.

Vulvovaginal tuberculosis is extremely rare. Ulcers with regular borders appear; these tend to merge and possess an irregular base and occasionally caseum. Advanced cases produce rectal or vaginal fistulae.

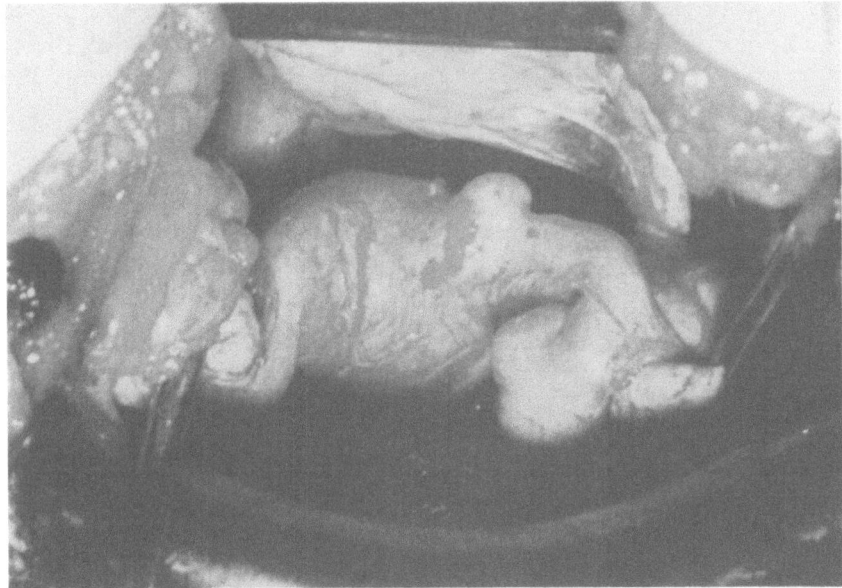

Figure 1 A 19-year-old girl with primary amenorrhea and biphasic BBT. Gross adhesions involving the adnexa. Both tubes are enlarged and occluded. The uterus is small and the ovaries are normal. Histology revealed tuberculous salpingitis

Histology

The histologic picture in florid cases characteristically exhibits a tubal lumen with caseum, thinned and confluent mucosal folds, and a tubal wall with confluent epithelioid granulomas, occasionally with caseum. The muscularis contains a heavy lymphocyte infiltration like in other affected organs (Figs. 2

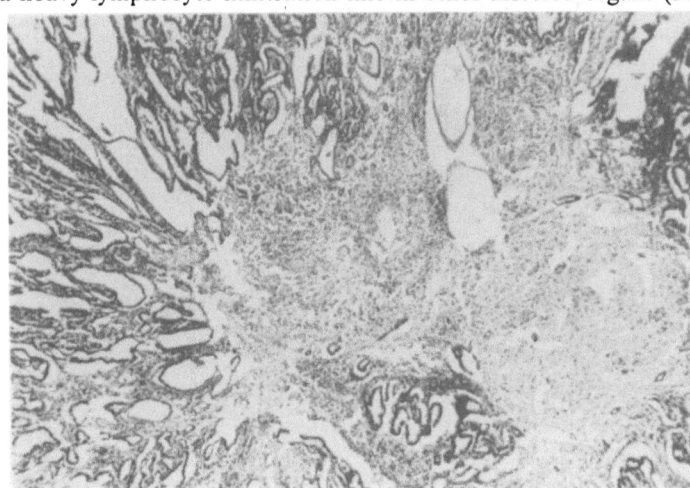

Fig. 2 Tuberculous salpingitis. There are several epithelioid granulomas with Langhan's cells. Tubal folds are shown on the left (×32)

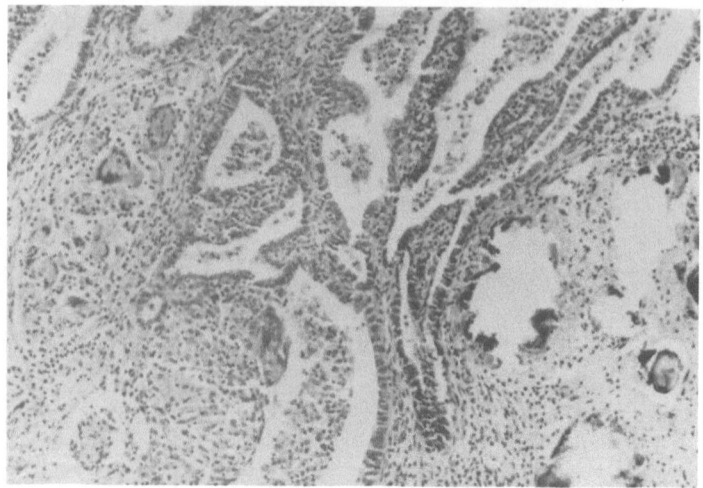

Fig. 3 Tuberculous salpingitis. Epithelioid granulomas and Langhan's cells (×80)

and 3). The syenchia of the tubal folds may produce intricate adenomatous patterns.

The specific microscopic lesion is the Köster follicle or the tubercle. It consists of many epithelioid cells surrounding Langhan's cells, occasionally with microcalcifications, caseum, or necrotic areas. A diffuse inflammatory reaction with many lymphocytes surrounds the clumping epithelioid cells.

Tubercles are usually located on the spongiose and compact layers of the endometrium, although Nogales (1979) reports an incidence of up to 40% in the basal layer. The tubercles occasionally invade the neighboring glands. In

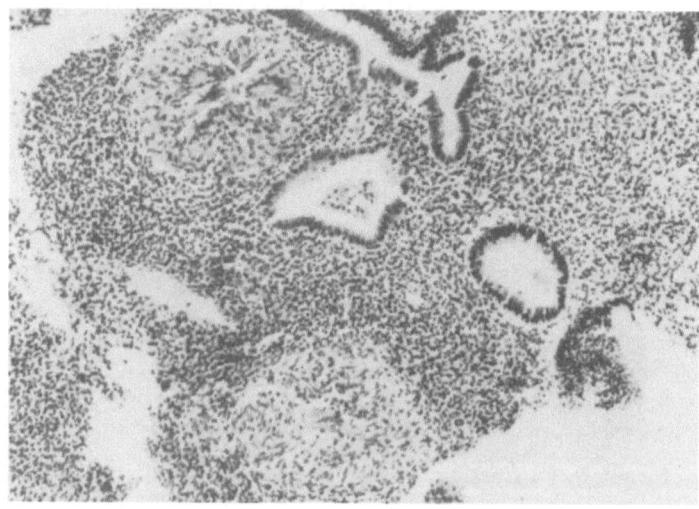

Fig. 4 Tuberculous endometritis with small typical Köster follicles: epithelioid and Langhan's cells surrounded by lymphocytes (×80)

6

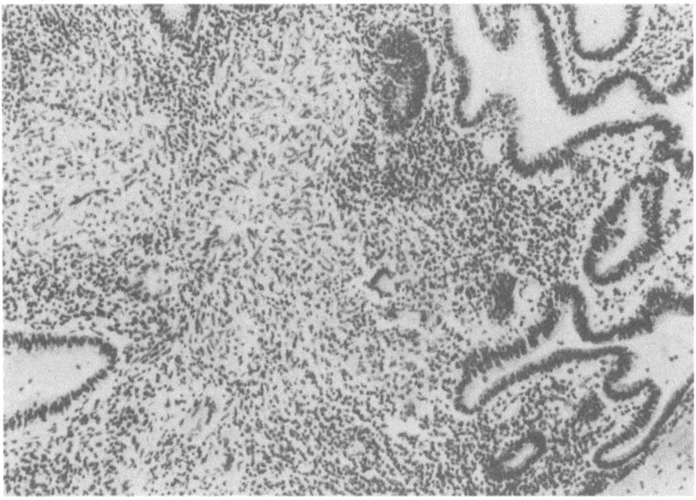

Fig. 5 Tuberculous endometritis. Epithelioid and Langhan's cells are close to endometrial glands (×80)

rare cases Schaumann bodies are present in the giant cells, but caseation is unusual (Figs. 4 and 5).

Functional reactions to endometrial tuberculosis are mainly seen in areas close to the Köster follicles. They appear in various degrees and patterns and are caused by an inactive gland, irregular maturation, or even deficient secretory patterns. These reactions are probably due to the local effects of the inflammatory foci, which suppress the endometrium's response. In advanced cases the mucosa is totally destroyed and replaced by granulomatous tissue containing areas of hyalinization and necrosis, which invade the underlying myometrium. This morphology was present in 20% of the advanced cases reported by Nogales in 1979.

Endometrial synechia and even cervical occlusion with pyometra are occasionally present in advanced cases. Follicular patterns with varying number of lymphoid follicles surrounding epithelioid cells and a giant cell are found in cervical tuberculosis (Figs. 6 and 7). At times, granulomas are not present and there is only a diffuse cervicitis with lymphocyte infiltration surrounding epithelioid cells. Sometimes foamy cells, nuclear atypia, and changes in cell polarity in which the goblet cells in the basal layers present a morphology resembling microglandular hyperplasia, are seen in association with tuberculosis of the cervix.

PREVALENCE AND INCIDENCE

In the past four decades there has been a significant decline in the incidence of genital tuberculosis. The prevalence of genital tuberculosis varies geographically and is closely related to the general prevalence of tuberculosis. Countries with high rates of pulmonary tuberculosis present parallel rates of genital tuberculosis.

7

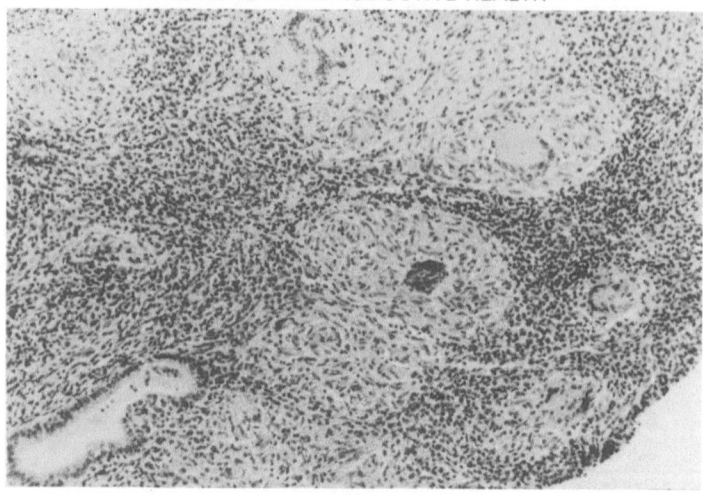

Fig. 6 Tuberculous cervicitis. There are several Köster follicles with epithelioid and giant cells surrounded by lymphocytes (×80)

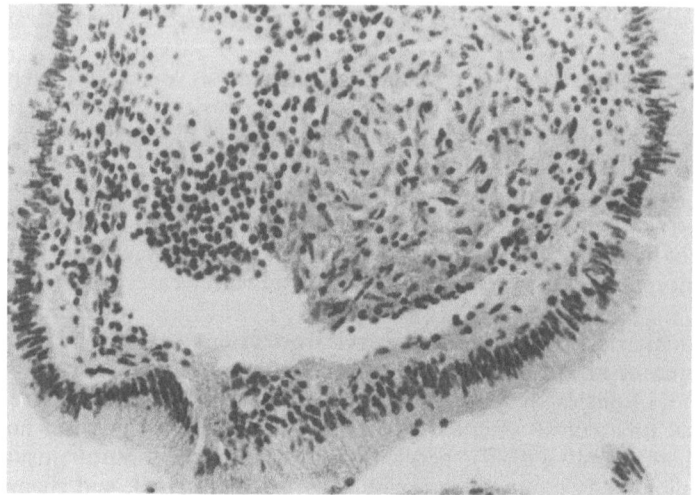

Fig. 7 Tuberculous cervicitis. Epithelioid granulomas with lymphocytes (×200)

In Spain the high incidence of pulmonary tuberculosis between 1940 and 1956 related to the effects of the civil war (1936–39) and World War II. Nogales observed an overall prevalence rate of 1.6% (1436 cases) of genital tuberculosis among 78,000 patients attending the gynecological department of the University of Madrid between 1947 and 1978. The highest rate, 5.5%, in this series was recorded in 1956, and it has continually declined since 1965, running parallel to pulmonary tuberculosis; the lowest rate of 0.27% was observed in 1977. In our department, a tenfold reduction has been recorded from 1.25% in 1969 to 0.12% in 1982.

In other countries, such as Rumania, the prevalence of women with tuberculosis is 0.25%. Estimates among gynecological admissions range from 0.05% in New Zealand to 0.002% in Sweden. Our research group detected a 0.17% prevalence among gynecological patients.

PREVIOUS EXPOSURE TO TUBERCULOSIS

A careful history reveals the presence of tuberculosis in the family or among immediate contacts in about 20% of cases. In about half of the cases a personal history of tuberculosis, usually pulmonary, cervical lymphadenitis, or abdominal, is obtained, although one-third of patients present evidence of lung lesions that are already healed. In our clinic, 60% of women with genital tuberculosis have a personal or family history of tuberculosis (Vanrell *et al.*, 1980).

AGE AND TIME OF ONSET

Genital tuberculosis occurs most frequently in women of reproductive age, that is, between 20 and 40 years old; only rarely is it diagnosed before puberty. Often many years elapse from the time of the primary infection with the tubercle bacilli, which frequently remains latent or has a very insidious course, to the time at which it is finally diagnosed.

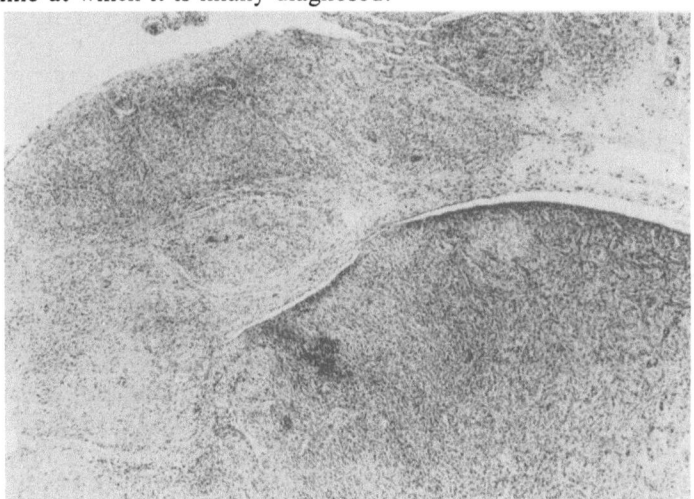

Fig. 8 Peritoneal tuberculosis. Perioophoritis (×40)

Until recently, it was generally accepted that genital tuberculosis rarely occurs after the menopause; Schaefer, for example, reports an incidence of only 4% in this group (1976). In our series, however, 17.2% of women over 50 have been diagnosed with the disease, and similar data have been reported in Madrid (Nogales *et al.*, 1969). Other reports of a high incidence of tuberculosis in postmenopausal women have appeared in the past decade, including 51% reported by Falk *et al.* There has also been a change in the age incidence from 6.5% in women aged 40 to 43.3% of women in their 50s (Sutherland, 1982). We have not been able to show changes in the age incidence among our patients.

INFERTILITY

Infertility is the most common and frequently the only symptom of genital tuberculosis. The frequency of primary infertility among patients with genital tuberculosis has been variously reported as 75% (Rozin, 1966); 85% (Schaefer, 1976); 94% (Nogales *et al.*, 1979); and 98% (Halbrecht, 1971).

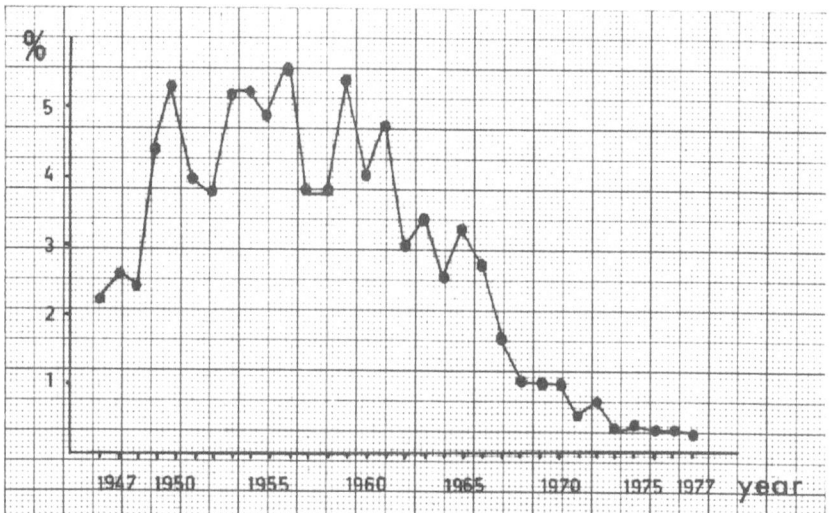

Fig. 9 Annual percentage of genital tuberculosis in the gynecologic pathology specimens, 1974–77 (Nogales *et al.*, 1978)

On the other hand, the frequency of genital tuberculosis among infertile women is affected by cultural as well as geographical considerations, and ranges from 0.7% in Australia (Rozin, 1968) to 17.4% in India (Malkani, 1966). In the United States it is below 1% and below 5% in Italy (Giarola, 1968). In our infertility clinic, there is a 5.5% prevalence of genital tuberculosis.

In our clinic material, however, only 40.4% of patients with genital tuberculosis had primary infertility; the remainder had experienced normal pregnancy, abortion, or ectopic pregnancy. Similar findings have been reported by Hutchins (1977) and an even lower prevalence of 12.2% with primary infertility was reported in Sweden (Falk *et al.*, 1980). Tubal occlusion is the obvious cause of infertility in these women who were unable to conceive. In the other cases, tubal transport and conception are impaired to varying degrees due to destruction of the tubal mucosa. Endometrial and ovarian involvement play a minor role in infertility.

Clinically overt cases of genital tuberculosis do occur; advanced infiltrative forms with palpable adnexal masses or associated peritoneal or intestinal involvement are occasionally detected. The available reports classify data according to its source: (1) surgical gynecological specimens (e.g. uterus and adnexa) obtained at laparotomy and (2) infertility material. An overall incidence of from 2 to 20% has been reported in the review of Schaefer (1976).

OTHER SYMPTOMS

In our clinical material more than 40% of women complained of moderate lower abdominal pain, over the hypogastrium and both iliac fossae. Occasionally, severe pain is reported and may be associated with dyspareunia and/or severe dysmenorrhea.

The menstrual cycle is usually unaffected, but some patients may present with dysmenorrhea and occasional bleeding abnormalities (Magnin *et al.*, 1981). Irregular bleeding and postmenopausal bleeding occur in 15% and 4%, respectively, of our patients with genital tuberculosis.

Amenorrhea varies from 3 to 5% in our study group and has been variously reported by others; 3% (Poland, 1965), 7% (Rozin, 1966), 25% (Aburel and Petrescou, 1971), and 10% (Legros and Bastien-Yvenou, 1978). The usual cause of amenorrhea is the total destruction of the endometrium subsequent to a fibrotic reaction and only rarely ovarian destruction and failure.

Other symptoms of tuberculosis, such as general malaise, anorexia, low-grade fever, nocturnal sweating, and weight loss, occur mainly in active cases of tuberculosis. These symptoms were present only in 2.1% of our patients with genital tuberculosis.

A negative tuberculin reaction indicates that there has been no contact with tubercle bacilli and therefore excludes the possibility of tuberculosis. Following the primary infection, there is a gradual reaction, depending on the degree of the immune response and showing a very intense positive tuberculin test in recent or active cases.

DIAGNOSIS

We have already noted that genital tuberculosis is frequently symptomless. Until recently, genital tuberculosis was thought to occur almost exclusively in infertile women of reproductive age, but menopausal forms have been diagnosed in women with children (Hutchins, 1977; Falk *et al.*, 1980; Sutherland, 1982).

The *physical examination* is usually negative, as in 90% of cases reported by Halbrecht in 1971 and in 50% of our own patients (Vanrell *et al.*, 1980). In advanced cases, masses can be detected on pelvic examination; these are relatively painless, of semi-solid consistency, and are usually adherent to the

11

uterus and pelvic wall. The diagnosis of genital tuberculosis requires special methods; these methods are discussed below.

Endometrial biopsy

The histological study of the endometrium, based on specimens obtained by suction or by D&C, is a most useful diagnostic tool, although it has two inherent limitations.

First, the incidence of false-negative reports is high, since tubal involvement occurs more frequently than endometrial and is undetected by this method (Fig. 9, Table 1). Endometrial biopsy generally attains a diagnostic accuracy of 50–80%, although in our department only 46% of cases are detected by this method (Vanrell *et al.*, 1980). Thus, when genital tuberculosis is suspected and endometrial biopsy results are negative, a D&C procedure should be performed under general anesthesia. Progestin therapy can be very useful prior to curettage in these cases. Second, the diagnostic value of epithelioid granuloma has been questioned by some researchers who claim that its presence corresponds to a nonspecific form of inflammation and that *Mycobacterium tuberculosis* must be identified to establish the diagnosis.

Despite these possible shortcomings, many pathologists support the value of endometrial biopsy, because other types of granuloma (sarcoidosis and Crohn's disease) rarely involve the genital tract and because the presence of tuberculous follicles, as typically found in the endometrium, always indicates an existing tuberculous salpingitis. The presence of lymphoid follicles only warrants further investigation before the diagnosis can be ascertained, although they are highly suggestive of tuberculosis (Nogales, 1979).

Endometrial biopsy should be obtained in the late premenstrual phase, at the time of the follicles' optimal development. The use of total curettage, as opposed to multiple biopsy sampling including cornual regions, encompasses some risks, which should be considered. Although D&C offers greater diagnostic accuracy, it induces pelvic peritonitis in as many as 6.4% of patients (Halbrecht, 1971); miliary dissemination has also been reported following cervical dilatation (Schaefer, 1976). Therefore, we customarily perform an endometrial biopsy and reserve full curettage for those cases in which insufficient material is obtained to substantiate a diagnosis.

Table 1. Distribution of tuberculous lesions in surgical gynecological specimens

	Number of cases	Organ involved	Percentage involved
Fallopian tubes	331	331	100
Endometrium	201	151	79
Myometrium	201	40	20
Cervix	41	10	24
Ovaries	335	37	11

From: Nogales *et al.* (1979). *Obstet. Gynecol.*, **53**, 422

Table 2. Incidence of genital tuberculosis in the gynecologic pathology specimens

Year	Total specimens (number of cases)	Tuberculous involvement	Percentage
1969	1114	14	1.25
1970	2074	12	0.57
1971	1998	14	0.70
1972	2156	19	0.88
1973	2263	19	0.83
1974	2478	9	0.36
1975	2786	8	0.28
1976	3099	12	0.38
1977	3484	14	0.40
1978	3366	9	0.26
1979	4218	4	0.09
1980	3948	4	0.10
1981	4214	6	0.14
1982	4013	5	0.12
Total	41,211	149	

From González-Merlo *et al.* (unpublished data)

Table 3 Age distribution of women with genital tuberculosis. Total 149 cases

Age	Percentage
<19	6.38
20–29	42.55
30–39	31.91
40–49	2.13
>50	17.02

From González-Merlo *et al.* (unpublished data)

Bacteriological investigation

The detection of acid-fast bacilli is the simplest method to diagnose genital tuberculosis, particularly in the presence of caseum. Bacteriological studies can be effected with tissue obtained by endometrial or tubal biopsy or by the collection of menstrual blood and discharge, including cervical mucus and uterine and vaginal secretions. Several methods are used: direct smear, culture, and guinea pig inoculation.

According to Halbrecht menstrual blood culture has an accuracy of up to 89.2% when used over nine or ten cycles. Only then can the investigations of menstrual blood culture be considered negative. In our department, only 30% of cultures of the menstrual blood were positive (Vanrell *et al.*, 1980), and several other researchers report similar findings including 20% by Legros and Bastien-Yvenou (1978), 40% by Magnin *et al.* (1981), and 52.7% by Aburel and Petrescu (1971).

Table 4 Manifestations of genital tuberculosis. Total 149 women

	Percentage
No symptoms	12.76
Pain	42.55
Abnormal menstrual bleeding	14.89
Infertility	40.42
Other symptoms	2.1

From González-Merlo *et al.* (unpublished data)

Table 5 Major radiologic signs on hysterosalpingogram in 36 cases of proved tuberculosis

Uterine hypoplasia	10
Intramural obstruction	11
Tubal beading	3
Rigid tubes (wire)	5
Tubal clubbing	9
Sactosalpinx	4
Hydrosalpinx	13
Intravasation	1

Modified from: Teixidor

In some instances guinea pig inoculation may yield the only positive result when other investigations are negative (Hok and Loen, 1967; Rozin, 1975, González-Ruiz, 1973). In our experience, this method was positive in 44% of cases and more reliable than menstrual blood cultures in 30%.

Hysterosalpingogram

Radiologic findings, although useful, can only suggest the presence of genital tuberculosis; other diagnostic evidence is necessary to establish the diagnosis.

The diagnostic criteria previously reported by Dalsace and García-Calderón (1958) and Rozin (1975) have been confirmed in a detailed radiologic study of 36 women with genital tuberculosis in whom the diagnosis was based on bacteriological and histological investigations (Teixidor, 1976). The following radiologic signs are very suggestive of genital tuberculosis (Table 5):

(1) Small uterus with diminished cavity (Fig. 10) and a long endocervical canal; filling defects and irregular contours are often present as well (Figs. 11–13).

(2) Rigid tubes, especially in the proximal portion: the so-called wiry tubes (Fig. 14).

(3) Cylindrical tubes, slightly dilated midportions and a distal bulbous dilatation due to occlusions; clubbing (Figs. 14 and 15).

(4) Tubes with irregular lumen, in which dilatation alternates with strictures: beading; minute fistulae (Figs. 16 and 20).

(5)   Bilateral intramural obstruction (Figs. 11 and 19).

(6)   Distal occlusion with ampullary dilatation (bilateral hydrosalpinx) (Figs. 17 and 18).

(7)   Intravasation (Figs. 16, 19 and 20).

The following signs are considered presumptive:

(1)   Unilateral tubal occlusion (Fig. 15).

(2)   Unilateral or bilateral tubal dilatation that allows the medium to escape into the peritoneum.

(3)   Unilateral distal dilatation with complete occlusion: hydrosalpinx.

(4)   Lack of definition of the distal ampullary regions due to flossy or irregular shadows.

(5)   Calcification of the pelvic lymph nodes, fallopian tubes, or ovaries (Figs. 10 and 21).

In our experience, only 43% of women with genital tuberculosis had one or more of the signs described above (Venrell and González-Merlo, 1980).

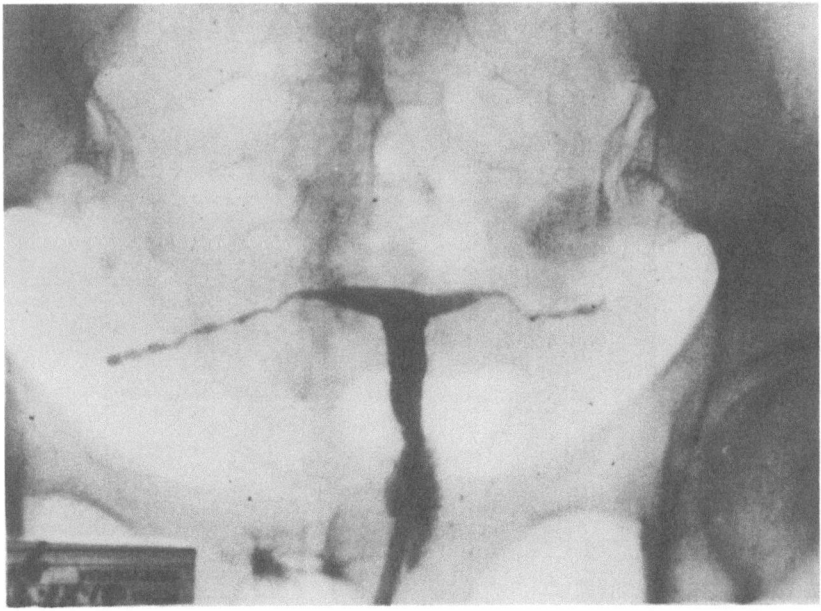

Fig. 10   HSG. A round 1.5 cm shadow compatible with a calcified lymphonide. There is a reduced uterine cavity with irregular contour. Tubal occlusion with beading. Biopsy at the time of laparotomy revealed tuberculous salpingitis

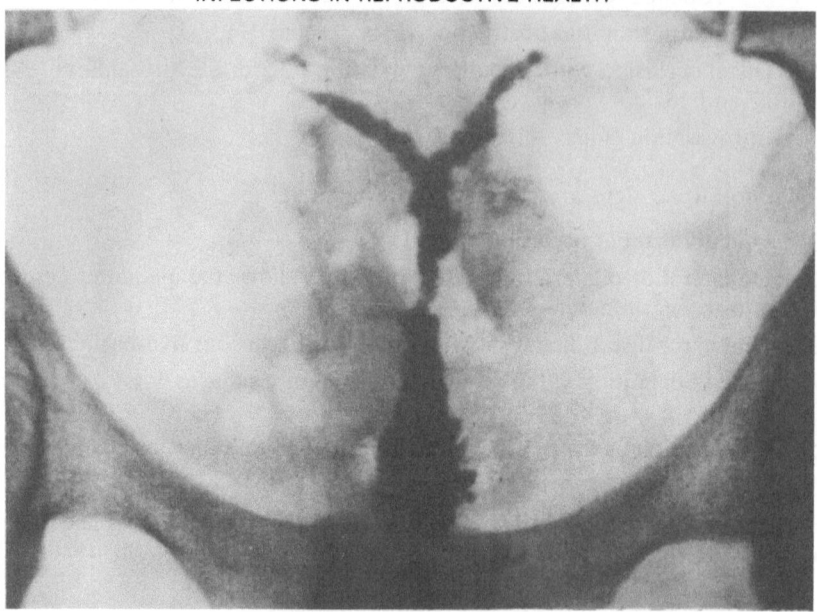

Fig. 11 HSG. Uterus bicornis with irregular cavum and proximal obstruction. Guinea pig inoculation of menstrual blood revealed genital tuberculosis

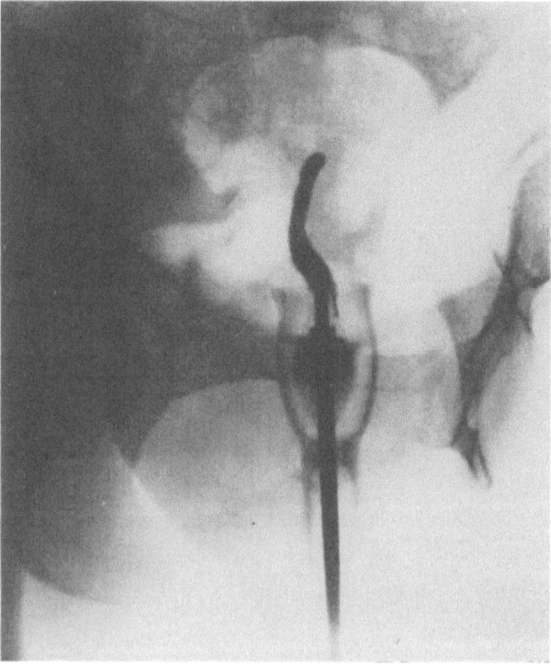

Fig. 12 HSG. Very deformed and reduced uterine cavity in a 19-year-old patient with biphasic BBT and primary amenorrhea. Laparoscopy showed dense pelvic adhesions involving the adnexa. Culture of the aspirate showed tuberculosis

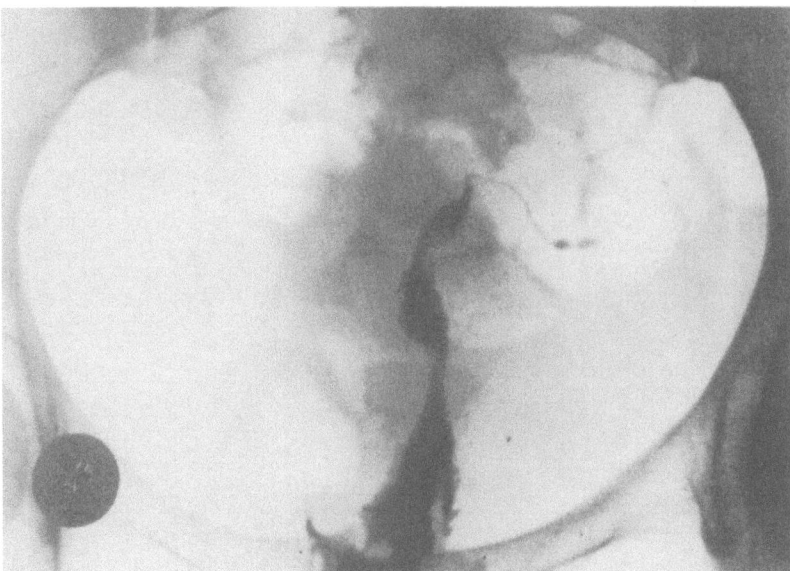

Fig. 13 HSG. A small deformed cavum filling with contrast only one horn and lack of filling on the left side. Only one tube is visualized; it shows rigidity and beading. Histology showed endometrial tuberculosis.

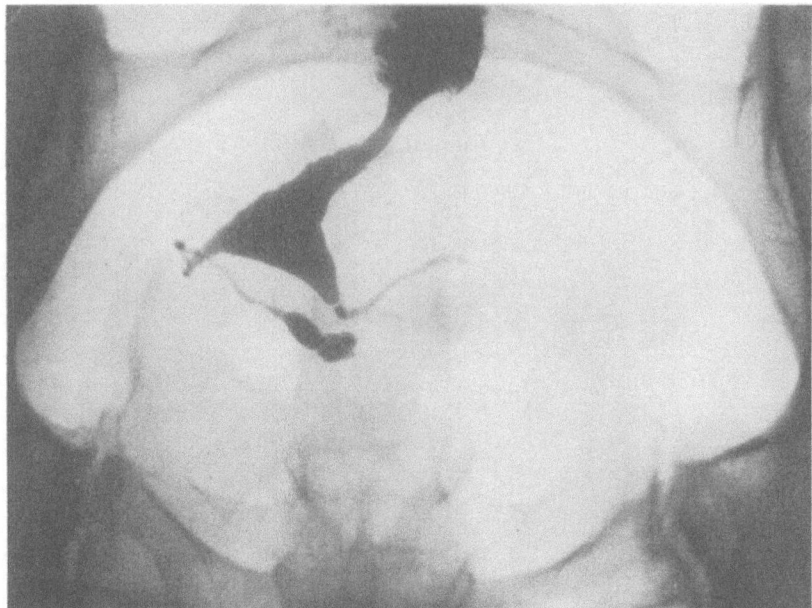

Fig. 14 HSG. The uterus is small. Both tubes are rigid with distal occlusion and dilatation. Endometrial tuberculosis on histology

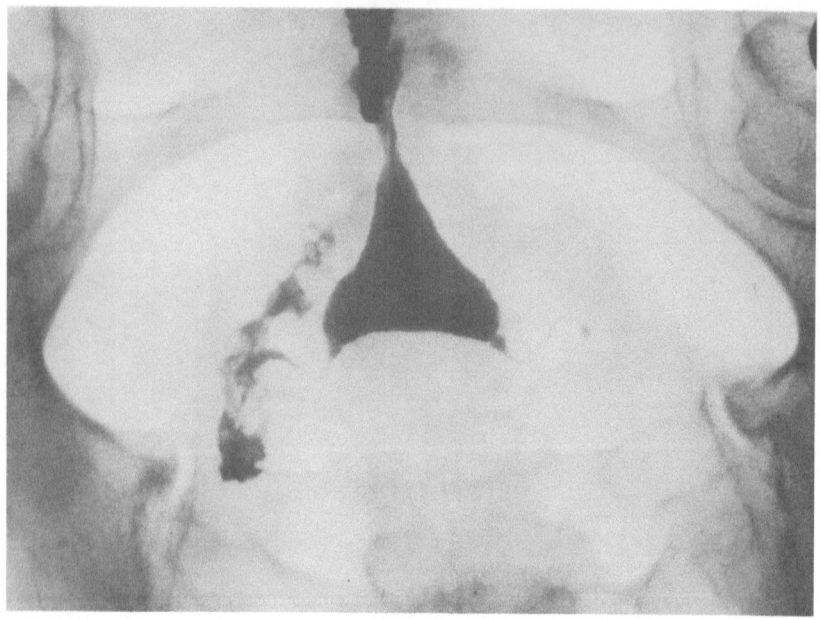

Fig. 15 HSG. Normal cavity. The right tube shows rigidities and occlusions in the mid-portion. The left tube is patent but slightly dilated. Endometrial histology: tuberculosis

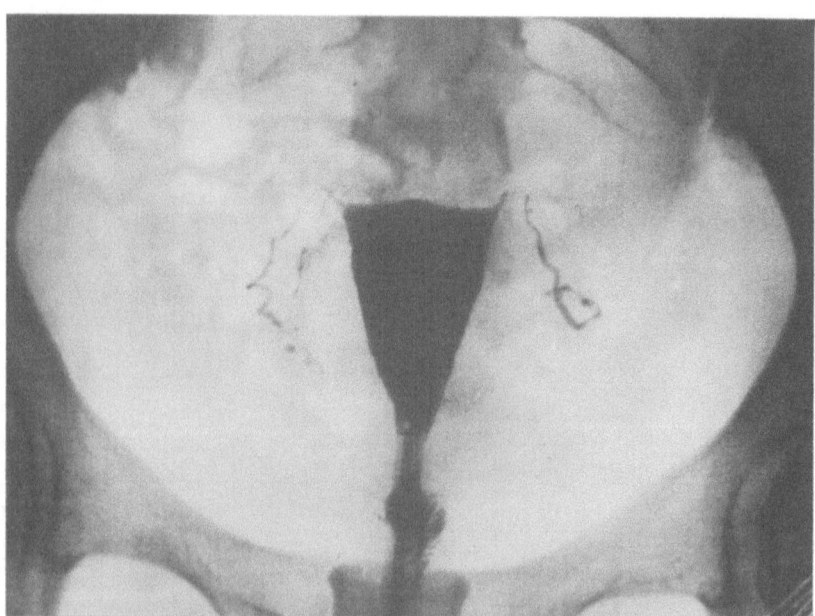

Fig. 16 HSG. Normal uterus. Both tubes with occlusion and beading. Intravasation. Endometrial histology: tuberculosis

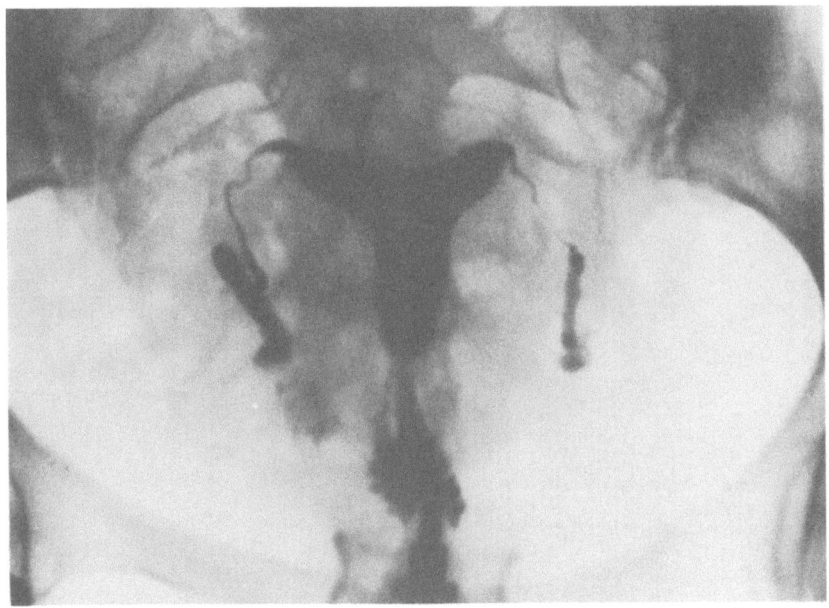

Fig. 17 HSG. Bilateral hydrosalpinx. Biopsy revealed tuberculous salpingitis

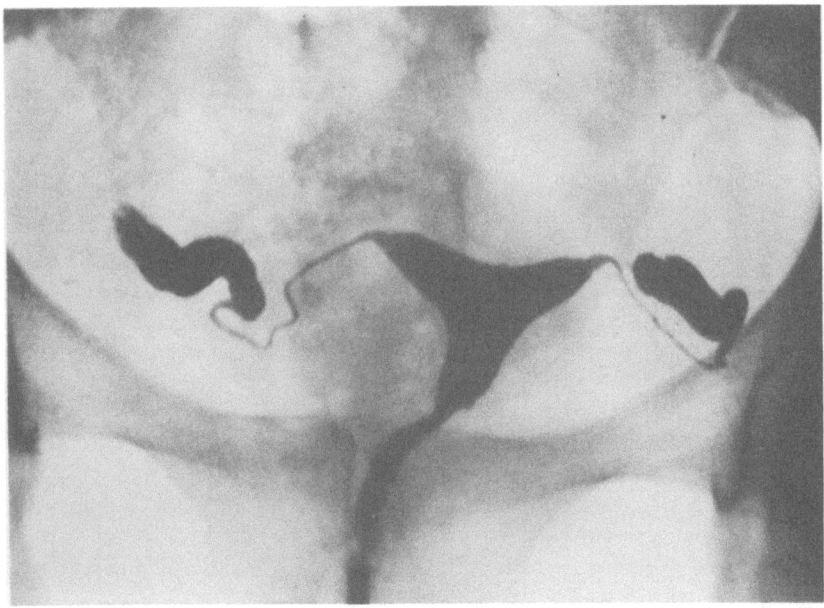

Fig. 18 HSG. Bilateral hydrosalpinx. Culture of menstrual blood detected tuberculosis

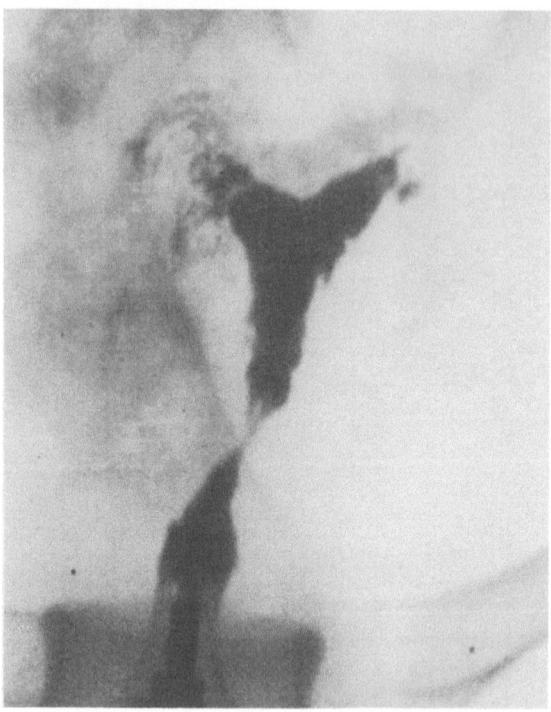

Fig. 19 HSG. Deformed cavum with irregular outline. Bilateral intramural occlusion. Intravasation. Endometrial histology: tuberculosis

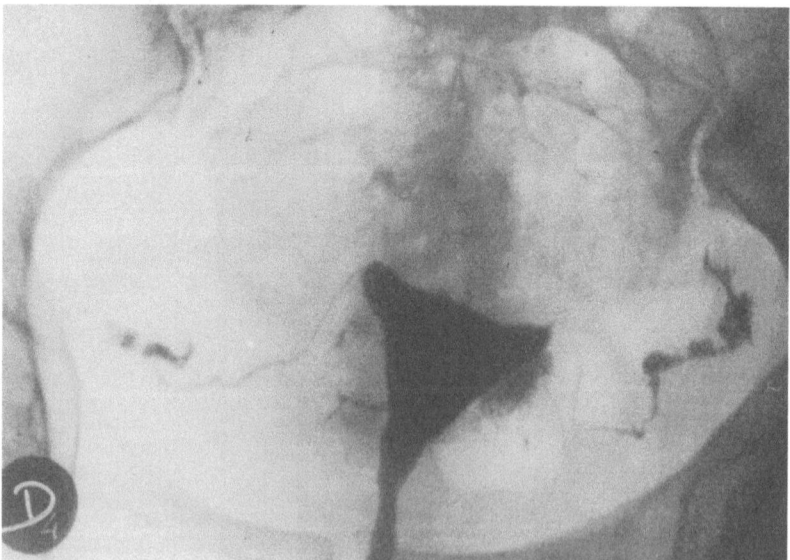

Fig. 20 Small uterus. Bilateral tubal rigidity and beading. Intravasation. Tuberculosis was diagnosed by endometrial biopsy

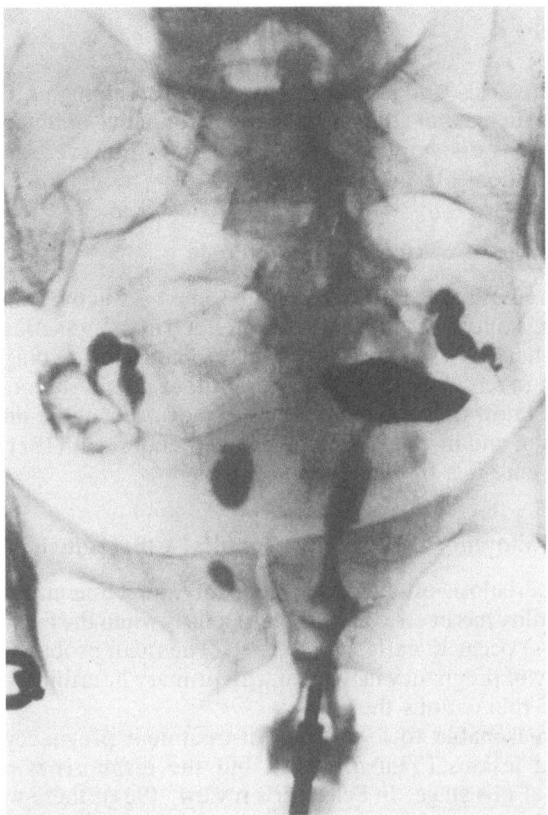

Fig. 21 HSG. Small uterus. The left tube shows distal occlusion and dilatation. The right tube is rigid but patency is conserved. There are two calcified lymph nodes

Laparoscopy

Laparoscopy can be useful when genital tuberculosis is suspected and other methods have failed to reveal its presence. The visualization of caseum or tubercles and sampling of tissue for histology or bacteriology can be effected. The main operative difficulty is due to adhesions. Only 7% of our cases have been diagnosed by samples obtained through laparoscopy.

Laparotomy

As already mentioned, genital tuberculosis can be completely overlooked, and it is not surprising that the diagnosis is only established by the study of the surgical specimens obtained at laparotomy. This has occurred in 45% of our cases.

PROGNOSIS

Genital tuberculosis and especially tuberculous salpingitis frequently leave permanent sequelae that seriously impair reproductive potential. Exacerbation or hematogenous dissemination to other organs, however, are rare, and this condition is seldom life-threatening.

Spontaneous cure of genital tuberculosis

Genital tuberculosis was formerly considered a destructive, chronic condition, with a high mortality rate, that only rarely ended in spontaneous cure (Rovinsky and Guttmacher, 1965). At present, many women who are diagnosed as having latent genital tuberculosis demonstrate no other manifestation than infertility. Although we know that spontaneous cures may occur, little information exists as to how often and in which cases it is likely. Halbrecht (1971) maintains that spontaneous cure is a frequent occurrence.

Pregnancy following treatment of genital tuberculosis

Although tuberculosis often leads to infertility, infection may occur after some degree of fertility has been achieved, particularly when the first (and subsequent pregnancy(ies) occur in early adolescence. The main problem lies in assessing the possibility of pregnancy in women with primary infertility who are receiving effective anti-tuberculous therapy.

It seems reasonable to look for post-treatment pregnancy in those cases with minimal lesions (Ylinen, 1961), but the diagnosis is only established infrequently at this stage. In Schaefer's review (1964), there were 155 cases of pregnancy, although this number diminished to less than 100 when our diagnostic criteria were applied. Included in his report were 125 ectopic pregnancies and 56 abortions. Halbrecht estimates that 18% of women conceive following treatment of genital tuberculosis, although 95% of these pregnancies will result in abortion or are ectopic. In our department, we have attended to women with three normal full-term pregnancies and three ectopic pregnancies among a group of 28 women who had minimal lesions before treatment.

TREATMENT

It is important to determine whether other active sites of tuberculosis, especially pulmonary and renal, are present before starting antituberculosis treatment. In most cases, when genital tuberculosis is diagnosed, the primary lesions can no longer be detected or have already healed.

Chemoantibiotic

Although very potent antituberculosis drugs are presently available, almost every case of genital tuberculosis would benefit from treatment with a combination of two drugs, preferably bactericidal in nature. Surgery should be restricted to very selective cases. Several therapeutic regimens are currently proposed; all of these are based on the observation that the best results can be obtained with the combination of two or three agents administered over 9 months to a year, as is the case in other forms of tuberculosis. Whenever possible culture and sensitivity should be made to avoid the risk of antibiotic resistance. Until recently, the combination of isoniazid, streptomycin, and PAS had been used with varying success rates. Sutherland (1977), reviewing 25 years' experience with this regimen, has reported high rates of recurrence or drug resistance, varying from 42% after 3 months' use of streptomycin and PAS to 12% after the triple combination during 18 months' to 2 years' treatment.

At present the combination of ethambutol and rifampin is considered the most useful regimen because of the low incidence of primary resistance. Isoniazid may be safely added to this regimen in a single morning dose of 300 mg daily. This combination is given for 3 months at the following dosages: rifampin, 450–600 mg daily 30 minutes before breakfast; ethambutol, 15 mg/kg daily after breakfast. Ethambutol is then withdrawn and treatment continued with rifampin and isoniazid for the remainder of the year. Some authors advise giving isoniazid and ethambutol only during the first year and then continuing indefinitely with isoniazid (Schaefer, 1976).

Follow-up of the treatment responses

Generally it is difficult to know if and when the cure has been achieved. Endometrial biopsy or D&C should be performed for histological and bacteriological investigation after 6 months' treatment. After treatment has been completed and negative results have been achieved for the biopsy or culture of menstrual blood, a hysterosalpingogram can be done. Since there are no criteria of certainty regarding the cure of genital tuberculosis, it is advisable to repeat cultures of menstrual blood every 3 months during the 2 years of treatment.

Toxic effects

Chemotherapeutic regimens should be carefully supervised to detect toxic effects. Ethambutol may induce optic neuritis and renal insufficiency (1% of patients receiving 25 mg/kg daily). Rifampin may produce itching, nausea, and, in rare instances, hemolytic anemia and oligoanuria. Since isoniazid may induce peripheral neuritis and hepatitis, it is convenient to provide neuroophthalmological follow-up and laboratory investigations at 2-month intervals.

SURGICAL TREATMENT

The surgical indications in cases of genital tuberculosis have been reduced by more than half since the advent of modern antituberculous therapy (Magnin et al., 1981). Surgery is only indicated when the disease persists or recurs after a year of a well-conducted treatment with the most effective available drugs, when pelvic masses are still present or growing after 6 months of treatment, or when pain persists in spite of prolonged treatment.

The extent of surgical excision may vary from bilateral salpingectomy to total hysterectomy and bilateral salpingo-oophorectomy. It is important that antituberculosis treatment be initiated before surgical treatment, preferably 6 months prior. This simplifies the surgical approach and reduces the risk of fistulae and residual abscesses. If the diagnosis is made at the time of laparotomy, samples should be taken to establish the diagnosis and any surgical attempt abandoned until the patient can be treated with an antituberculous regimen for 4–6 months. This therapy should be maintained for 1 year following the operation.

Tuboplasty

There should be no attempt to restore tubal patency in genital tuberculosis; it is bound to fail due to the extensive damage of the tubal mucosa associated with occlusion. Many authors have reported unfavorable results in this type of case (Brun and Saurel, 1974; Semchyshyn and Cecutti, 1975; Ballon et al., 1975; Rozin, 1975; and Schaefer, 1976). On the other hand we have obtained three normal full-term pregnancies in three women undergoing salpingolysis for adhesions due to minimal grade of tuberculosis, as revealed by the intraoperative biopsy.

References

Aburel, E. and Petrescou, V. (1971). *La Tuberculose Génitale de la Femme*. (Paris, Masson)
Ballon, S., Clewell, W. and Lamb, E. (1975). Reactivation of silent pelvic tuberculosis by reconstructive tubal surgery. *Am. J. Obstet. Gynecol.*, **122**, 991
Brun, G. and Saurel, J. (1974). La tuberculose génitale de la femme. *Bordeaux Méd.*, **15**, 2217
Dalsace, J. and García-Calderón, J. (1958). *Tuberculosis uterotubárica*. In Dalsace, J. and García-Calderón, J. (eds.). *Ginecología radiológica* (Barcelona: L. Miracle)
Falk, V., Ludviksson, K. and Agren, G. (1980). Genital tuberculosis in women: Analysis of 187 newly diagnosed cases from 47 Swedish hospitals during the ten year period 1968 to 1977. *Am. J. Obstet. Gynecol.*, **138**, 974
Giarola, A. and Agostini, G. (1978). Tuberculose génitale et stérilité. *Gynécologie*, **29**, 291
González-Merlo, J. (1983). Tuberculosis genital. In J. González-Merlo (ed.). *Ginecología*. Third edition p. 457. (Salvat Editores, S.A. Barcelona)
González-Merlo, J. and Márquez, M. (1972). Endometritis tuberculosa. In J. González-Merlo y M. Márquez (eds.). *Patología del Endometrio*, p. 166. Editorial Científica Médica Barcelona
González-Ruiz, J. (1973). Tuberculosis genital femenina y esterilidad. Estudio de 120 casos. p. 138 Thesis, Barcelona
Halbrecht. I. (1971). Tuberculosis of the female genital organs. Clinical forms, diagnostic methods and results of treatment. In Joel, Ch.: *Fertility Disturbances in Men and Women*, p. 381 (Basel: S. Karger)
Hok, T. T. and Loen, L. K. (1967). The isolation of tubercle bacilli from endocervical mucus of infertile women. *Am. J. Obstet. Gynecol.*, **99**, 307
Hutchins, C. I. (1977). Tuberculosis of the genital tract: A changing picture. *Br. J. Obstet. Gynecol.*, **84**, 534
Legros, R. and Bastien-Yvenou, C. (1978). Tuberculose utéroannexielle. Etude rétrospective durant les 20 dernières années. *J. Gynecol. Obstet. Biol. Reprod.*, **7**, 1235
Magnin, G., Bremond, A., Rochet, Y. (1981). La tuberculose génitale de la femme. *Encycl. Méd. Chir. Paris. Gynecologie*, **490A**[10] **(3)**, 1981

TUBERCULOUS INFECTIONS OF THE FEMALE GENITAL TRACT

Malkani, P. K. (1966). Epidemiology of genital tuberculosis in India. In E. T. Rippmann, R. Wenner (eds.), *Latent Female Genital Tuberculosis* (Basel: S. Karger)

Nogales, F., Parache, J. and Martínez, H. (1969). Pathologische Anatomie der Genitaltuberkulose. Bericht über 1205 Fälle. *Gynäk. Rdsch.*, **7**, 81

Nogales, F., Tarancon, I. and Nogales, Jr. F. (1979). The pathology of female genital tuberculosis. A 31-year study of 1436 cases. *Obstet. Gynecol.*, **53**, 422

Poland, B. (1965). Female pelvic tuberculose with special reference to infertility. *Am. J. Obstet. Gynecol.*, **91**, 350

Rovinsky, J. J. and Gutmacher, A. F. (1965). *Medical and Gynecologic Complications of Pregnancy* (Baltimore: Williams & Wilkins)

Rozin, S. (1975). Genital tuberculosis. In S. J. Behrman, and R. W. Kistner (Eds.). *Progress in Infertility*, 2nd ed. p. 189 (Boston: Little, Brown)

Schaefer, G. (1964). Full term pregnancy following genital tuberculosis. *Obstet. Gynecol. Surv.*, **19**, 81

Schaefer, G. (1976). Female genital tuberculosis. *Clin. Obstet. Gynecol.*, **19**, 223

Semchyshyn, S. and Cecutti, A. (1975). Abdominal pregnancy complicated by genital and renal tuberculosis and hemolytic anemia. *Fertil. Steril.*, **26**, 1142

Sutherland, A. M. (1977). Twenty-five years experience of the drug treatment of tuberculosis of the female genital tract. *Br. J. Obstet. Gynecol.*, **84**, 881

Sutherland, A. M. (1982). Postmenopausal tuberculosis of the female genital tract. *Obstet. Gynecol.*, **59**, 54S

Teixidor, N. (1976). Estudio antómico-radiológico de la tuberculosis genital femenina. Thesis, Barcelona

Vanrell, J. A., Balasch, J., Deulofeu, P. *et al.* (1980). Tuberculosis genital en estériles asintomáticas. X World Congress of Fertility and Sterility, Madrid

Ylinen, O. (1961). Genital tuberculosis in women. *Acta Obstet. Gynecol. Scand. Suppl.*, **40**, 2

2
Genitourinary tuberculosis in men

D. L. COHN and F. N. JUDSON

Gonococci, *Chlamydia*, and Gram-negative rods are much more common genitourinary pathogens than is *Mycobacterium tuberculosis*. The incidence of genitourinary tuberculosis in the United States has declined in recent decades. Moreover, the existing disease has changed as better microbiologic and radiographic techniques have led to more rapid and specific diagnosis and effective antituberculous chemotherapy has improved outcome. In the past, surgery and other supportive measures were the mainstays of treatment; at present cure is usual.

Nonetheless, genitourinary tuberculosis continues to occur in developed as well as less developed countries. Because the clinical manifestations of this condition are generally nonspecific, tuberculous infection must remain in the differential diagnosis of a large number of genitourinary tract disorders. In particular, the recent influx of Southeast Asian refugees and other immigrants ensures that tuberculosis will be present in the United States for years to come. Hence, concerned clinicians need to understand the clinical manifestations, diagnosis, treatment, and prevention of genitourinary tuberculosis in men.

EPIDEMIOLOGY

In 1979, 27,669 new cases of active tuberculosis were reported in the United States, of which extrapulmonary tuberculosis comprised 14.9% (Centers for Disease Control, 1981). A total of 664 cases of genitourinary tuberculosis were reported, which accounted for 16.1% of extrapulmonary disease and 2.4% of all types of tuberculosis. Genitourinary tuberculosis was the third most common form of extrapulmonary tuberculosis after lymphatic and pleural disease (CDC, 1981).

The incidence of genitourinary tuberculosis was 0.30 cases per 100,000, compared to a rate of 12.6 cases per 100,000 for all forms of tuberculosis. As with most other forms of tuberculosis, the frequency of disease for genitourinary tuberculosis increased with age, ranging from 0.03 cases per 100,000 for ages

27

0–4 to 0.67 cases per 100,000 for persons over 65 (CDC, 1981). Christiansen (1974) reported an age range of 18–59 years, with a mean of 29 in 72 men with genitourinary tuberculosis, and Simon *et al.* (1977) reported a range of 19–85 years, with a mean of 45. Although these authors note that genitourinary tuberculosis is twice as common among men, this observation may only reflect higher overall infection rates in men (CDC, 1981).

A comparison of autopsy data for genitourinary tuberculosis in the era preceding the advent of chemotherapy and the time since supports the concept of decreased absolute and relative morbidity and mortality from genitourinary tuberculosis. Of 5424 autopsies performed on men at Bellevue Hospital between 1935 and 1944, 21% of patients with tuberculosis as a secondary cause of death and 26% of patients with tuberculosis as the primary cause of death had genitourinary tuberculosis. In contrast, of 4260 autopsies performed between 1952 and 1960 at the same institution, genitourinary tuberculosis was noted in 7% of patients with tuberculosis as a secondary cause and in 11% of patients with tuberculosis as the primary cause of death (Rosenberg, 1963). Similarly, Gow (1971) has noted a decreased mortality from genitourinary tuberculosis as chemotherapy has become more effective, with mortality rates progressively declining from 7.9% between 1946 and 1952, to 4.6% from 1953 to 1963, and finally to 2.2% from 1964 to 1969.

TRANSMISSION AND PATHOGENESIS

In almost all cases, initial infection with *M. tuberculosis* occurs through the lungs. Following inhalation into alveoli of droplet nuclei containing tubercle bacilli, organisms are phagocytosed by, and multiply within, macrophages. The infection spreads via the lymphatic system to regional lymph nodes and, finally, the blood, through which seeding of other organs takes place. During ensuing weeks the host develops cell-mediated immunity, with the subsequent arresting of bacillary multiplication and healing by fibrosis and calcification, although progressive primary disease occurs in a small percentage of cases (approximately 5%). Tuberculosis disease occurs in most individuals as a reactivation of initially infected anatomical sites (Danneberg, 1982).

The time between the initial infection in a pulmonary or extrapulmonary site and the subsequent development of genitourinary tuberculosis ranges from 2 to 36 years (Christiansen, 1974; Simon *et al.*, 1977; Cinman, 1982). One of the more striking reported examples of reactivation of genitourinary tuberculosis was TB epididymitis in a 41-year-old man who had had tuberculosis of the wrist at age 5 (Christiansen, 1974).

It is generally accepted that the initial event in the pathogenesis of genitourinary tuberculosis is the hematogenous seeding of the kidneys at the time of bacillemia. This concept is supported by autopsy evidence revealing bilateral lesions in over 90% of cases although clinically apparent disease was present in only one kidney. The glomerulus is the initial site of infection; a tuberculoma forms or ulceration takes place and spreads into the medulla and collecting system. Infection of the ureter, bladder, prostate, seminal vesicles, and epididymis then most likely develops by direct extension through contaminated urine (Medlar *et al.*, 1949). Some authors are of the opinion that tuberculous epididymitis is secondary to hematogenous seeding. This belief is based on findings that the disease is frequently found in the globus minor, which has a greater blood supply than other parts of the epididymis, can be bilateral, and occasionally is noted when pathologic assessment of the kidneys fails to reveal a focus of past or present infection (Gow, 1971; Ross *et al.*, 1961).

Only rarely has genitourinary tuberculosis been documented to be sexually transmitted. Lattimer *et al.* (1954) reported a localized ulceration in the fourchette of a 33-year-old woman that was associated with lymphadenopathy and proved to be due to *M. tuberculosis*. Her husband had a past medical history of tuberculous epididymitis and, at the time of her diagnosis, was found to have cavitary renal tuberculosis, tuberculosis prostatitis, and positive urine and semen cultures for *M. tuberculosis*. Sexual transmission to the female was attributed to the heavy inoculum of organisms in the untreated male's ejaculate and the repeated trauma induced by sexual contact. There are only eight other cases in the literature documenting this mode of transmission, all but one of which occurred in the prechemotherapy era (Lattimer *et al.*, 1954).

The infectiousness of urine from patients with genitourinary tuberculosis is of a very low order. Vasquez and Lattimer (1959) found that 22% of children who were household contacts of adults with positive urine cultures but no evidence of pulmonary tuberculosis were tuberculin positive compared to a 10% tuberculin positivity rate in the general population; this study, however, lacked matched controls. Even though patients with genitourinary tuberculosis excrete low numbers of tubercle bacilli in their urine, the chance of aerosolization of urine into infective droplet nuclei is highly unlikely, and there are no good epidemiologic data to support the concept that urine is a vehicle for transmission.

CLINICAL MANIFESTATIONS

Although the kidney is the most common site of involvement in genitourinary tuberculosis, it is not unusual for more than one organ in the genitourinary system to show some evidence of disease. The most common presenting symptoms are dysuria, frequency, hematuria, nocturia, urgency, and flank pain (Table 1). Constitutional symptoms, such as fever and weight loss, are seen less often, as are suprapubic pain and gross pyuria. Parenchymal disease in the kidney can include granulomas, diffuse or focal calcification, masses, cavitation, infundibular stenosis or stricture, calicectasis, or scarring.

Ureteral disease manifests clinically as obstruction, most often due to stricture formation, but it can also arise secondary to edema and spasm (Rees and Holland, 1970; Murphy *et al.*, 1982). Strictures are usually unilateral; they tend to be short and localized but can be multiple and are most often seen at the ureterovesical junction (Murphy *et al.*, 1982; Claridge, 1970). Due to the ongoing inflammatory response, ureteral stricture can occur during and after successful medical treatment of genitourinary tuberculosis; therefore, patients should have radiographic follow-up for this complication.

Bladder involvement is rare, but in long-standing cases can be seen as a

Table 1 Presenting symptoms of genitourinary tuberculosis

Symptom	Frequency (%)
Dysuria	30–53
Frequency	41–60
Hematuria	18–38
Nocturia	20–37
Urgency	6–20
Flank pain	10–60
Fever	2–18

thickened bladder wall or contracted bladder. A paravesicular tuberculoma mimicking a tumor has been reported (Kumar *et al.*, 1981)

Tuberculous epididymitis is the most common form of genital tuberculosis. Patients present with painless scrotal swelling, appreciated as a mass that grows insidiously over the course of months. Pain occurs in 12% of cases, secondary hydrocoele in 5%, and sinus tracts less frequently (Farnell and Thomas, 1983; Reeve *et al.*, 1974). The disease is bilateral in up to 34% of cases, and the vas deferens is thickened in 50% (Ross *et al.*, 1961). It may be difficult, if not impossible, to distinguish epididymal from testicular swelling in some cases.

Tuberculosis of the testis, on the other hand, is rare; when seen it is usually due to direct invasion by contiguous epididymitis. There are only a few reported cases of isolated testicular tuberculosis (Riehle and Jayaraman, 1982; Stanisic *et al.*, 1978).

Tuberculosis of the prostate has a nonspecific presentation. It can present as an incidental finding on biopsy in patients with systemic symptoms and no other evidence of genitourinary tuberculosis (O'Dea *et al.*, 1978), but it has also been frequently associated with epididymitis (Veenema and Lattimer, 1957). There is no classic physical finding; some infected prostates are small and fibrotic, others soft due to caseous centers, and still some others have frank nodules.

Penile tuberculosis, which is a very rare disease entity, consists of chronic indurated, nonhealing ulcers that may be associated with nodules (Lewis, 1946; Agarwalla *et al.*, 1980; Venkataramaiah *et al.*, 1982). Before the advent of chemotherapy the vast majority of cases were due to ritual circumcision that resulted in primary inoculation (Lewis, 1946). Other cases of primary disease were thought to be sexually transmitted. Rare cases have been reported as secondary extension from urethral involvement associated with more widespread genital tract disease. Even more unusual are a few cases possibly due to hematogenous seeding of the corpus cavernosum.

Tuberculous urethritis is also an unusual clinical manifestation. It presents as dysuria, urinary retention, periurethral abscess, or multiple perineal urinary fistulas (Raghavaiah, 1979) and is invariably associated with involvement elsewhere in the genitourinary tract. Urethritis is thought to be rare because bacteria are supposedly washed away by the urinary stream, and it is possible that the condition only occurs in patients with preexisting urethral pathology.

Other unusual presentations of genitourinary tuberculosis in the male include a perineal mass possibly secondary to lymphatic spread (Stanisic *et al.*, 1978), rectovesicocutaneous fistula (Hashmonai *et al.*, 1982), hemospermia (Yu *et al.*, 1977), and nephrobronchial fistula (Blight, 1980).

Complications of genitourinary tuberculosis vary widely and depend on the extent and location of disease prior to the initiation of chemotherapy. Renal dysfunction, as measured by decreased glomerular filtration, has been noted in up to 58% of patients, although significant uremia occurs in only 5%. Alterations in concentrating ability occur in 84% of patients, demonstrating the common medullary localization of lesions (Wisnia *et al.*, 1978). Hypertension is rare (Gow, 1971). Patients with genitourinary tuberculosis may be more susceptible to urinary tract infections with other bacteria because of underlying anatomical damage (Christiansen, 1974; Simon *et al.*, 1977).

Before chemotherapy became available, infertility was noted as a sequela of genitourinary tuberculosis, especially when prostatic and seminal vesicle involvement was significant (Veenema and Lattimer, 1957). Most patients were sterile, as measured by failure to conceive after the diagnosis was established, decreased volume of ejaculate, azoospermia, oligospermia, and/or decreased sperm motility.

DIAGNOSIS

When the clinical presentation is consistent with genitourinary tuberculosis, a history of exposure, especially to a household contact, or a past history of tuberculous infection should raise the possibility of genitourinary tuberculosis. Abnormal chest radiographs that are consistent with old healed disease are seen in 50–70% of patients with genitourinary disease, and active disease with positive sputum cultures is occasionally noted (Christiansen, 1974; Kollins *et al.*, 1974; Teklu and Ostrow, 1976). Tuberculin skin tests are positive in 90–100% of patients with genitourinary tuberculosis. Urinalysis reveals hematuria in 12–77%, pyuria in 46–89%, and proteinuria in 13–80% of cases (Christiansen, 1974; Simon *et al.*, 1977; Kollins *et al.*, 1974; Teklu and Ostrow, 1976).

The diagnosis is firmly established by isolating *M. tuberculosis* from an infected site. Positive urine cultures confirm the diagnosis in most situations, but purulent material from sinus tracts or tissue specimens (e.g. prostatic biopsies or resected epididymis) may also grow the organism. At times a presumptive diagnosis is established by finding caseating or noncaseating granulomas in tissue sections, and this is supported by response to anti-tuberculous chemotherapy. In general, urine specimens for acid-fast smears are not recommended, since saprophytic nontuberculous mycobacteria can contaminate specimens resulting in false-positive smears. A well collected, concentrated, morning urine specimen is preferable to a 24-hour collection (Kenney *et al.*, 1960).

Several radiographic abnormalities appear on intravenous pyelography, including focal calcifications in the kidney, parenchymal masses, cortical scarring, medullary cavitation, nonvisualization, calyceal and pelvic dilatation, papillary destruction, and ureteral stricture with and without hydronephrosis. Other morphologic abnormalities include beaded, corkscrew, and pipestem ureters;

prostatic and seminal vesicle calcification; and contracted bladder with a thickened wall.

TREATMENT

Chemotherapy with isoniazid (INH) and rifampin for 9 months is currently recommended in the treatment of pulmonary tuberculosis (CDC, 1980). Six-month regimens have also been used successfully and are currently under investigation in the United States (Snider *et al.*, 1982; Cohn *et al.*, 1983). Official recommendations for the use of short-course chemotherapy in the treatment of extrapulmonary disease have not been established due to lack of controlled data. The relatively small burden of organisms (compared to pulmonary disease) suggests that short-course regimens should be effective for treatment of extrapulmonary tuberculosis (Dutt and Stead, 1982). This is especially true for treatment of genitourinary tuberculosis since high levels of most antituberculous medications concentrate in the urine, and probably in the genitourinary organs as well.

Many older reports document successful treatment of genitourinary tuberculosis with varying combinations of INH, para-aminosalicylic acid, streptomycin, and ethambutol, but stress the importance of treatment over 18–24 months (Gow, 1963; Wechsler and Lattimer, 1975; Lattimer and Ehrlich, 1968). However with the addition of rifampin, shorter regimens have been used and appear to be effective as well. Gow (1976) has successfully treated genitourinary tuberculosis with INH, rifampin, and ethambutol for 3 months followed by INH and rifampin for an additional 3–6 months. More recently, he has treated with INH, rifampin, and pyrazinamide for 2 months, followed by INH and rifampin for 2–4 months (Gow, 1979, 1981). Mallo *et al.* (1978) have demonstrated sterilization of renal cavities with treatment for 6–8 months with INH, rifampin, and ethambutol. At the current time we believe that standard chemotherapy for genitourinary tuberculosis caused by sensitive organisms should be INH and rifampin for 9 months; however, when Gow's results are corroborated by other investigators with appropriate periods of follow-up, 4–6 months regimens should become standard.

Surgical therapy for genitourinary tuberculosis has changed dramatically since the advent of effective chemotherapy. In the past, removal of a destroyed nonfunctioning kidney was often performed but the necessity to perform this procedure has declined in the post-chemotherapy era (Lattimer and Ehrlich, 1968; Flechner and Gow, 1980). Although some debate remains, current indications for nephrectomy include a nonfunctioning kidney associated with persistent abscess and/or sinus tract, hypertension, persistent intractable pain, hemorrhage, or inability to rule out renal carcinoma (Narayana, 1982; Gow, 1979; Flechner and Gow, 1980). Ureteral strictures can usually be dilated, but at times reimplantation procedures are necessary (Gow, 1971; Murphy *et al.*, 1982; Kerr *et al.*, 1970). An enterocystoplasty may be required for severe cases of bladder contracture (Kerr *et al.*, 1970). Epididymitis generally responds to medical therapy alone, but some authors recommend epididymectomy if there is poor response after 2 months of medical therapy or carcinoma or seminoma cannot be ruled out (Skutil and Gow, 1977). Tuberculosis of the prostate or seminal vesicles never requires surgical intervention.

The use of steroids is controversial, although Gow (1981) advocates their use in the early intensive phase of chemotherapy to prevent stricture formation. There are no controlled data to properly answer this question.

References

Agarwalla, B., Mohanty, G. P., Sahu, L. K. *et al.* (1980). Tuberculosis of the penis: report of 2 cases. *J. Urol.*, **124**, 927

Blight, E. M. (1980). Nephrobronchial fistula due to tuberculosis. *Urology*, **15**, 526

CDC (1980). Guidelines for short-course tuberculosis chemotherapy. *Morbid. Mortal. Weekly Rep.*, **28**, 97

CDC (1981). *Tuberculosis in the United States, 1979*. Publication No. 82–8322 (Atlanta: Center for Disease Control)

Christiansen, W. I. (1974). Genitourinary tuberculosis: review of 102 cases. *Medicine*, **53**, 377.

Cinman, A. C. (1982). Genitourinary tuberculosis. *Urology*, **20**, 353

Claridge, M. (1970). Ureteric obstruction in tuberculosis. *Br. J. Urol.*, **42**, 688

Cohn, D. L. , Catlin, B. J., Sbarbaro, J. A. *et al.* (1983). Evaluation of a four-drug six-month directly-administered regimen for treatment of tuberculosis. *Am. Rev. Resp. Dis. Suppl.*, **127**, 192

Danneberg, A. M. (1982). Pathogenesis of pulmonary tuberculosis. *Am. Rev. Resp. Dis. Suppl.*, **125**, 25

Dutt, A. K. and Stead, W. W. (1982). Present chemotherapy for tuberculosis. *J. Infect. Dis.*, **146**, 698

Farnell, B. and Thomas P. (1983). Tuberculosis of the epididymis. *Can. Med. Assoc. J.*, **128**, 1296

Flechner, S. M. and Gow, J. G. (1980). Role of nephrectomy in the treatment of nonfunctioning or very poorly functioning unilateral tuberculous kidney. *J. Urol.*, **123**, 822

Gow, J. G. (1963). Genitourinary tuberculosis: A study of 700 cases. *Lancet.*, **2**, 261

Gow, J. G. (1971). Genitourinary tuberculosis: A study of the disease in one unit over a period of 24 years. *Ann. Roy. Coll. Surg. Engl.*, **49**, 50

Gow, J. G. (1976). Genitourinary tuberculosis: A study of short course regimens. *J. Urol.*, **115**, 707

Gow, J. G. (1979). Genitourinary tuberculosis: A 7-year review. *Br. J. Urol.*, **51**, 239

Gow, J. G. (1981). The management of genitourinary tuberculosis. *J. Antimicrob. Chemother.*, **7**, 590

Hashmonai, M., Bolkier, M. and Schramek, A. (1982). Tuberculous recto-vesico-cutaneous fistula. *Br. J. Urol.*, **54**, 324

Kenney, M., Loechel, A. B. and Lovelock, F. J. (1960). Urine cultures in tuberculosis. *Am. Rev. Resp. Dis.*, **82**, 564

Kerr, W. K., Gale, G. L., Struthers, N. W. *et al.* (1970). Prognosis in reconstructive surgery for urinary tuberculosis. *Br. J. Urol.*, **42**, 672

Kollins, S. A., Hartman, G. W., Carr, D. T. *et al.* (1974). Roentgenographic findings in urinary tract tuberculosis. *Am. J. Roentgenol.*, **121**, 487

Kumar, S. Chandrasekar, D., Rao, M. S. *et al.* (1981). Solitary paravesical tuberculoma masquerading as bladder carcinoma. *Tubercle*, **62**, 143

Lattimer, J. K., Colmore, H. P., Sanger, G. *et al.* (1954). Transmission of genital tuberculosis from husband to wife via the semen. *Am. Rev. Tuberc.*, **69**, 618

Lattimer, J. K. and Ehrlich., R. M. (1968). Present aspects of genitourinary tuberculosis. *Adv. Tuberc. Res.*, **16**, 32

Lewis, E. L. (1946). Tuberculosis of the penis: a report of 5 new cases and a complete review of the literature. *J. Urol.*, **56**, 737

Mallo, N., Dalet, F. and Villavicencio, H. (1978). Treatment of renal tuberculosis: Microbiological study of 271 renal tuberculous cavities. *Eur. Urol.*, **4**, 269

Medlar, E. M., Spain, D. M. and Holliday, R. W. (1949). Post mortem compared with clinical diagnosis of genitourinary tuberculosis in adult males. *J. Urol.*, **51**, 1078

Murphy, D. M., Fallon, B., Lane V. *et al.* (1982). Tuberculous stricture of the ureter. *Urology*, **20**, 382

Narayana, A. S. (1982). Overview of renal tuberculosis. *Urology*, **19**, 231

O'Dea, M. J., Moore, S. B. and Greene, L. F. (1978). Tuberculous prostatitis. *Urology*, **11**, 483

Raghavaiah, N. V. (1979). Tuberculosis of the male urethra. *J. Urol.*, **122**, 417

Rees, R. W. M. and Hollands, F. G. (1970). The ureter in renal tuberculosis. *Br. J. Urol.*, **42**, 693

Reeve, H. R., Weinherth, J. L. and Peterson, C. J. (1974). Tuberculosis of the epididymis and testicle presenting as a hydrocele. *Urology*, **4**, 329

Riehle, R. A. and Jayaraman, K. (1982). Tuberculosis of testis. *Urology*, **20**, 43

Rosenberg, S. (1963). Has chemotherapy reduced the incidence of genitourinary tuberculosis? A comparison based on autopsy material from Bellvue Hospital. *J. Urol.*, **90**, 317

Ross, J. C., Gow, J. G. and St. Hill, C. A. (1961). Tuberculosis epididymitis: a review of 170 patients. *Br. J. Surg.*, **48**, 663

Simon, H. B., Weinstein, A. J., Pasternak, M. S. *et al.* (1977). Genitourinary tuberculosis: Clinical features in a general hospital population. *Am. J. Med.*, **63**, 410

Skutil, V. and Gow, J. G. (1977). Urogenital tuberculosis: the present state in Europe. *Eur. Urol.*, **3**, 257

Snider, D. E., Rogowski, J., Zierski, M. *et al.* (1982). Successful intermittent treatment of smear-positive pulmonary tuberculosis in six months: a cooperative study in Poland. *Am. Rev. Resp. Dis.*, **125**, 265

Stanisic, T. H., Kolbusz, W. and Carter, M. (1978). Unusual presentation of genital tuberculosis. *Urology*, **12**, 351

Teklu, B. and Ostrow, J. H. (1976). Urinary tuberculosis: a review of 44 cases treated since 1963. *J. Urol.*, **115**, 507

Vasquez, G. and Lattimer, J. K. (1959). Danger to children of infection from exposure to urine containing tubercle bacilli. *J. Am. Med. Assoc.*, **171**, 29

Veenema, R. J. and Lattimer, J. K. (1957). Genital tuberculosis in the male: Clinical pathology and effect on fertility. *J. Urol.*, **78**, 65

Venkataramaiah, N. R., Raalte, J. A. and Dutte, S. N. (1982). Tuberculous ulcer of the penis. *Postgrad. Med. J.*, **58**, 59

Wechsler, M. and Lattimer, J. K. (1975). An evaluation of the current therapeutic regimen for renal tuberculosis. *J. Urol.*, **113**, 760

Wisnia, L. G., Kukolj, S., de Santa Maria, J. L. *et al.* (1978). Renal function damage in 131 cases of urogenital tuberculosis. *Urology*, **11**, 457

Yu, H. Y. Y., Wong, K. K., Lim, T. K. *et al.* (1977). Clinical study of hemospermia. *Urology*, **10**, 562

3
Pelvic actinomycosis

D. H. GREMILLION and M. GALBRAITH

INTRODUCTION

Actinomycosis is an indolent, slowly progressing infection with anaerobic Gram-positive organisms. Clinicians should be familiar with it as it has been emphasized in recent reviews. The first microscopic description of the organism was by Von Graefe in 1854; the organisms were first isolated in 1875 by Cohn. The disease state was described later, first in cattle (1877) and subsequently in humans (1878).

Human actinomycosis is not common, and the effective, early use of antibiotics has further reduced the frequency of invasive, systemic disease. Even more uncommon is actinomycosis of the female pelvic organs; only 213 cases had been reported as of 1970 and less than 300 cases by 1976.

EPIDEMIOLOGY

Actinomycosis is sporadic but worldwide in its occurrence; there are no recorded epidemics. There is no race or age predilection; however, two-thirds of the cases in one large series were between the ages of 30 and 60 years (Brown, 1973). Until recently it was thought that males developed actinomycosis 3 to 5 times more frequently than females. The recent apparent increase among females in association with IUCD use may change this relationship.

MICROBIOLOGY

Bacteria of the family *Actinomyces* are anaerobic, Gram-positive, branching, pleomorphic, rod-like non-acid-fast cells. Morphologic and microbiologic features of the genus *Actinomyces* are summarized in Table 1. Their improper identification as fungi has resulted from a tendency to form long branching filaments and from the fungus-like appearance of the characteristic 'sulfur

35

Table 1. Microbiologic and morphologic features of *Actinomyces*

Gram-positive rods
  Non-motile
  Non-sporeforming
  Non-acid-fast
Strict anaerobes
Tendency to form long branching filaments in pus
Sulfur granules
Lack nuclear membrane, mitochondria and chitin
Contain muramic acid and lysine

granule' seen so commonly in properly prepared anatomic specimens. *Actinomyces* organisms lack a nuclear membrane, mitochondria and chitin, all of which are present in fungi. Moreover, their cell walls contain muramic acid and lysine which are not found in fungal cell walls. Another finding of differential and clinical importance is that the *Actinomyces* are affected by penicillin, whereas fungi are not. *Actinomyces israelii* is a strict anaerobe and grows slowly; 4 days are required for a colony to reach the size of 2–4 mm. Brain–heart infusion agar with 5% defibrinated sheep blood is routinely used for isolation, but thioglycolate broth is also suitable. Of the seven species of *Actinomyces* (Table 2), only *A. israelii* is commonly associated with human disease. *A. bovis* does not occur in man.

Table 2 Species of the genus *Actinomyces* and clinical relationships

Species	Disease	Habitat
A. bovis (1879)	Cattle actinomycosis	Dental plaque, oral cavity, tonsil
A. israelii	Human actinomycosis Lacrimal canniculitis	Dental plaque, oral cavity, tonsil
A. naeslundii (1951)	Human actinomycosis Lacrimal canniculitis	Dental plaque, oral cavity, tonsil
A. suis	Human actinomycosis Lacrimal canniculitis	Dental plaque, oral cavity, tonsil
A. viscosus	Human actinomycosis Lacrimal canniculitis	Dental plaque, oral cavity, tonsil
A. odontolyticus	Human actinomycosis Lacrimal canniculitis	Dental plaque, oral cavity, tonsil
A. propionicus	Human actinomycosis Lacrimal canniculitis	Dental plaque, oral cavity, tonsil
A. eriksonii	Lung abscess	Dental plaque, oral cavity, tonsil, intestinal tract

A characteristic feature of the purulent secretions obtained from *Actinomyces* infections is the 'sulfur granule'. These are hard discrete yellow grains which are visible and large enough (40–400 μm) to be trapped by the gauze of surgical dressings. Microscopically 'sulfur granules' appear as dense masses of bacteria. Although they are considered characteristic, they were present in only 7% of 181 cases in one large study (Brown, 1973). Other pathogens may also produce 'sulfur granules', notably *Staphylococcus aureus*, *Nocardia* species and *Strepto-*

myces species. Only *A. odontolyticus* does not form granules. *Actinomyces* can be recovered from carious teeth and the oral cavity as well as the intestinal tract of healthy persons. The organism should be regarded as a saprophyte or commensal of low virulence which requires special conditions to cause disease.

Isolation of *Actinomyces* from the inanimate environment has not been described, and all infections with this organism must be presumed to originate with the host's own microflora. Concurrent isolation of additional aerobic and anaerobic pathogens is frequent along with actinomycosis. In Brown's series (1973) other aerobic and anaerobic bacteria were detected in 30% of cases. The associated growth of *Actinobacillus actinomycetemcomitans* is well known, but at present thought to be of little clinical significance.

CLINICAL MANIFESTATIONS

The predominant areas of infections are cervicofacial, thoracic, and abdominal (Table 3). In each instance the disease generally takes the form of a chronic, painful, indurated swelling which spreads to adjacent structures. Less commonly, there is hematogenous spread to remote sites. Individual lesions are characterized by chronic suppuration, often with fistulae draining pus and sulfur granules, extensive necrosis and fibrosis of surrounding tissues. Lesions may be mistaken for tumors because they are generally slowly growing and firm.

Table 3 Clinical forms of actinomycosis (percentages)

	Cope, 1949	Brown, 1973
Cervicofacial	63	32
Thoracic	15	33
Abdominal	22	28
Pelvic	—[a]	2
Other	—[a]	5

[a] Data not reported

Of those cases involving the abdomen, only a small number affect the female organs. In a study done three decades ago at the Mayo Clinic, only 10 of 122 cases (8%) of abdominal actinomycosis involved the female genital tract (Putman *et al.*, 1950). In a series of 181 cases reported 20 years later (Brown, 1973), only 28% were abdominal; of these, only 4 (8%) were of pelvic origin. Fewer than 250 cases of female genital tract actinomycosis had been reported by 1970 (Surur, 1974). Between 1970 and 1980, however, this number had increased to approximately 400. In all likelihood this figure underestimates the true number of cases.

The ovaries are most commonly affected, with concurrent salpingo-ovarian involvement next in frequency. Less frequently involved are the corpus uteri, vulva, cervix and fallopian tubes alone. Bilateral involvement of adnexa has been reported to occur in 44% of cases (Paalman *et al.*, 1949). The right adnexa are affected twice as commonly as the left (38% vs 17%, respectively). This observation suggests the possibility of contiguous spread to the right adnexa from cecal and appendiceal sites since these are the most common locations of abdominal involvement. In a review of 151 cases of pelvic actinomycosis, 91% arose from a contiguous GI focus, often a ruptured appendix (MacCarthy, 1955).

ACTINOMYCOSIS ASSOCIATED WITH IUCD USE

Use of intrauterine contraceptive devices (IUCDs) has expanded the clinical awareness of pelvic actinomycosis. The first cases reported were fatal tubo-ovarian abscesses in patients using metal IUCDs (Barth, 1928; Tietze, 1930). IUCDs came into much more widespread clinical use in the early 1960s, and many reports of IUCD associated actinomycosis followed. At present, the disease may be considered rare although, as noted above, the currently reported cases may understate the true incidence. Since the first report in the modern era (Brenner and Archring, 1967), occasional case reports or series have appeared with fewer than 400 cases appearing in the western literature. A recent prospective study of 9191 patients using IUCDs identified 36 (0.4%) with *Actinomyces* on vaginal smear; of these 36, 9 (25%) had aggressive disease (Bhagavan and Gupta, 1978). These investigators considered aggressive disease to be present when *Actinomyces* colonization occurred in the presence of active clinical signs of infection (fever, discharge). Other studies have detected somewhat higher rates of *Actinomyces* colonization in IUCD wearers ranging from 8% (Hager *et al.*, 1979) to 20% (Jones and Buschman, 1979). Invasive disease was less frequent in the latter studies, however.

Apparently the risk of actinomycosis with IUCD use is quite low, but in the subgroup of patients colonized with *Actinomyces* as detected by smear or culture, the risk of invasive disease may be present and IUCD removal is warranted. Patients with IUCD-associated actinomycosis often present with findings of acute pelvic inflammatory disease; fever, chills, vaginal discharge, pain, intermenstrual bleeding and menorrhagia. In one study, however, half of the cases were asymptomatic (Bhagavan and Gupta, 1978) and were detected only by smear.

Almost all types of IUCDs have been associated with pelvic actinomycosis. Most have been in place over 2 years when disease occurs (Majmudar, 1980), but cases occurring as soon as 2 months after insertion have been reported (Hager *et al.*, 1979).

COMPLICATIONS

Complications of pelvic actinomycosis are not common and are limited to hematogenous dissemination or direct extension by contiguous spread to surrounding structures. Hematogenous dissemination has rarely been reported. In one notable case a brain abscess due to *Actinomyces israelii* occurred 4 years after hysterectomy for pelvic actinomycosis in a patient who received no antibiotics (de la Monte *et al.*, 1982). The liver is the most frequent visceral organ involved with hematogenous spread. Contiguous spread has been reported more frequently; this may involve the urinary bladder (King and Lam, 1978), ureters (House, 1981), retroperitoneal space (Willscher *et al.*, 1978) or abdominal cavity (O'Brien, 1975). Presentation with urinary symptoms or obstructive uropathy may result. Deaths due to pelvic actinomycosis are rare. Only two deaths were reported in the antibiotic era: one occurred in a 28-year-old female with intraabdominal rupture of a large tubovarian abscess and two IUCDs *in situ* (Hager *et al.*, 1979) and the other in a 26-year-old woman with a ruptured adenexal abscess (Doberneck, 1982).

PATHOGENESIS

The oxidation–reduction potential of viable tissues is the most effective host defense against anaerobic bacteria. When anaerobes are exposed to reduced oxygen levels – as is the case in the presence of injury, necrosis, or foreign bodies – they proliferate and invade surrounding tissue. Violation of tissue planes and barriers characterizes *Actinomyces* infection. Oropharyngeal and pulmonary actinomycosis probably result from the colonization of carious teeth and tonsillar crypts. Vaginal colonization likewise accounts for much of the reported pelvic actinomycosis, although spread from adjacent abdominal structures was previously thought more common. All organs may be involved if bloodstream invasion occurs. Remarkably, spread to regional lymph nodes is rare.

Colonization of the vagina in IUCD users appears to play an important role in the pathogenesis of pelvic actinomycosis. First identified in pap smears by light microscopy (Gupta *et al.*, 1976), subsequent investigations have documented vaginal colonization in IUCD users with rates ranging from 1% (Valicenti *et al.*, 1982) to 25% (Sykes and Shelley, 1981). *Actinomyces* has not generally been found in non-IUCD users in spite of many studies assessing the normal vaginal flora. A notable exception is a recent study employing pepsin digestion and rhodamine conjugation of anti-*Actinomyces* antibody to reduce nonspecific staining (Pine *et al.*, 1981). These authors report 39% colonization in IUCD users compared to 13% in non-IUCD users, a difference which was not statistically significant but which is of considerable clinical interest because it implies that *Actinomyces* can be found in the vaginas of women not wearing IUCDs. Routine light microscopy and anaerobic culture do not reliably demonstrate *Actinomyces*. A direct fluorescent antibody technique using antibody labeled with fluorescein or rhodamine detects *Actinomyces* more reliably but suffers from frequent false-positives.

According to some the duration of IUCD use determines the risk of colonization and subsequent infection, with the incidence increasing after 2 years of use (Valicenti *et al.*, 1982; Spence *et al.*, 1978). However, no association of infection with duration of use was found in a prospective evaluation of 293 patients in Britain (Duguid *et al.*, 1980). Orogenital sexual contact may facilitate vaginal colonization with *Actinomyces* (Gupta *et al.*, 1978). Although certain types of IUCD are more commonly associated with *Actinomyces* infection, this may be a function of their frequency of use (Spence *et al.*, 1978). The protective effect of metal devices suggested by one investigator (Duguid *et al.*, 1980) has not been validated by other studies.

Some investigators speculate that calcium deposits on the IUCD surface enhance colonization by providing a 'niche' for attachment and growth of *Actinomyces* (Johnson *et al.*, 1976; Schmidt *et al.*, 1980; Gonzales, 1981). A crust of calcium and organic debris forms on the IUCD. Both the microorganisms and the host are postulated as sources of the calcium, but it is clear that calcium precipitates in the absence of microorganisms. Calcium is present in uterine fluid and its precipitation on foreign bodies may be facilitated by changes in pH during the menstrual cycle. Deposits can be detected as soon as 6 months after IUCD insertion and increase with duration of use, leading some investigators to recommend biennial replacement.

DIAGNOSIS

A high index of suspicion is the clinician's best asset in diagnosing pelvic actinomycosis. Only 19 of 181 cases (10%) reported in one series were suspected (Brown, 1973). The diagnosis should be considered in any female with an IUD *in situ* or recently removed who presents with pelvic inflammatory disease, a tumor-like mass or vaginal discharge.

Tissue samples suspected of containing *Actinomyces* should be transported to the microbiology laboratory as soon as possible under anaerobic conditions. Cultures should be observed for 2 weeks or more before being called negative. Even under the best of conditions and using the latest culture techniques, recovery of *Actinomyces* is disappointing. *Actinomyces* often exists in a setting of mixed aerobic and anaerobic flora which may overgrow the fastidious *Actinomyces* and obscure its identification. Examining purulent secretions by Gram-stain and tissue by hematoxylin and eosin stain or Brown and Brenn stain may reveal the organism in mycelial or bacillary form. Direct fluorescent antibody testing of purulent secretions is very effective but not generally available. Colonization is best detected on routine pap smear with detection rates of 70–95% reported by experienced investigators (Valicenti *et al.*, 1982; Spence *et al.*, 1978).

Clinically silent abdominal abscesses due to *Actinomyces* occur and should be sought when abdominal or pelvic actinomycosis is diagnosed. Gallium-67 scanning, ultrasound, or computerized axial tomography may have a role in identifying unsuspected pelvic abscess sites and in guiding surgeons to prospective sites for drainage.

TREATMENT

Systemic or pelvic actinomycosis responds well to penicillin or tetracycline therapy. Penicillin should be administered parenterally in doses of 4–12 million units daily. Follow-up oral penicillin VK for several months is usually recommended after parenteral penicillin. Tetracycline is considered the therapy of choice by many investigators because of the rapid clinical response it gives and the convenience of an oral route of administration. Clindamycin is an alternative choice antibiotic in patients allergic to penicillin and intolerant of tetracycline. Long-course therapy is necessary. Other antibiotics show suitable activity *in vitro*, including chloramphenicol, erythromycin, lincomycin, minocycline and doxycycline. Clinical studies to document their effectiveness is lacking, however. Duration of antibiotic therapy is not well established by clinical trials but has usually been maintained for 3–4 weeks after resolution of all clinical signs of disease. Actinomycosis has a tendency to relapse, and patients should be followed carefully after treatment has ended.

In our opinion, asymptomatic patients with IUCDs and vaginal *Actinomyces* colonization should have the IUCDs removed and an alternative form of contraception recommended. If *Actinomyces* cannot be detected following the next menstrual cycle, another IUCD may be reinserted. It is our opinion that antibiotics need not be given if signs of pelvic infection are not present, although reports of late complications have been published (Hager *et. al.*, 1978).

Hyperbaric oxygen has been used with success in some refractory cases. Its use remains controversial, however. Increased oxygenation of tissues may facilitate wound healing and lead to death of strict anaerobic organisms. Comparative studies have not been done, but limited clinical trials are promising especially in refractory cases (Manheim *et al.*, 1969).

Surgical debridement of devitalized tissues is often necessary because of poor penetration of antibiotics. Abdominal and pelvic forms of the disease are usually associated with abscesses that require surgical drainage. Older literature indicates cure following adequate drainage and debridement only.

SUMMARY

Actinomycosis is an uncommon infection of the female genital tract with fewer than 300 cases reported by 1976. The responsible organism is a strict anaerobe. Until relatively recently it had been thought to be a fungus because of its branching morphology. When the female genital tract is involved, disease often arises from a contiguous gastrointestinal focus or from colonized IUCDs. Colonization of IUCDs with *Actinomyces* may be an indication for removal. Pelvic actinomycosis may be complicated by direct extension to surrounding structures or by hematogenous spread to remote sites such as the liver or brain. Obstructive uropathy may result from direct extension to the nearby ureters or bladder. Although complications may be severe, deaths are rare. Penicillin is the antibiotic of choice. When given in high doses for prolonged periods of time treatment with penicillin is very successful, but therapy often requires a coordinated program of drainage and debridement of devitalized tissue.

The views expressed are solely those of the authors and not those of the United States Air Force or the Department of Defense.

References

Barth, H. (1928). Uber parametritis Actinomycotica ahre Entstehung. *Arch. Gynecol.*, **134,** 310

Berardi, R. S. (1979). Abdominal actinomycosis. *Surg. Gynecol. Obstet.*, **149,** 257

Bhagavan, B. S. and Gupta, P. K. (1978). Genital actinomycosis and intrauterine contraceptive devices: cytopathologic diagnosis and clinical significance. *Human Pathol.*, **9**, 567

Bhagavan, B. S., Ruffier, J. and Shinn, B. (1982). Pseudo-actinomycotic radiate granules in the lower female genital tract: Relationship to the Splendore–Hoeppli phenomenon. *Human Pathol.*, **13**, 898

Brenner, R. W. and Archring, S. W. (1967). Pelvic actinomycosis in the presence of an endocervical contraceptive device. *Obstet. Gynecol.*, **29**, 71

Brown, J. R. (1973). Human actinomycosis: a study of 181 subjects. *Human Pathol.*, **4**, 319

Brown, R. and Bancewicz, J. (1982). Ureteric obstruction due to pelvic actinomycosis. *Br. J. Surg.*, **69**, 156

Burkman, R. T. (1981). Association between intrauterine devices and pelvic inflammatory disease. *Obstet. Gynecol.*, **57**, 269

Cope, V. S. (1949). Visceral actinomycosis. *Ann. Roy. Col. Surg. Med.*, **5**, 394

de la Monte, S. M., Gupta, P. K. and White, C. L. (1982). Systemic Actinomyces infection: a potential complication of intrauterine contraceptive devices. *J. Am. Med. Assoc.*, **248**, 1876

Doberneck, R. C. (1982). Pelvic actinomycosis associated with use of intrauterine devices. *Am. Surg.*, **48**, 25

Duguid, H. L., Parratt, D. and Traynor, R. (1980). Actinomyces-like organisms in cervical smears from women using intrauterine contraceptive devices. *Br. Med. J.*, **2**, 534

Edelman, D. A., Berger, G. S. and Keith, L. G. (1982). The use of IUDs and their relationship to pelvic inflammatory disease: A review of epidemiologic and clinical studies. *Curr. Prob. Obstet. Gynecol.*, vi (3), 5

Gonzalez, E. R. (1981). Calcium deposits on IUCDs may play a role in infections. *J. Am. Med. Assoc.*, **245**, 1625

Gupta, P. K., Erozan, Y. S. and Frost, J. K. (1978). Actinomyces and the IUD: An update. *Acta Cytol.*, **22**, 281

Gupta, P. K., Hollander, D. H. and Forst, J. K. (1976). Actinomyces in cervico-vaginal smears: an association with IUCD usage. *Acta Cytol.*, **20**, 295

Gupta, P. K. and Woodruff, J. D. (1982). Actinomyces in vaginal smears. *J. Am. Med. Assoc.*, **247**, 1175

Hager, W. D., Douglas, B., Majmudar, B. *et al.* (1979). Pelvic colonization with actinomyces in women using intrauterine contraceptive devices. *Am. J. Obstet. Gynecol.*, **135**, 680

Hager, W. D. and Majmudar, B. (1978). Pelvic actinomycosis in women using intrauterine contraceptive devices. *Am. J. Obstet. Gynecol.*, **133**, 60

House, M. J. (1981). Abdominal actinomycosis: A complication of laparoscopy? *Br. J. Obstet. Gynecol.*, **88**, 459

Johnson, A. B., Maness, R. F. and Wheeler, R. G. (1976). Calcareous deposits formed on IUDs in human exposures. *Contraception*, **14**, 507

Jones, M. C. and Buschman, B. O. (1979). The prevalence of actinomyces-like organism found in cervico-vaginal smears of 300 IUCD users. *Acta Cytol.*, **23**, 282

Karbour, A., Harger, J., Ryan, J. *et al.* (1980). The significance of the presence of actinomycetes in Papanicolaou's smears of IUD users. *Acta Cytol.*, **24**, 76

King, D. T. and Lam, M. (1978). Actinomycosis of the urinary bladder: Association with an intrauterine contraceptive device. *J. Am. Med. Assoc.*, **240**, 1512

Lomax, C. W., Harbent, G. M. and Thornton, W. N. (1976). Actinomycosis of the female genital tract. *Obstet. Gynecol.*, **48**, 341

Luff, R. D., Gupta, P. K., Spence, M. R. *et al.* (1978). Pelvic actinomycosis and the intrauterine contraceptive device: A cyto-histomorphologic study. *Am. J. Clin. Pathol.*, **69**, 581

MacCarthy, J. (1955). Actinomycosis of the female pelvic organs with involvement of the endometrium. *J. Pathol.*, **69**, 176

Majmudar, B. (1980). Actinomycosis and the IUCD. *S. Med. J.*, **73**, 835

Manheim, S. D., Chondray, C., Ludwig, A. *et al.* (1969). Hyperbaric oxygen in the treatment of actinomycosis. *J. Am. Med. Assoc.*, **210**, 552

Mead, P. B., Beechman, J. B. and Maeck, J. (1976). Incidence of infections associated with the intrauterine contraceptive device in an isolated community. *Am. J. Obstet. Gynecol.*, **125**, 79

O'Brien, P. K. (1975). Abdominal adendometrial actinomycosis associated with an intrauterine device. *Can. Med. Assoc. J.*, **112**, 596

Paalman, R. J., Dockerty, M. B. and Mussey, R. D. (1949). Actinomycosis of the ovaries and fallopian tubes. *Am. J. Obstet. Gynecol.*, **58**, 419

Pine, L., Malcolm, G. B. and Curtis, E. M. *et al.* (1981). Demonstration of Actinomyces and Arachina species in cervicovaginal smears by direct staining with species-specific fluorescent-antibody conjugate. *J. Clin. Microbiol.*, **13**, 15

Putman, H. C., Dockerty, M. B. and Waugh, J. M. (1950). Abdominal actinomycosis: an analysis of 122 cases. *Surgery*, **28**, 781

Richter, G. O., Pratt, J. H., Nichols, D. R. *et al.* (1972). Actinomycosis of the female genital organs. *Minn. Med.*, **55**, 1003

Schmidt, W. A., Bedrossian, C. W., Ali, V. *et al.* (1980). Actinomycosis and IUCDs: The clinicopathologic entity. *Diag. Gynecol. Obstet.*, **2**, 165

Schuffer, M. A., Elguezubal, A., Sultana, M. *et al.* (1975). Actinomycosis infections associated with intrauterine contraceptive devices. *Obstet. Gynecol.*, **45**, 67

Spence, M. R., Gupta, P. K., Frost, J. K. *et al.* (1978). Cytologic detection and clinical significance of Actinomyces israelii in women using intrauterine contraceptive devices. *Am. J. Obstet. Gynecol.*, **131**, 295

Surur, F. (1974). Actinomycosis of the female genital tract. *N.Y. St. Med. J.*, **74**, 408

Sykes, G. S. and Shelley G. (1981). Actinomyces-like structures and their association with IUCDs: pelvic infection and abnormal cervical cytology. *Br. J. Obstet. Gynecol.*, **88**, 934

Targum, S. D. and Wright, N. H. (1974). Association of the intrauterine device and pelvic inflammatory abscess: a retrospective pilot study. *Am. J. Epidemiol.*, **100**, 262

Taylor, E. S., McMillan, J. H., Greer, B. E. *et al.* (1975). The intrauterine device and tubo-ovarian abscess. *Am. J. Obstet. Gynecol.*, **123**, 338

Tietze, K. (1930). Actinomycosis of the Uterus, *Diech. Med. Wsche.*, **vi**, 1307

Valicenti, J. F., Pappas, A. A., Craber, C. D. *et al.* (1982). Detection and prevalence of IUCD-associated actinomyces colonization and related mortality: a prospective study of 69,925 cervical smears. *J. Am. Med. Assoc.*, **247**, 1149

Willscher, M. K., Mozden, P. J. and Olsson, C. A. (1978). Retroperitoneal fibrosis with ureteral obstruction secondary to *Actinomyces israelii. Urology*, **12**, 569

Editor's note: Interested readers should consult the additional references in the postscript to the Preface of this volume.

L. KEITH

4
Toxoplasma in pregnancy

M. S. RAHMAN and J. RAHMAN

INTRODUCTION

Toxoplasmosis is an infectious disease caused by the protozoan parasite *Toxoplasma gondii*. This disease has extremely variable clinical manifestations, and because most patients are asymptomatic the disease goes unrecognized. In some patient groups, however, including neonates and immunosuppressed patients, toxoplasmosis may cause life-threatening illness. The importance of *T. gondii* to obstetricians lies in its ability to produce clinically unrecognizable disease in the mother and to potentially infect the unborn child (Hume, 1972; Desmonts and Couvreur, 1974). Approximately 3300 infants are born with congenital toxoplasma infection each year in the United States (Wilson *et al.*, 1980). The incidence of congenital toxoplasmosis resulting in fetal damage is approximately 1 in 8000 births in the United States (Sever, 1980).

THE PARASITE AND ITS PATHOGENESIS

Toxoplasma gondii is an obligate intracellular parasite. It is now recognized that *T. gondii* is a coccidia-like organism and a member of the toxoplasmida within the subphyllum sporozoa.

Members of the cat family are the definitive host of this parasite, which has a life cycle in cats similar to that of the malarial parasite in mosquitoes. Man and animals other than felines serve as intermediary hosts. *T. gondii* may reside in a host in one of three forms: as a trophozoite, within tissue cysts, or as an oocyst. The trophozoites are crescent-shaped or round cells that are about $3 \times 7 \, \mu$m in size with a well-defined nucleus. The trophozoite stage of *T. gondii* accompanies the acute stage of the infection. During this stage the organism is capable of invading all nucleated mammalian cells. It multiplies rapidly within cells by endodyogeny or budding, leading to cell rupture and further dissemination. The host eventually develops antibodies to the parasite, killing the free trophozoites. Only the intracellular organisms survive; they become dormant and form tissue cysts. The tissue cysts are usually round or spindle-shaped and are 10–100 μm in diameter; they may contain as many as 3000 organisms. Tissue cysts may be formed virtually in any organ of the host as early as 8 days after infection and may persist throughout the life of the host. Skeletal muscle, brain, and ocular tissues are the most frequent sites of tissue-cyst formation. The appearance of tissue cysts marks the latent phase of the infection.

The cat and other felines become infected by ingesting tissue cysts from the muscle tissue of captured rodents and birds or in raw meat. The cysts are resident to the gastric secretions of the stomach, in contrast to the free trophozoites, which are easily destroyed. When the cysts reach the small intestine the trophozoites are released; they then undergo asexual and sexual stages of development in the epithelium of the gut. The end result is the formation of oocysts, which are excreted in the feces of the cat. Given favorable temperature and humidity, oocysts sporulate in 3–4 days to become infectious for humans and other domestic animals. Oocysts are capable of surviving for many months and are resistant to many chemical agents, including ordinary disinfectants. Arid conditions, extreme heat, and freezing temperatures destroy them.

EPIDEMIOLOGY

T. gondii has a worldwide distribution. It infects all orders of mammals, some birds, and probably some reptiles. Once considered a rare disease, toxoplasmosis is now recognized to be a significant public health hazard. Infection is transmitted to man by eating raw or undercooked meat that contains cysts. Some studies have found 25% of pork, 10% of mutton, and <1% of beef samples to contain toxoplasma cysts (Anderson, 1979). Infection may also occur when oocysts excreted by recently infected cats and other felines have been ingested. Cats that hunt and scavenge for their food may contaminate the environment by their feces and, therefore, constitute an important source of infection. Domesticated cats that eat only canned and dried foods do not represent a health hazard. On rare occasion, the ingestion of chicken eggs or raw milk may be a source of toxoplasma infection. Flies and cockroaches may also act as vectors in the transportation of the viable cysts (Wallace, 1973). Blood transfusion and organ transplantation may also transmit the infection. Laboratory workers may acquire toxoplasmosis accidentally as a result of self-inoculation.

An important mode of disease transmission is by the maternofetal route. Women who acquire the acute infection during pregnancy expose their developing fetus to the risk of transplacental infection.

The incidence of seropositivity for toxoplasmosis increases with age, and both sexes are equally affected. The rate of infection varies from 5% to 94%, depending upon the geographical location.

In general, warm and moist climates seem to favor the spread of infection, while the prevalence of infection is lower in the cold or hot and arid areas. Low rates of toxoplasmosis are reported from Arizona (Feldman, 1968), northern Norway (9.5%), Iceland, and the extreme northern parts of the USSR (4.2%) (Nekrasova, 1975). In contrast, higher rates of infection are recorded from some tropical regions such as El Salvador (93%) (Remington *et al.*, 1970), Tahiti (77%) (Feldman and Miller, 1956), and Paris (87%) (Desmonts *et al.*, 1965). An incidence of 31.2% has been reported for western Saudi Arabia (Basalamah and Serebour, 1981). Clearly there appear to be other climatic and ecologic factors that may affect the organism's ability to flourish.

The incidence of primary maternal infection during pregnancy is reported to be 8 per 1000 pregnancies in Paris (Desmonts and Couvreur, 1965), 7 per 1000 in Saudi Arabia (Basalamah and Serebour, 1981), 6.4 per 1000 in the United States (Sever, 1966), and 2.2 per 1000 in London (Kader, 1980).

IMMUNITY

In acquired toxoplasmosis the initial immune response is marked by the formation of IgM antibodies within 7–14 days after primary infection; peak levels are reached by 20 days (Monif, 1982). A gradual decline in the titers of IgM accompanies the production of specific antibodies of the IgG type. In chronic infections the antibody is exclusively IgG type. The acute infection may be distinguished from the chronic type on the basis of immunoglobulin levels.

CLINICAL MANIFESTATIONS

The clinical manifestations of toxoplasma infection in adults are extremely variable and may mimic a variety of other infectious diseases, particularly those of viral origin, such as infectious mononucleosis or cytomegalovirus infection.

Maternal infection

Acquired maternal infection may be so mild as to escape detection. When symptoms do occur, the clinical picture is most commonly that of lymphadeno-pathy accompanied only occasionally by malaise, fever, and skin rash. Posterior cervical, supraclavicular, and suboccipital lymph nodes are most commonly affected. Occasionally lymph nodes all over the body may be involved, although unilateral involvement is not unusual. The enlarged nodes are firm, discrete, and usually tender. The distinctive histologic feature of affected nodes is marked reticular cell hyperplasia in the germinal center.

Severe maternal infection is uncommon. The clinical picture relates to the organ system involved, and may be associated with headache, vomiting, mental depression, myalgia, pneumonia, hepatitis, myocarditis, encephalitis, delirium, and even convulsions.

Transmission of infection to the fetus

The parasite is most likely to be transmitted from mother to fetus when the mother has acquired primary infection during the pregnancy. Under these circumstances approximately one-third of the fetuses become infected (Desmonts and Couvreur, 1974). In contrast fetal infection rarely occurs when maternal infection precedes the pregnancy. The risk of fetal infection also varies with the trimester of pregnancy during which the mother becomes infected, the highest incidence occurring in the last trimester, although in this case the disease in the newborn remains subclinical. If the mother is infected during the first half of the pregnancy, the fetus is affected less frequently, but the disease in the neonate is more severe. The difference in the severity of clinical disease in the newborn may be due to the relative immaturity of the fetal immune system at the time of the parasitemia.

Fetal infection

In severe cases congenital toxoplasmosis can lead to the death of the fetus. At the other extreme, the apparent effect of the infection may be so minimal that the fetus appears completely normal at birth; only at a later age do signs of chorioretinitis, mental retardation, hearing loss, or other nervous system problems appear. A prospective study from Paris of 542 women who acquired the disease in pregnancy found that approximately two-thirds of the viable infants with congenital toxoplasmosis were asymptomatic in the neonatal period (Desmonts and Couvreur, 1979). The severe form of the disease in infants may manifest as fever, convulsions, hydrocephaly or microcephaly, chorioretinitis, intracranial calcification, hepatosplenomegaly, jaundice, thrombocytopenia, lymphadenopathy, and temperature instability.

Very little information is available regarding the outcome of children with subclinical or asymptomatic congenital *Toxoplasma* infection. The results of one recent study indicate that nearly all of these children develop adverse sequelae months or years later (Wilson *et al.*, 1980). In a follow-up study up to a mean age of 8.5 years of 24 children born with subclinical congenital infection, 22 (92%) ultimately developed adverse sequelae. Chorioretinitis, mental retardation, deafness, and other nervous system problems were the most common disabilities (Wilson *et al.*, 1980).

DIAGNOSIS

The diagnosis of toxoplasmosis may be established by one of these methods:

(1) isolating the parasite from the blood, cerebrospinal fluid, or biopsy material through animal inoculation;

(2) demonstrating the presence of protozoa microscopically in tissue sections;

(3) applying serological methods.

Inoculation techniques are time-consuming, and most hospital laboratories do not have facilities to perform this procedure. Since infection with *T. gondii* tends to be subclinical, serologic methods are the most effective and are commonly used for the diagnosis of the disease in clinical practice. *Toxoplasma* infection produces both IgM and IgG antibodies. The large IgM molecule does not cross the placenta, whereas IgG is passively transferred through the placenta to the fetus.

Of the many serologic tests currently available, the Sabin–Felman dye test (DT), the immunofluorescent antibody test (IFAT), and the indirect hemagglutination test (IHT) are most commonly employed to detect IgG antitoxoplasma antibodies. Although the DT involves the use of living organisms, it is sensitive and highly specific and has no known cross-reaction in man. The loss of ability of the toxoplasmas to stain with alkaline methylene blue in the presence of serum containing antibodies forms the basis of the dye test.

The more recently developed IFAT technique is the most widely used because it is easily and economically performed and because it does not involve living organisms. It appears to measure the same antibodies as does the DT and has a similar diagnostic range and sensitivity. Antibodies are detectable by both these tests within 1–2 weeks after primary infection, and high titers (greater than 1 : 1000) are present for 6–8 weeks. Titers decline during the subsequent months but can remain detectable for life. In some cases titers as high as 1 : 1000–1 : 4000 persist for months or years after the acute infection.

The IHT detects antibodies that rise later than the DT and IFAT. The peak level of antibodies occurs as long as 6 months after the infection and remains elevated even longer. Indirect hemagglutination antibodies may not be detectable early after the acute infection, and a negative test may therefore be misleading in the diagnosis of acute acquired toxoplasmosis and fetal infections. A negative test is useful, however, for population surveys.

The complement fixation test (CFT) detects antibodies that appear later than those demonstrated by the DT and IFAT methods and, therefore, becomes negative earlier. A positive CFT does not in itself indicate a recent infection, but a negative test that is turning positive or increasing in titers in conjunction with stable high DT and IFAT titers indicates active or recent infection.

The IgM-fluorescent antibody test is a valuable method for the diagnosis of acute toxoplasmosis because the initial antibody response to toxoplasma infection mostly involves IgM molecules (Remington and Desmonts, 1973). The test relies on the earlier appearance and disappearance of IgM antibodies, in contrast to the DT and IFAT methods, which are based on the delayed IgG response. The presence of IgM antibodies in the infant indicates intrauterine synthesis of IgM by the infected fetus, because these antibodies do not cross the placental barrier, as do IgG antibodies. Thus, the detection of IgM antibodies in the cord or fetal blood is a direct indication of congenital toxoplasmosis. A negative IgM–IFAT test, however, does not exclude congenital *Toxoplasma* infection, and repeated testing in the suspected neonates may result in a positive test at a later date. A false-positive IgM–IFAT may result from the presence of rheumatoid factor or contamination of cord blood samples by maternal blood that contains IgM *Toxoplasma* antibodies. Therefore, the presence of rheumatoid factor and maternal blood in the sample must be excluded when IgM–IFAT is positive.

The enzyme-linked immunosorbent assay (ELISA) has recently been used with success in the serodiagnosis of a variety of infections. The ELISA technique can be modified to detect both the IgG and IgM antibodies. Naot and Remington (1980) described a 'double-sandwich' IgM–ELISA method, which is based on the method used by Duermeyer and Van der Veen (1978) for hepatitis A virus. They consider it to be a highly specific and sensitive test for the detection of IgM antibodies to *Toxoplasma*. It may well be that this IgM–ELISA method will prove a significant addition to the presently available serologic methods for the diagnosis of acute *Toxoplasma* infection in adults and congenital toxoplasmosis in children.

TOXOPLASMOSIS AND ABORTION

The relationship between *Toxoplasma* infection and abortion has not been adequately defined. It is generally believed that acute maternal infection during early pregnancy frequently leads to spontaneous abortion. In the series of Couvreur and Desmonts (1962), three of the four women who acquired the infection before the 4th month, terminated their pregnancy in abortion. Whether or not chronic toxoplasmosis causes abortion is a matter of extreme controversy. On the one hand, there is a significantly higher incidence of abortion in women with *Toxoplasma* antibodies (Jones *et al.*, 1969; Zieghelboim *et al.*, 1968; Eckerling *et al.*, 1968) as compared to those with no antibodies. On the other hand, Sever (1968) could find no such correlation between positive serology in women with prior history of abortions.

A close association between toxoplasmosis and habitual abortion was reported in studies of 70 patients (Langer, 1963) and 47 patients (Werner *et al.*, 1963), respectively. No correlation was found in 73 habitual aborters studied by Kimbal *et al.* (1971). Likewise, in a controlled study of 123 patients of habitual abortion, Rahman and Rahman (1982) found no association with toxoplasmosis.

Similarly, isolating the organism from the aborted tissues has produced conflicting results. A high percentage of recoveries was reported by Langer (1963), but Kimbal *et al.* (1971) could not isolate the parasite from 42 abortuses. We also were unable to demonstrate placental involvement with *Toxoplasma* in any of our seven cases.

At present, the rate at which chronic toxoplasmosis causes abortion is difficult to ascertain. It obviously varies in different geographical areas and social and cultural situations.

TOXOPLASMOSIS AND STILLBIRTH/PREMATURE LABOR

The association of positive serology for toxoplasmosis and stillbirth was reported by Zieghelboim *et al.* (1968), whereas no such correlation was found by either Jones *et al.* (1966) or Sever (1968). The role of toxoplasmosis in cases of premature delivery is also disputed.

TREATMENT

Maternal infection

Routine chemotherapy of acquired *Toxoplasma* infection in the nonpregnant woman is rarely indicated unless there is severe involvement of the central nervous system, heart, lungs, or other vital organs, or if the acute infection occurs in an immunosuppressed patient.

An infection that had been acquired long before conception has no effect on the fetus and warrants neither chemotherapy nor therapeutic abortion. Reliable guidelines for managing an acutely infected woman during pregnancy have not been developed. There is evidence that treatment of the acutely infected mothers during pregnancy may prevent the development of infection in the fetus. A reduction of approximately 50% of congenital infections was reported in the offspring of 388 acutely infected mothers treated with spiramycin during pregnancy (Desmonts and Couvreur, 1979) as compared to the untreated group. Similar results were obtained by workers who used pyrimethamine and sulphonamides (Kraubig, 1965).

The rationale for treating the primary maternal infection is to prevent the spread of the disease to the fetus. Once the fetus is infected, however, maternal treatment with spiramycin does not affect the development of the disease in the fetus because spiramycin does not cross the placenta. There are no reliable data currently available regarding the effect of pyrimethamine and sulphonamides in such circumstances.

If seroconversion or a rise in the antibody titer is documented in the first trimester of pregnancy, approximately one-third of the fetuses will be affected. Since there is no reliable way of determining if the fetus is infected or not, termination of pregnancy should be considered.

Most physicians do not consider chemotherapy for first-trimester maternal infection safe. *Pyrimethamine is a potential teratogen and should not be used during the period of organogenesis.* Spiramycin, a macrolide antibiotic similar in action to erythromycin and less toxic than pyrimethamine, has been used on a large series of patients and at all stages of pregnancy without apparent adverse effects on the fetus (Desmonts and Couvreur, 1974). The usual dose of spiramycin is 2 g/day in divided doses over a period of 3 weeks.

Maternal infection acquired during the second trimester of pregnancy should be treated regardless of the severity of the disease. The patient must be informed of the potential danger and toxicity of the drug therapy and written consent must be obtained before treatment is initiated.

The treatment is pyrimethamine (Daraprim), a folic acid antagonist, and sulphonamides. A combined therapy with these drugs has generally been preferred. The standard treatment in adults consists of 25 mg/day pyrimethamine for 3 weeks, after a loading dose of 50 mg, and 4 g/day sulphadiazine in divided doses, for 3 weeks. This combination of therapy has a synergistic effect against trophozoites. Unfortunately, there is no effective therapy currently available against the cystic form of the disease. Pyrimethamine therapy may result in folic acid deficiency in the mother and may produce bone-marrow depression, leading to agranulocytosis, thrombocytopenia, and megaloblastic anemia. Administratation of folinic acid (6 mg/day i.m.) is effective in preventing bone-marrow depression. It should be prescribed as a routine, along with pyrimethamine. Therapy should be monitored by biweekly estimations of complete blood count and platelet count.

Maternal infection occurring in the third trimester of pregnancy is best treated with combined pyrimethamine and sulphonamides, in similar doses.

Sulphonamide therapy should be discontinued at least 2–3 weeks prior to the expected date of delivery to avoid the danger of kernicterus developing in the neonate.

The value of prophylactic chemotherapy for latent *Toxoplasma* infection in patients with previous history of obstetric problems has been contested. Some authors recommended prophylactic antitoxoplasma chemotherapy for women with latent infection with dye test titers of 1 : 64 and above (Langer, 1966; Eckerling *et al.*, 1968). Others are unable to substantiate the beneficial effect of prophylactic therapy (Kabelitz and Kabelitz, 1961; Zieghelboim *et al.*, 1968). Sharf *et al.* (1973) treated 38 women with a previous history of obstetric problems and a dye test antibody titer of 1 : 64 or greater with prophylactic pyrimethamine and triple sulpha before and during a subsequent pregnancy. A fourfold reduction in the antibody titer to negative titers was achieved in 78.9% of these cases, and 71% of births were normal, thus establishing a relationship between latent *Toxoplasma* infection and abortion, premature delivery, and stillbirth. Sharf *et al.* seem to be convinced of the value of prophylactic chemotherapy for latent toxoplasmosis.

Treatment of congenitally infected babies

The infant with congenitally acquired toxoplasmosis requires treatment, irrespective of the magnitude of the disease. The recommended treatment regimen consists of pyrimethamine, 1 mg/kg body weight, daily, for 3–4 days, followed by 0.5 mg/kg per day in a single dose for 21–30 days. The maximum dose per day should not exceed 25 mg; along with pyrimethamine, sulphonamides or triple sulphonamides, 100 mg/kg per day in four daily doses and folinic acid 5 mg, twice a week, should be administered. These drugs are particularly toxic to young infants and therapy must be monitored with biweekly complete blood and platelet counts. Treatment may need to be repeated two or three times during the first year, depending on the evidence of exacerbation of the disease process.

PREVENTION

Interrupting the chain of transmission of *T. gondii* infection is the most important aspect in the prevention of the disease. Physicians who care for women of child-bearing age should advise them of the specific hygienic precautions that minimize the risk of infection. Since ingestion of raw and undercooked meat is the most common source of infection, pregnant women should be advised to eat meat that has been thoroughly cooked at temperatures in excess of 66 °C. Freezing meat to below 20 °C for 24 hours will also destroy the tissue cyst form of the parasite. Women at risk should wash their hands thoroughly after handling raw meat or coming into contact with cats. Pet cats of patients should not be allowed access to natural prey or refuse. Gloves should be worn when handling potentially contaminated litter pans. Fruits and vegetables may be contaminated with oocysts and should be thoroughly washed before consumption.

Therapeutic abortion and the introduction of more effective drug therapies could be the most reliable means of reducing the incidence of congenital toxoplasmosis. Unfortunately, therapeutic abortion is not practical when the maternal infection is discovered in the second half of pregnancy. More than half of the congenitally infected infants are born of mothers who acquired the infection in the second half of pregnancy (Desmonts and Couvreur, 1979). If the acute maternal infection is discovered in the second and third trimesters of pregnancy, either from clinical manifestations or from serologic testing, antitoxoplasma chemotherapeutic agents should be instituted in the hope of preventing congenital infection.

CONCLUSION

The outcome of a pregnancy complicated by *Toxoplasma* infection can be so destructive and the late manifestations of subclinical infection are so variable that the need for effective preventive measures is paramount. Recent studies have shown that nearly all children born with subclinical infection subsequently develop adverse sequelae (Wilson *et al.*, 1980). The cost–effectiveness of routine serologic screening of pregnant mothers for the prevention of congenital toxoplasmosis is currently being investigated in the United Kingdom and in the United States. Until additional data define the efficacy of such a program, prenatal testing of all women, such as is conducted for rubella infection, seems to be a logical approach. In addition, less expensive and more easily performed testing procedures to diagnose acquired and recrudescent toxoplasmosis are urgently required.

SUMMARY

The acquired maternal *Toxoplasma* infection has extremely variable clinical manifestations and may mimic a variety of other infectious diseases. The infection may be so mild that it remains undetected. Severe maternal infection is uncommon and the clinical picture varies according to the organ system involved.

Fetal infection rarely occurs when the maternal infection precedes the pregnancy, but approximately one-third of the fetuses are infected when the mother acquires the primary infection during the pregnancy. The risk of fetal infection varies with the trimester of the pregnancy during which the mother becomes infected. The highest incidence of fetal involvement is in the last trimester, yet the disease is subclinical. Fetal infection occurs less frequently if the primary maternal infection occurred during the first half of pregnancy, but the disease in the neonate is more severe. The difference in the severity of clinical disease in the newborn may be due to the relative immaturity of the fetal immune state at the time of parasitemia in the early pregnancy as compared to late pregnancy.

The most adverse effect of congenital toxoplasmosis is death of the fetus causing miscarriage or still-birth. Nearly all infants born with the subclinical or asymptomatic congenital *Toxoplasma* infection develop adverse sequelae months or years later. Chorioretinitis, mental retardation, deafness and other nervous system problems are the commonest disabilities.

The causal relationship between toxoplasmosis and abortion is not established. Acute maternal infection during early pregnancy is more likely to cause spontaneous abortion. Whether the chronic infection causes abortion is debatable. Conflicting results have been reported from studies from different parts of the world. However, it is generally agreed that no definite correlation exists between the chronic maternal infection and habitual abortions. Chronic toxoplasmosis as a cause of abortion may depend upon the geographical area and social and cultural habits of the population. Likewise, no definite association between chronic maternal infection and still-birth or premature labor has been established.

There is strong evidence that the treatment of acutely infected mothers with spiramycin or pyrimethamine during pregnancy reduces the incidence of congenital infection by approximately 50%. However the potential teratogenic effect of chemotherapeutic agents in the first trimester of pregnancy must be borne in mind. Therapeutic termination of pregnancy should be considered if acute maternal infection occurs in the first trimester. Infants born with congenital toxoplasmosis should receive chemotherapy irrespective of the severity of the disease.

References

Anderson, S. (1979). *Toxoplasma gondii*. In G. L. Mandell, G. R. Douglas Jr, and J. E. Bennett (eds.), *Principles and Practice of Infectious Diseases*, p. 2127. (New York: Wiley & Sons)

Basalamah, A. H. and Serebour, F. E. K. (1981). Toxoplasmosis in pregnancy. *Saudi Med. J.*, **2**, 125

Couvreur, J. and Desmonts, G. (1962). Congenital and maternal toxoplasmosis: a review of 300 congenital cases. *Dev. Med. Child Neurol.*, **4**, 519

Desmonts, G. and Couvreur, J. (1974). Congenital toxoplasmosis: a prospective study of 378 pregnancies. *N. Engl. J. Med.*, **290**, 1110

Desmonts, G. and Couvreur, J. (1979). Congenital toxoplasmosis: a prospective study of the off-spring of 542 women who acquired toxoplasmosis during pregnancy: Pathophysiology of congenital disease. In: O. Thalhammer, K. Baumgarten and A. Pollak (eds.), *Perinatal Medicine*, p. 51 (Stuttgart: Thieme)

Desmonts, G., Couvreur, J. and Ben Rachid, S. (1965). Le toxoplasma, la mère et l'enfant. *Arch. Fr. Pediatr.*, **22**, 1183

Desmonts, G., Couvreur, J., Alison, F., Baudelot, J., Gerbeaux, J. and Lelong, M. (1965). Etude épidemiologique sur la toxoplasmose: de l'influence de la cuisson des viandes du boucherie sur la fréquence de l'infection humaine. *Rev. Fr. Etudes Clin. Biol.*, **10**, 952

Duermeyer, W. and Van der Veen, J. (1978). Specific detection of IgM-antibodies by ELISA, applied in hepatitis-A. *Lancet*, **2**, 684 .

Eckerling, B., Neri, A. and Eylan, E. (1968). Toxoplasmosis: a cause of infertility. *Fertil. Steril.*, **19**, 883

Feldman, H. A. (1968). Toxoplasmosis. *N. Engl. J. Med.*, **279**, 1370

Feldman, H. A. and Miller, L. T. (1956). Serological study of toxoplasmosis prevalence. *Am. J. Hyg.*, **64**, 320

Hume, O. S. (1972). Toxoplasmosis and pregnancy. *Am. J. Obstet. Gynecol.*, **114**, 703

Jones, M. H., Sever, H. L., Baker, T. H. *et al.* (1966). Toxoplasmosis, antibody level and pregnancy outcome. *Am. J. Obstet. Gynecol.*, **95**, 809

Jones, M. H., Sever, J. L., Baker, T. H. *et al.* (1969). Toxoplasmosis and abortion. *Am. J. Obstet. Gynecol.*, **104**, 919

Kabelitz, B. and Kabelitz, H. J. (1961). Indications and results of drug treatment in acquired toxoplasmosis. *Z. Trop. Parasitol.*, **12,** 179

Kader, N. (1980). TORCH infections: a significant health hazard to pregnant women. *Postgrad. Doct. (MEE)*, **3,** 222

Kimbal, A. C., Kean, B. H. and Fuchs, F. (1971). The role of toxoplasmosis in abortion. *Am. J. Obstet. Gynecol.*, **111,** 219

Kraubig, H. (1965). Die Bedeutung der Toxoplasmose fuer die Geburts-hilfe. *Gynaecologia*, **159,** 185

Langer, H. (1963). Repeated congenital infection with toxoplasma gondii. *Obstet. Gynecol.*, **21,** 318

Langer, H. (1966). Toxoplasmose prakitische Fragen und Ergebiusse. In H. Kirchhoff and H. Kraubig, p. 123 (Stuttgart: Thieme)

Monif, G. R. G. (1982). Protozoa – Toxoplasma gondii (Toxoplasmosis). In *Infectious Diseases in Obstetrics and Gynaecology*, p. 278. (Philadelphia: Harper & Row)

Naot, Y. and Remington, J. S. (1980). An enzyme-linked immunosorbent assay for detection of acute acquired toxoplasmosis. *J. Infect. Dis.*, **142,** 757

Nekrasova, L. I. (1975). The prevalence of toxoplasmosis in the extreme north of the USSR Medskaya, *Parazit.*, **43,** 666 (English summary in *Abstracts on Hygiene*, **50,** 217)

Rahman, M. S. and Rahman, J. (1982). *Relationship between Abortion and Infection with Toxoplasma Gondii and Listeria Monocytogenes.* I International Symposium on Reproductive Health Care, Maui, Hawaii

Remington, J. S., Efron, B., Cavanaugh, E. *et al.* (1970). Studies on Toxoplasmosis in El Salvador. Prevalence and incidence of Toxoplasmosis as measured by Sabin–Feldman dye test. *Trans. Roy. Soc. Trop. Med. Hyg.*, **64,** 252

Remington, J. S. and Desmonts, G. (1973). Congenital toxoplasmosis: variability in the IgM-fluorescent antibody response and some pit-falls in diagnosis. *J. Pediatr.*, **83,** 27

Sever, J. L. (1966). Perinatal infections affecting the developing fetus and newborn. In H. Eichenwald (ed.), *Prevention of Mental Retardation through Control of Infectious Diseases*, p. 56 (Washington: U.S. Government Printing Office)

Sever, J. L. (1968). *Perinatal Toxoplasmosis: Clinical and Serological Studies.* VIII International Congress on Tropical Medicine and Malaria, Teheran

Sever, J. L. (1980). Toxoplasmosis. In J. T. Quennan (ed.), *Management of High Risk Pregnancy*, p. 395 (New Jersey: Medical Economics Company)

Sharf, M., Eibschitz, I. and Eylan, E. (1973). Latent toxoplasmosis and pregnancy. *Obstet. Gynecol.*, **42,** 349

Wallace, G. D. (1973). Intermediate and transport hosts in the natural history of toxoplasma gondii. *Am. J. Trop. Med. Hyg.*, **22,** 456

Werner, H., Schmidtke, L. and Thomaschek, G. (1963). Toxoplasma-infektion and schwanger-schaft: Der histologische nachweis des intrauterinen infektionsweges. *Klin. Wschr.*, **41,** 96 (*Trop. Dis. Bul.*, **60,** 787)

Wilson, C. B. and Remington, J. S. (1980). What can be done to prevent congenital toxoplasmosis? *Am. J. Obstet. Gynecol.*, **138,** 357

Wilson, C. B., Remington, J. S., Stagno, S. *et al.* (1980). Development of adverse sequelae in children born with subclinical congenital toxoplasma infection. *Pediatrics*, **66,** 767

Zieghelboim, J., Maekett, G. A., Teppa, P. *et al.* (1968). Reproductive wastage and toxoplasma antibodies. *Am. J. Obstet. Gynecol.*, **101,** 839

5
Infections in the African continent

O. P. ARYA

Infections causing infertility and pregnancy wastage can be divided into those which are principally sexually acquired and those acquired nonvenereally.

SEXUALLY TRANSMITTED DISEASES

Among sexually transmitted diseases (STDs), gonorrhea, chlamydial infection and syphilis are the major causes of infertility and pregnancy wastage, respectively. No reliable national statistics on these diseases are available from any African country, and what data there are greatly underreport the true picture. Nonetheless information is being gathered from prevalence surveys for selected population groups carried out by experienced personnel with appropriate laboratory support. The results of these surveys (Tables 1–9) show considerable variation between countries and between population groups within a country.

Gonorrhea

The general lack of appropriate diagnostic and treatment facilities in Africa leads to patients remaining untreated, being treated inadequately or employing self-medication. Inappropriate treatment practices have resulted in alarmingly high rates of both uncomplicated and complicated gonorrhea (Tables 1–5). Although many patients are treated by private doctors in the larger cities, the true incidence of gonorrhea is likely to be much higher than that shown in Table 1 for some urban areas, and indeed several times higher than in industrialized countries. For example, the estimated number of gonorrhea cases in the Ugandan capital of Kampala was 60 000 in 1972 (Lomholt, 1976), compared with 53 439 cases in the whole of England in the same year (Department of Health and Social Security, 1973). At the same time, the incidence in the semiurban area of Kasangati, Uganda (Table 1) was as high as in some big American cities (American Social Health Association, 1972).

Of interest is the fact that the incidence of gonorrhea was as high as 30%

Table 1 Number of gonorrhea and early syphilis cases seen in some sexually transmitted disease clinics in Africa

Author(s)	Year of study	Country	Place	Population	Clinic	Number of cases		
						Gonorrhea	Early Syphilis	Congenital Syphilis
Arya and Bennett, 1976	1972	Uganda	Kasangati (semi-urban)	12 000	Kasangati Health Centre	264	27	
Lomholt, 1976	1972	Uganda	Kampala	350 000	Mulago Hospital	19 000	2000	40
Ratnam, 1980	1978 (6 months)	Zambia	Lusaka	560 000	University Teaching Hospital	3076[a]	504[a]	
Verhagen, 1974	1971	Kenya	Nairobi	500 000	Pumwani	15 000		

[a] Derived from percentages in the original paper

among some educated groups such as university students in selected African countries (Table 2). A high proportion of men acquire the infection from prostitutes of whom in one study (Meheus *et al.*, 1974) more than 51% were found to be harboring *Neisseria gonorrheae*.

Gonorrhea rates as high as 17% have been found amongst women attending antenatal, family planning, and gynecology clinics in some African countries (Table 3). Most of these women were asymptomatic and thus constitute a large reservoir of infection. According to the World Health Organization (WHO), up to 20% these women eventually develop serious complications such as pelvic inflammatory disease (PID), including postpartum and postabortal sepsis, ectopic pregnancy and infertility (WHO, 1978). Some infants go on to develop ophthalmia neonatorum.

Table 2 Incidence/prevalence of gonorrhea in selected population groups (male university students, prostitutes, food and liquor handlers) in Africa

Authors/dates	Country	Place	Group studied	Number at risk	Number studied	Number infected	(%)
Arya and Bennett, 1967	Uganda	Kampala	University students	1200	–	224	(19)
Meheus, 1973	Rwanda	Butare	University students	413	–	126	(30)
Meheus *et al.*, 1974	Rwanda	Butare	Prostitutes	–	86	44	(51)
Nsanze *et al.*, 1982	Kenya	Nairobi	Prostitutes	–	41	8	(20)
Ongom *et al.*, 1976	Uganda	Kampala	Food and liquor handlers	–	632	54	(8)
Widy-Wirski *et al.*, 1982	Central African Republic	Bangui	University students	Not known	–	Not known	(31)

Pelvic inflammatory disease

Several authors have reported PID as a major medical problem in Africa. Forty per cent of the acute admissions to the gynecology wards of teaching hospitals in Kenya (Carty *et al.*, 1972), 25% in Uganda (Grech *et al.*, 1973), 44% in Rhodesia (Brown and Cruickshank, 1976) and 40% in Ethiopa (Perine *et al.*, 1980) resulted from a diagnosis of acute pelvic infection. Ectopic pregnancy, often a direct result of gonococcal pelvic infection, has been a common surgical emergency among African women (Carty *et al.*, 1972). Although the polymicrobial etiology of pelvic infection is now recognized in Africa (Peıine *et al.*, 1980), the bacteriologic focus until recently has been on *N. gonorrheae* (Table 4). In Africa, as in other non-African nations, there appears to be a correlation between the age of sexual debut and an increased risk of PID (Muir and Belsey, 1980). Over 83% of the patients with PID in a Ugandan study (Grech *et al.*, 1973) had their first sexual experience before the age of 16.

Table 3 Prevalence of gonorrhea in antenatal clinic, family planning clinic and gynecology clinic attenders in Africa

Authors/dates	Country	Place	Antenatal clinic			Family planning clinic			Gynecology clinic		
			Number studied	Number infected	(%)	Number studied	Number infected	(%)	Number studied	Number infected	(%)
Finlayson et al., 1974	S. Africa	Western Cape	1276	68	(5)				945	50	(5)
Hall and Whitcomb, 1978	S. Africa	Soweto				186	19	(10)			
Hoosen et al., 1981	S. Africa		312	31	(10)						
Hopcraft et al., 1973	Kenya	Nairobi				200	35	(17)			
Hopcraft et al., 1973	Kenya	Kiambu (rural)				50	7	(14)			
Mandara et al., 1980	Tanzania	Dar es Salaam				405	29	(7)			
Meheus et al., 1980	Swaziland	Manzini	51	2	(4)	52	1	(2)			
Nasah et al., 1980	Cameroon	Yaounde	720	106	(15)	134	18	(13)			
Nsanze et al., 1982	Kenya	Nairobi	54	–	(–)	57	10	(17)			
Osoba and Onifade, 1973	Nigeria	Ibadan	208	7	(3)						
Ratnam and Chatterjee, 1980	Zambia	Lusaka	163	19	(12)						
Vink and Moodley, 1980	S. Africa								100	11	(11)
Weissenberger et al., 1977	Zimbabwe	Salisbury	50	1	(2)	100	12	(12)	118	13	(11)
Widy-Wirski et al., 1982	Central African Republic	Bangui	Not known		(9)						

60

Little information exists on the frequency of postabortal or postpartum infection in Africa where these events are thought to be common antecedents of infertility. Nevertheless, in one Ugandan study (Grech *et al.*, 1973), of the 86 patients admitted with acute pelvic infection, nine (10%) became infected in puerperium and in eight (9%) the onset of infection followed abortion. In Addis Ababa, Ethiopia, puerperal sepsis was the cause for admission in 132 (10%) of the 1329 women admitted to the gynecology wards (Perine *et al.*, 1980); of the remaining admissions 397 (30%) had PID.

Table 4 Prevalence of gonorrhea in postpartum women and patients with pelvic inflammatory disease (PID) in Africa

Authors/dates	Country	Place	PID patients			Postpartum women		
			Number studied	Number infected	(%)	Number studied	Number infected	(%)
Brown and Cruickshank, 1976	Rhodesia	Salisbury	50	2	(4)			
Carty *et al.*, 1972	Kenya	Nairobi	58	25	(43)			
Grech *et al.*, 1973	Uganda	Kampala	86	33	(38)			
Nasah *et al.*, 1980	Cameroon	Yaounde	25	3	(12)	296[a] 42[c]	30 9	(10) (21)
Perine *et al.*, 1980	Ethiopia	Addis Ababa	100	19	(19)	200[a] 67[b]	18 19	(9) (28)
Ratnam *et al.*, 1980	Zambia	Lusaka	100	46	(46)			

[a] = Asymptomatic
[b] = Hospitalized with puerperal sepsis
[c] = Symptomatic

A field study in rural Eastern Uganda (Arya *et al.*, 1973) found the gonococcal isolation rate to be twice as high in pregnant women (40%) as in nonpregnant women (20%). This observation, coupled with more recently noted high rates of gonorrhea in pregnant women elsewhere in Africa – see (Table 3) and also pointed out by other investigators (Muir and Belsey, 1980) – suggests a potential role of *N. gonorrheae* and possibly other sexually transmitted agents in the etiology of puerperal sepsis and postabortal infection. This proposition was confirmed in the recent Ethiopian study (Perine *et al.*, 1980; Table 4), reporting a 28% isolation rate of *N. gonorrheae* from women hospitalized with puerperal sepsis.

Gonococcal ophthalmia neonatorum and vulvovaginitis

One of the consequences of untreated gonococcal infection during pregnancy is ophthalmia neonatorum, infection of the newborn infant's eyes by direct contact with infected cervical or vaginal secretions during delivery. This tragic condition is frequently encountered where gonorrhea is common, and may serve as a reasonable indicator of the prevalence of gonorrhea in the community. Ophthalmia neonatorum accounted for 25% of the inpatient admissions at one provincial hospital's eye department in Uganda, and *N. gonorrheae* was the causative agent in at least 22% (Otiti, 1975). In another Ugandan study in the Mulago Teaching Hospital, *N. gonorrheae* was isolated from 25 (73%) of 34 babies with ophthalmia neonatorum in a period of just 3 months (Onyango-Ogony and Hetland-Eriksen, 1975). In a recent study of 278 neonates seen in 1 month in Bangui, Central African Republic (Meheus *et al.*, 1982), 27 (10%) were found to have conjunctivitis; *N. gonorrheae* was the cause in 26% of the cases. In another study of 61 Nigerian children with acute purulent conjunctivitis, *N. gonorrheae* was isolated in 44% of the cases (Amoni, 1979). Although hospital-based these high figures confirm the epidemiological importance of gonococcal infection in various communities.

Gonococcal vulvovaginitis is also common in areas such as those described above. Sixteen of the 17 Nigerian children aged 2 to 9 years presenting with vaginal discharge at the University College Hospital Ibadan, were culture-positive for *N. gonorrheae* (Osoba and Alausa, 1974).

Infertility

In many parts of Africa up to 30% of the women suffer from infertility (WHO, 1975). Almost two-thirds of one gynecologist's time in an East African country was spent seeing cases of infertility (Mati *et al.*, 1973). After reviewing the available data, a WHO Scientific Group (WHO, 1981) concluded that 'globally, it was difficult to separate the problem of infertility from that of sexually transmitted diseases'.

The sequelae of gonococcal infection in the female include endosalpingitis resulting in partial or complete tubal occlusion; those in the male include epididymitis and epididymal occlusion.

Since gonorrhea is a major cause of PID in Africa, it is also an important cause of infertility. The association between gonorrhea infection and infertility has been demonstrated in several field surveys. Some of the findings from a survey of two Ugandan districts, Teso in the East with low fertility (crude birth rate of 37 per 1000), and Ankole in the West with high fertility (crude birth rate of 55 per 1000) are shown in Table 5. Comparisons between fertile and infertile men and women have been described elsewhere (Arya *et al.*, 1973; Arya and Taber, 1975; Arya *et al.*, 1980a) and show gonorrhea-associated correlates to be significantly more common among the infertile than fertile men and women. In a Kenyan study of 379 couples with infertility, the main cause was tubal occlusion following PID in 73% of the females (Mathews *et al.*, 1981). Earlier in the same hospital, gonococci had been isolated from 43% of the cases of PID (Carty *et al.*, 1972).

In vitro *susceptibility of* N. Gonorrheae

Inappropriate treatment practices, self-treatment, and the availability of antibiotics without prescription in many towns and cities of Africa have led to the

Table 5 Gonococcal infection and its correlates in men and women in the Teso and Ankole Districts of Uganda

Total studied	Teso Number	(%)	Ankole Number	(%)	Significance of difference (p)
Men	270		166		
Past history of urethral discharge	150	(56)	18	(11)	<0.001
Present history of urethral discharge	25	(9)	3	(2)	<0.01
Urethral discharge present	32	(12)	13	(8)	–
Epididymis thickened	74	(27)	7	(4)	<0.001
Epididymis thickened bilaterally	16	(6)	1	(0.6)	<0.001
Gonococci in urethral material	24	(9)	7	(4)	–
Women	295		168		
Pelvic infection	56	(19)	10	(6)	<0.001
Gonococci in cervix	54	(18)	4	(2)	<0.001

emergence of gonococcal strains with decreased sensitivity to penicillin and other antibiotics. Since such strains account for up to 80% of the gonococcal infections in some parts of Africa (Arya *et al.*, 1980b), the treatment of this condition is becoming more difficult and expensive. To make matters worse penicillinase-producing *N. gonorrheae* (PPNG) strains which are completely resistant to penicillin require treatment with alternative drugs costing many times more than penicillin, and thus add to the burden of the already over-stretched resources of the poor countries of Africa (WHO, 1978). These new strains are becoming more prevalent in developing countries at a much faster rate than in the industrialized nations. No accurate statistics on their incidence or prevalence are available from Africa, but in Ibadan, Nigeria, and possibly in neighboring Ghana and the Ivory Coast, places frequently mentioned as heavily infected (WHO, 1983), these strains account for 30–50% of all gonococcal infections (Osoba, personal communications; Perine *et al.*, 1983). This situation clearly will result in more treatment failures with increased risk of complications developing.

Urethral stricture

Urethral strictures in men are seen frequently in areas where gonorrhea is common and control measures inadequate. For example, in Mulago Hospital, Kampala, Uganda, 750 new cases of urethral stricture were registered yearly (Bewes, 1973). Griffith (1963) demonstrated a correlation between gonorrhea, urethral stricture, and the general fertility rate in Uganda. The gonorrhea figures were, however, based on diagnoses of questionable accuracy.

Chlamydial and 'nonspecific' genital infections

Whereas considerable information has become available during the last decade on the incidence and prevalence of gonococcal infections in many parts of Africa, little is known of the other sexually transmissible agents associated with PID.

'Nonspecific' genital infections are now the commonest sexually transmitted diseases in the industrialized nations. Although not widely recognized in Africa, they have also been reported in the clinics where patients are carefully examined and laboratory diagnosis is possible. For example, 31% of all new cases of urethral discharge among male university students in Kampala, Uganda, over a period of 6 years were nongonococcal (Arya, 1972). In a Nigerian study of 442 men (Osoba, 1972b), 271 (61%) were found to be suffering from nongonococcal urethritis (NGU). The latter rather high figure was thought to be due partly to widely practiced self-treatment with antibiotics and partly to patients having received penicillin from general practitioners before referral to the clinic. In Swaziland, on the other hand, only 5–20% of urethritis cases have been found to be nongonococcal (Meheus *et al.*, 1980).

Chlamydia trachomatis, considered to be the causative agent in over 50% of men having NGU in the western countries (Taylor-Robinson and Thomas, 1980), is also frequently associated with acute epididymitis (Berger *et al.*, 1978) and PID (Westrøm, 1980). Among women in Sweden, nongonococcal pelvic infection has been found to be more frequently associated with tubal occlusion than gonococcal infection (Westrøm, 1980). Information from Africa regarding this condition is scanty. Chlamydia isolation rates in the few published African studies have been much lower than in the West, i.e. 4–9% in Kenya (Table 6). However, type-specific antichlamydial antibodies were present in much higher proportions. They are present in over 45% of female STD patients in Addis Ababa, Ethiopia (Forsey *et al.*, 1982), in over 70% of women in Kenya (Nsanze *et al.*, 1982) in 10–35% of various population groups studied in Ibadan, Nigeria (Darougar *et al.*, 1982) and in 71% of STD patients in Swaziland (Meheus *et al.*, 1980).

The incidence of chlamydial ophthalmia in Africa is also unknown. However, in two studies of neonatal conjunctivitis in the Central African Republic (Meheus *et al.*, 1982) and Gambia (Mabey and Whittle, 1982), *C. trachomatis* was isolated in 19% and 35% of the cases respectively (Table 6).

Syphilis

Syphilis is a serious problem in a number of African countries. Once again, however, the data are inadequate and largely based on selected study populations. Whether acquired or congenital, syphilis is easy to diagnose in its early stages. In Mulago Hospital, Kampala, Uganda in 1972 (Table 1) 2000 cases of early acquired syphilis and 40 cases of early congenital syphilis were seen compared with 1187 and 15 cases respectively in the whole of England in the same year (Department of Health and Social Security, 1973). Equally high rates have recently been described in Zambia (Tables 1 and 7) where 7.5% of

Table 6 *Chlamydia trachomatis* isolation rates in selected populations in some African countries

Population groups	Gambia[a]			Kenya[b]			Swaziland[c] Central African Republic[d]		
	Number studied	Chlamydia-positive	(%)	Number studied	Chlamydia-positive	(%)	Number studied	Chlamydia-positive	(%)
Antenatal clinic	87	6	(7)	54	3	(6)			
Family planning clinic				57	2	(4)			
STD clinic				58	4	(7)			
Prostitutes				41	2	(5)			
Male patients with gonorrhea	59	8	(14)	112	10	(9)	70[c]	1	(1)
Male patients with NGU	19	4	(21)				5[c]	1	(20)
Female contact of men with NGU	33	6	(18)						
Gynecology clinic with symptoms	22	3	(14)						
Infants with ophthalmia neonatorum	37	13	(35)				27[d]	5	(19)

[a] Mabey and Whittle, 1982
[b] Nsanze et al., 1982
[c] Meheus et al., 1980
[d] Meheus et al., 1982

200 neonates admitted into the intensive care unit during 1 month were found to have syphilis (Bhat *et al.*, 1982).

Once the infectious stage of syphilis is past, the diagnosis is essentially based on serological tests. It then often becomes difficult to differentiate venereal syphilis from nonvenereal treponematosis such as yaws, which was endemic in much of Africa until the mass treatment campaign in the 1950s and 1960s and which is reappearing in some areas (WHO, 1982). In some studies the incidence

Table 7   Syphilis in Zambia: seroreaction rates in pregnant women[a] and neonates[b]

Group of patients	Total	No. RPR, TPHA-Reactive	(%)
Antenatal patients	202	25	(12)
Patients whose pregnancies resulted in:			
abortions	240	45	(19)
stillbirth	100	42	(42)
Patients admitted for delivery	464	30	(7)
Neonates admitted to intensive care unit	200	15	(7)[c]

[a] Ratnam *et al.*, 1982
[b] Bhat *et al.*, 1982
[c] Diagnosed congenital syphilis

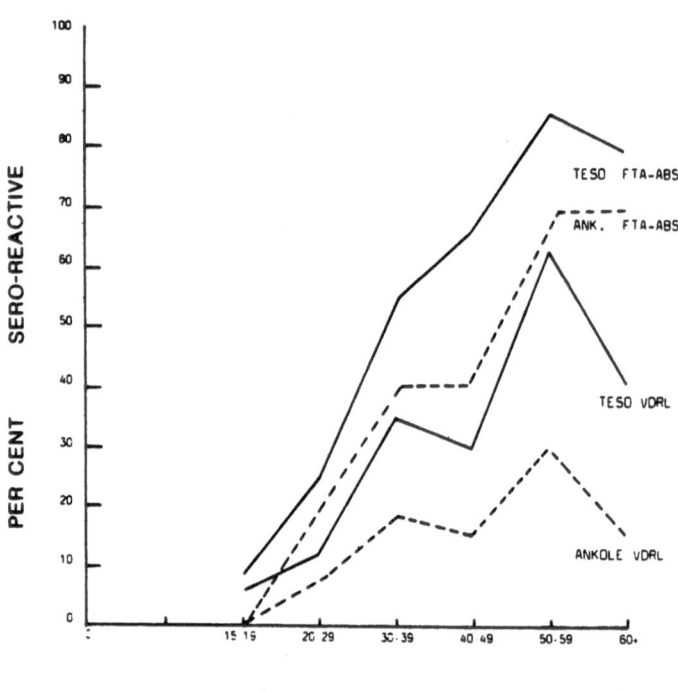

AGE GROUPS (YEARS)

Fig. 1   Age-specific seroreaction rates in the Teso and Ankole districts of Uganda

Table 8 Seroreaction rates in antenatal clinic and family planning clinic attenders, and blood donors

Authors/dates	Year of study	Country	Place	Number studied (test performed)	Number positive	(%)
Blavy and Diakhate, 1982	1982	Senegal	Dakar	2230[b] (TPHA)	245	(11)
Friedmann and Wright, 1977	1976	Ethiopia	Addis Ababa	337[a] (FTA-200)	37	(11)
Meheus et al., 1975	1975	Rwanda	Butare	862[a] (VDRL)	28	(3)
Meheus et al., 1980	1978	Swaziland	Manzini	103[d] (RPR)	10	(10)
Osoba, 1972a	1968–70	Nigeria	Ibadan	8024[a] (VDRL)	158	(2)
Rampen, 1978	1975	Malawi	Malawi	22,560[c] (Kahn)	1389	(6)
Ursi et al., 1981	1979	Swaziland		90[d]	30	(33)

[a] Antenatal clinic attenders
[b] Blood donors
[c] a+b
[d] a+family planning clinic attenders

Table 9 Seroreaction rates and past history of genital sores in Teso and Ankole districts of Uganda

	Teso	(%)	Ankole	(%)	Significance of difference (p)
Males					
FTA (Abs) positive	71/116	(61.2)	41/113	(36.3)	<0.001
VDRL positive	33/85	(38.8)	15/97	(15.5)	<0.001
Past history of genital sores	61/270	(22.6)	6/166	(3.6)	<0.001
Females					
FTA (Abs) positive	57/115	(49.6)	50/166	(30.1)	<0.01
VDRL positive	22/87	(25.3)	18/143	(12.6)	<0.05

of syphilis may therefore have been overstated (Tables 7 and 8). Field surveys in the Ugandan districts of Teso with low fertility and Ankole with high fertility (Arya et al., 1975), showed positive serological tests in significantly more men and women from Teso than from Ankole (Table 9). It is highly likely that many of these men and women, especially the older ones, had had yaws. The age distribution of the seroreactors supports this premise (Fig. 1). The finding that positive serology increases with age along with VDRL reactivity rates which are lower than the FTA (ABS) positive rates, favors the hypothesis that many of these observations are due to pre-existing yaws, VDRL antibody having faded away with time. There also was evidence that some positive reactions, notably in the Teso district, were probably due to venereal syphilis. The serology was positive in 85% of the men who gave a past history of genital sores, compared with 52% who did not (p <0.01). Of all the Teso women who reported having had one or more abortions, serological tests were positive in 88% compared with 43% who did not report prior abortion (p <0.01). Among the 45 couples whose serological results were available, pregnancy losses were reported only by those six of the 20 couples in whom sera of both spouses gave positive results. These findings strongly support the possibility of some of these men and women having had venereal syphilis.

Other sexually transmissible agents

Although evidence exists that *Mycoplasma hominis* can cause salpingitis and *ureaplasma urealyticum* may account for a proportion of the cases of NGU (Taylor-Robinson and McCormack, 1980), no information on these conditions is available from Africa. Likewise, at present, no information exists on the epidemiological importance of *herpes simplex virus* and *cytomegalovirus* infections in Africa. The prevailing opinion is that none of the remaining sexually transmitted conditions such as *granuloma inguinale*, *chancroid*, and possibly also *lymphogranuloma venereum* are of epidemiological significance in relation to their possible effects on reproductive function.

NONVENEREAL INFECTIONS

Tuberculosis

Little is known of the contribution of genital tuberculosis to infertility in Africa. However, it is probably relatively unimportant. In a recent study in Kenya only two endometrial cultures were positive out of 163 cases investigated for infertility (Mathews *et al.*, 1981).

Mumps

Mumps orchitis, if bilateral, may cause infertility, but its epidemiological importance in this respect is thought to be insignificant (WHO, 1975).

Leprosy

Although lepromatous leprosy may have some effect on male infertility, there is no epidemiological information on the association of infertility with leprosy in Africa (WHO, 1975).

Brucellosis, histoplasmosis, listeriosis, relapsing fever, rickettsial infections, and toxoplasmosis

These may all rarely cause pregnancy wastage. *Malaria* may cause abortion and premature labour. *Trypanosomiasis* and *filariasis* have been claimed to affect male and female fertility. In all these conditions no epidemiologic studies have defined the risks (Adadevoh, 1974; WHO, 1975).

Schistosomiasis

Schistosome eggs have been found in the male and female reproductive organs. In a recent Nigerian study ova of *Schistosoma haematobium* were identified in the urines of 19 (42%) of 45 males with urethral discharge (Bello and Idiong, 1982). However, the importance of schistosomes in the causation of infertility or pregnancy wastage is unknown (Belsey, 1976).

PRACTICES WHICH PREDISPOSE TO INFECTION

Female circumcision

Female circumcision, practiced in a number of African and Middle Eastern countries and often performed by untrained personnel, has been reported to be an important factor in the etiology of PID in Sudan (Rushwan, 1980); however, its contribution to infertility remains to be determined.

Primitive midwifery

Primitive midwifery, including native medication, instrumentation, douching, and unskilled induced abortions are all common in selected areas of Africa and are likely to be followed by severe puerperal or postabortal sepsis (WHO, 1975). Pathogens may include *N. gonorrheae*, *C. trachomatis* and other organisms. There are no epidemiologic data from Africa in this respect backed by comprehensive microbiologic investigations.

References

Adadevoh, B. K. (ed.) (1974). *Sub-fertility and Infertility in Africa*, p. 15. (Ibadan, Nigeria: Caxton Press)

American Social Health Association (1972). *Today's VD Control Problem*. (New York: ASHA)

Amoni, S. (1979). Acute purulent conjunctivitis in Nigerian children in Zaria. *J. Pediatr. Ophthalmol. Strabismus*, **16,** 308

Arya, O. P. (1972). Some highlights on the etiology of the nongonococcal urethral discharge in males in Kampala, Uganda. *E. Afr. Med. J.*, **49,** 817

Arya, O. P. and Bennett, F. J. (1967). Venereal disease in an elite group (university students) in East Africa. *Br. J. Vener. Dis.*, **43,** 275

Arya, O. P. and Bennett, F. J. (1976). Role of the medical auxiliary in the control of sexually transmitted disease in a developing country. *Br. J. Vener. Dis.*, **52,** 116

Arya, O. P., Nsanzumuhire, H. and Taber, S. R. (1973). Clinical, cultural and demographic aspects of gonorrhoea in a rural community in Uganda. *Bull. WHO*, **49,** 587

Arya, O. P. and Taber, S. R. (1975). Correlates of venereal disease and fertility in rural

Uganda. (Geneva: World Health Organization). Unpublished document WHO/VDT/RES/ 75, 339; WHO/VDT/RES/GON/75.96

Arya, O. P., Taber, S. R. and Nsanze, H. (1980a). Gonorrhoea and female infertility in rural Uganda. *Am. J. Obstet. Gynecol.*, **138**, 929

Arya, O. P., Osoba, A. O. and Bennett,. F. J. (1980b). *Tropical Venereology*. p. 12. (Edinburgh: Churchill Livingstone)

Bello, C. S. and Idiong, D. U. (1982). Schistosoma urethritis: pseudogonorrhoeal disease in northern Nigeria. *Trop. Doct.*, **12**, 141

Belsey, M. A. (1976). The epidemiology of infertility: a review with particular reference to Sub-Saharan Africa. *Bull. WHO*, **54**, 319

Berger, R. E., Alexander, E. R., Manda, G. D. *et al.* (1978). Chlamydia trachomatis as a cause of acute 'idiopathic' epididymitis. *N. Engl. J. Med.*, **298**, 301

Bewes, P. C. (1973). Urethral stricture. *Trop. Doct.*, **3**, 77

Bhat, G. J., Hira, S. K., Ratnam, A. V. *et al.* (1982). Congenital syphilis in Lusaka. III. Incidence in the neonatal intensive care unit. *E. Afr. Med. J.*, **59**, 374

Blavy, G. and Diakhate, L. (1982). Occurrence of syphilis in blood donors in Dakar and the importance of new serological detection methods. *Bull. Soc. Pathol. Exot. Fil.*, **75**, 360

Brown, I. M. and Cruickshank, J. G. (1976). Etiological factors in pelvic inflammatory disease in urban blacks in Rhodesia. *S. Afr. Med. J.*, **50**, 1342

Carty, M. J., Nzioki, J. M. and Verhagen, A. R. (1972). The role of gonococcus in acute pelvic inflammatory disease in Nairobi. *E. Afr. Med. J.*, **49**, 376

Darougar, S., Forsey, T., Osoba, A. O. *et al.* (1982). Chlamydial genital infection in Ibadan, Nigeria. *Br. J. Vener. Dis.*, **58**, 366

Department of Health and Social Security (1973). *On the State of the Public Health* (London: HMSO). The Annual Report of the Chief Medical Officer for 1972

Finlayson, M. H., Gibbs, B. and Brede, H. D. (1974). Diagnosis and incidence of *Neisseria gonorrhoeae* in Cape coloured females in the western Cape: laboratory aspects. *S. Afr. Med. J.*, **48**, 259

Forsey, T., Darougar, S., Dines, R. J. *et al.* (1982). Chlamydial genital infection in Addis Ababa, Ethiopa: a seroepidemiological survey. *Br. J. Vener. Dis.*, **58**, 370

Friedmann, P. S. and Wright, D. J. M. (1977). Observations on syphilis in Addis Ababa. *Br. J. Vener. Dis.*, **53**, 276

Grech, E. S., Everett, J. V. and Mukasa, F. (1973). Epidemiologic aspects of acute pelvic inflammatory disease in Uganda. *Trop. Doct.*, **3**, 123

Griffith, H. B. (1963). Gonorrhoea and fertility in Uganda. *Eugenics Rev.*, **55**, 103

Hall, S. M. and Whitcomb, M. A. (1978). Screening for gonorrhoea in family planning acceptors in a developing community. *Public Health*, **92**, 121

Hoosen, A. A., Ross, S. M. and Mulla, M. J. *et al.* (1981). The incidence of selected vaginal infections among pregnant urban blacks. *S. Afr. Med. J.*, **59**, 827

Hopcroft, M., Verhagen, A. R., Ngigi, S., *et al.* (1973). Genital infections in developing countries: experience in a family planning clinic. *Bull. WHO*, **48**, 581

Lomholt, G. (1976). Venereal problems in a developing country. *Trop. Doct.*, **6**, 7

Mabey, D. C. and Whittle, H. C. (1982). Genital and neonatal chlamydial infection in a trachoma endemic area. *Lancet*, **2**, 300

Mandara, N. A., Takulia, S., Kanyawana, J. *et al.* (1980). Asymptomatic gonorrhoea in women attending family planning clinic in Dar es Salaam, Tanzania. *Trop. Geog. Med.*, **32**, 329

Mathews, T., Mati, J. K. and Fomulu, J. N. (1981). A study of infertility in Kenya: results of investigation of the infertile couples in Nairobi. *E. Afr. Med. J.*, **58**, 288

Mati, J. K. G., Anderson, G. E., Carty, M. J. *et al.* (1973). A second look into the problems of primary infertility in Kenya. *E. Afr. Med. J.*, **50**, 94

Meheus, A. (1973). Incidence et prévalence des maladies veneriennes dans des populations selectionnes en region urbaine au Rwanda. *Ann. Soc. Belge Méd. Trop.*, **53**, 179

Meheus, A., Ballard, R., Dalmini, M. *et al.* (1980). Epidemiology and etiology of urethritis in Swaziland. *Int. J. Epidemiol.*, **9**, 239

Meheus, A., De Clerq, A. and Prat, R. (1974). Prevalence of gonorrhoea in prostitutes in a central African town. *Br. J. Vener. Dis.*, **50**, 50

Meheus, A., Delgadillo, R., Widi-Wirski, R. *et al.* (1982). Chlamydia ophthalmia neonatorum in central Africa. *Lancet*, **2**, 882

Meheus, A., Eylenbosch, W. and Ndibwani, A. (1975). Serological evidence of syphilis in different population groups in Rwanda. *Trop. Geog. Med.*, **27**, 165

Meheus, A., Friedman, F., Van Dyck, E. *et al.* (1980). Genital infections in prenatal and family planning attenders in Swaziland. *E. Afr. Med. J.*, **57**, 212

Muir, D. G. and Belsey, M. A. (1980). Pelvic inflammatory disease and its consequences in the developing world. *Am. J. Obstet. Gynecol.*, **138**, 913

Nasah, B. T., Nguematcha, R., Eyong, M. *et al.* (1980). Gonorrhoea, trichomonas and candida among gravid and nongravid women in Cameroon. *Int. J. Gynaecol. Obstet.*, **18**, 48

Nsanze, H., Waigwa, S. R. N., Mirza, N. *et al.* (1982). Chlamydial infections in selected populations in Kenya. In Mårdh, P.-A., Holmes, K. K., Oriel, J. D. *et al.* (eds.) *Chlamydial Infections* (Fernstrom Foundation Series), p. 421. (Amsterdam: Elsevier)

Ongom, V. L., Wamboka, J. W., Nakagwa, E. *et al.* (1976). The prevalence of venereal diseases among food and beverage handlers in public places in Kampala, Uganda. *E. Afr. Med. J.*, **53**, 389

Onyango-Ogony, P. J. and Hetland-Erikson, J. (1975). Purulent ophthalmia neonatorum at Mulago Hospital. *E. Afr. Med. J.*, **52**, 640

Osoba, A. O. (1972a). Serological tests for syphilis among hospital patients in Ibadan: 1968–1970. In West African Council for Medical Research (eds.), *Proceedings of the First Medical Research Seminar, Lagos*, p. 49. (Nigeria: West African Council for Medical Research)

Osoba, A. O. (1972b). Epidemiology of urethritis in Ibadan. *Br. J. Vener. Dis.*, **48**, 116

Osoba, A. O. and Alausa, K. O. (1974). Vulvovaginitis in Nigerian children. *Niger. J. Pediatr.*, **1**, 26

Osoba, A. O. and Onifade, A. (1973). Venereal diseases among pregnant women in Nigeria. *W. Afr. Med. J.*, **22**, 23

Otiti, M. L. (1975). Ophthalmia neonatorum in Mbale Hospital, Uganda. *E. Afr. Med. J.*, **52**, 644

Perine, P. L., Duncan, M. E., Krause, D. W. *et al.* (1980). Pelvic inflammatory disease and puerperal sepsis in Ethiopia. *Am. J. Obstet. Gynecol.*, **138**, 969

Perine, P. L., Totten, P. A., Knapp, J. S. *et al.* (1983). Diversity of gonococcal plasmids, auxotypes and serogroups in Ghana. *Lancet*, **1**, 1051

Rampen, F. (1978). Venereal syphilis in tropical Africa. *Br. J. Vener. Dis.*, **54**, 364

Ratnam, A. V. (1980). Sexually transmitted diseases in Lusaka. *Med. J. Zambia*, **14**, 71

Ratnam, A. V. and Chatterjee, T. K. (1980). Sexually transmitted diseases in pregnant women in Lusaka. *Med. J. Zambia*, **14**, 75

Ratnam, A. V., Din, S. N. and Chatterjee, T. K. (1980). Gonococcal infection in women with pelvic inflammatory disease in Lusaka, Zambia. *Am. J. Obstet. Gynecol.*, **138**, 965

Ratnam, A. V., Din, S. N., Hira, S. K. *et al.* (1982). Syphilis in pregnant women in Zambia. *Br. J. Vener. Dis.*, **58**, 355

Rushwan, H. (1980). Etiologic factors in pelvic inflammatory disease in Sudanese women. *Am. J. Obstet. Gynecol.*, **138**, 877

Taylor-Robinson, D. and McCormack, W. M. (1980). The genital mycoplasmas. *N. Engl. J. Med.*, **302**; 1003, 1063

Taylor-Robinson, D. and Thomas, B. J. (1980). The role of *Chlamydia trachomatis* in genital-tract and associated diseases. *J. Clin. Pathol.*, **33**, 205

Ursi, J. P., Van Dyck, E., Van Houtte, C. *et al.* (1981). Syphilis in Swaziland. *Br. J. Vener. Dis.*, **57**, 95

Verhagen, A. R. H. B. (1974). Gonorrhoea. In Vogel, L. C. *et al.* (eds.) *Health and Disease in Kenya*, p. 375. (Nairobi: East African Literature Bureau)

Vink, G. and Moodley, J. (1980). Gonorrhoea in black women attending a gynecological outpatient department. *S. Afr. Med. J.*, **58**, 901

Weissenberger, R., Robertson, A., Holland, S. *et al.* (1977). The incidence of gonorrhoea in urban Rhodesian black women. *S. Afr. Med. J.*, **52**, 1119

Westrøm, L. (1980). Incidence, prevalence, and trends of acute pelvic inflammatory disease and its consequence in industrialized countries. *Am. J. Obstet. Gynecol.*, **138**, 880

Widy-Wirski, R., D'Costa, J., Biddle, J. *et al.* (1982). *Antimicrobial susceptibility of gonococci in the Central African Republic. Bull. WHO*, **60**, 959

World Health Organization. (1975). *The epidemiology of infertility*, Technical report No. 582. (Geneva: WHO)

World Health Organization. (1978). *Neisseria gonorrhoeae and gonococcal infections*, Technical report No. 616. (Geneva: WHO)

World Health Organization. (1981). *Nongonococcal urethritis and other selected sexually transmitted diseases of public health importance.* Technical report No. 660. (Geneva: WHO)

World Health Organization. (1982). *Treponemal infections*, Technical report No. 674. (Geneva: WHO)

World Health Organization. (1983). Surveillance of β-lactamase-producing *Neisseria gonorrhoeae* (PPNG). *Wkly. Epidemiol. Rec.*, **58**, 5

6
Puerperal sepsis with special reference to India

M. KOCHHAR

DEFINITION

Puerperal sepsis is infection of the genital tract after delivery or abortion. This infection may originate at the placental site or within lacerations of the cervix, vagina, or perineum. The genital tract may be involved alone or there may be spread to other sites. It is important to remember that pyrexia in the puerperium may also arise from infections of the breast, urinary tract, lungs, or any of a number of other medical or surgical conditions, including malaria and typhoid (still fairly common in India and other developing countries).

According to the Joint Committee on Maternal Welfare, the diagnosis of puerperal sepsis can be established if a fever of 38 °C (100.4 °F) persists after the first 24 hours and within 10 days postpartum. This standard is commonly employed in the United States (Williams, 1979). In England and Wales the puerperal pyrexia regulations (1951) define puerperal sepsis as 'any febrile condition occurring in a woman in whom temperature of 100.4 °F (38 °C) or more has occurred within 14 days after confinement or miscarriage'. The same definition also applies in India.

British Obstetrics and Gynaecological Practice (2nd edn) defines puerperal pyrexia as 'a rise of temperature to 100.4 °F (38 °C) or more, maintained for 24 hours or recurring during that period, in the first 21 days after confinement or miscarriage but excluding the first 24 hours'.

Despite the advent of antibiotics and modern obstetric practices, puerperal sepsis remains a major cause of maternal mortality and morbidity, not only in India but in other developing countries as well. Although mortality due to puerperal sepsis has all but been eliminated in developed nations, morbidity after cesarean section and vaginal delivery is not uncommon, and infection remains an important cause of maternal death (Tomkinson *et al.*, 1979). For example, in New York City one maternal death occurs per 1000 deliveries by cesarean section, and infection is the second leading cause of maternal death

(Richard and Schwarz, 1980). Septicemia is present in 11.7% of cases and pelvic abscess in 9.4% (Cunningham et al., 1978).

In developed countries, sepsis in obstetrics is mainly associated with cesarean section; 8.6% of patients with endometritis following cesarean section develop pelvic thrombitis. In a series of 3500 cesarean sections in New South Wales the infection rate was 13% (six times greater than vaginal delivery), as reported by the Maternal and Perinatal Mortality Committee (1969). In San Antonio, Texas, a prospective study revealed that 38.5% of women who delivered via cesarean section developed endometritis as compared to 1.2% after vaginal delivery (Gibbs, 1980). Another study also found that the rate of endometritis after cesarean section was five to ten times greater than after vaginal delivery (Sweet and Ledger, 1973).

At Kasturba Hospital, 50% of patients undergoing cesarean section had fever for more than 48 hours, and 20% had wound sepsis. These percentages are far from ideal. Although maternal mortality due to cesarean section has declined considerably in our area, maternal morbidity remains high. Most postpartum complications are related to sepsis, despite the use of broad-spectrum antibiotics and other preventive measures. In 1981–82, 40% of cesarean births were accompanied by some form of infection as determined by fever, endometritis, wound infection, urinary tract infection, peritonitis, and thrombophlebitis (Vohra et al., 1983).

Table 1 Comparison of maternal mortality due to sepsis in different countries[a]

Author	Countries	Period	Maternal mortality per 100 000 deliveries	Percentage of mortality due to sepsis
Chi et al.	Indonesia	1977–78[b]	390	22.2
Rao	India	1978–79	753	18.0
Narone	Zambia	1977–78	88	12.3
Ojo	Ghana/Nigeria	1962–71	820	7.0
Ojo	Hong Kong	1971	140	4.4
Shingawa	Sweden	1975	2.0	0.002
Shingawa and Katagiri	Japan	1977	23	2.0
Shingawa and Katagiri	United States	1975	13	—
Shingawa and Katagiri	England and Wales	1975	13	—

[a] From the Proceedings of 2nd International Seminar on Maternal and Perinatal Mortality, Pregnancy Termination and Sterilization, Bombay, India, 1975.
[b] From the Proceedings of 3rd International Seminar on Maternal and Perinatal Mortality, Pregnancy Termination and Sterilization, New Delhi, India, 1980.

Table 1 compares maternal mortality in different countries and the percentage of maternal mortality that is due to sepsis. Maternal mortality in India varies between 278 and 3499 per 100 000 deliveries, and 18% of this (on the average) is due to sepsis (Rao et al., 1977). Table 2 shows the maternal mortality due to sepsis in different parts of India. Mortality is higher in hospitals dealing with referred and high-risk cases.

Table 2 Maternal mortality in different parts of India[a]

Author	City	Year	Percentage of maternal mortality due to sepsis
Chowdhary	Eden Hospital, Calcutta	1979	21.0
Devi	Maternity Hospital, Hyderabad	1978	25.0
Engineer	Lucknow	1970–73	8.0
Hingorani	AIIMS, Delhi	1963–78	19.0
Kochhar	Kasturba Hospital, Delhi	1982	23.0
Mukherjee and Kotwani	LNJPH, Delhi	1980	24.0
Narula et al.	Kamla Nehru Memorial Hospital, Allahbad	1955–79	25.0
Rao and Mallika	Madras	1974–75	13.0

[a] From the Proceedings of 3rd International Seminar on Maternal and Perinatal Mortality, Termination and Sterilization, at All India Institute of Medical Sciences, Delhi, India, 1980.

HISTORICAL BACKGROUND

Puerperal infection is mentioned in the works of Hippocrates and Galen. In the seventeenth century Willis wrote on the subject of *febris puerperium*; the English term puerperal fever was first employed by Strofher in 1716. The work of Semmelweiss linking puerperal sepsis with unsanitary practices and Pasteur's cultivation of *Streptococcus* put to rest many older theories concerning the origin and nature of puerperal fever. The contagiousness of puerperal infection was first shown by John Leake (1772); in 1843, Oliver Wendell Holmes demonstrated that at least the epidemic forms of the infection could be traced to lack of proper antiseptic precautions on the part of physicians and nurses (Williams, 1979). The introduction of sulfonamides for the treatment of streptococcal infection in 1935, and their subsequent application in obstetrics (Colebrook and Kenny, 1936) has proven one of the greatest advances of the century (Donald, 1979). Death from sepsis now is rare among Western nations, and most women recover with prompt treatment. If not diagnosed and treated properly, however, puerperal sepsis may lead to secondary infertility and chronic pelvic inflammatory disease.

ETIOLOGY AND PREDISPOSING FACTORS

If the fetal membranes have been ruptured for a prolonged period prior to the onset of labor, or if a woman has undergone numerous vaginal examinations performed under less than aseptic conditions, the risk of puerperal infection is greatly increased. Instrumental delivery, manual removal of the placenta, episiotomy, and multiple lacerations of the vulva also increase the chances of serious postpartum infection. Puerperal infection is more common in women from lower socioeconomic classes. Anemia during pregnancy, inadequate prior nutrition, diabetes and toxemia, as well as any illness that compromises systemic resistance, are important predisposing factors. Maternal anemia is a particularly important concern in developing countries. At Kasturba Hospital, 20% of cases of puerperal sepsis were associated with moderate to severe anemia.

Infection is likely to complicate a prolonged labor, especially if the amniotic membrane has been ruptured for many hours. In one retrospective study of military dependents, the incidence of intrauterine infection was found to increase from 11% when there was no labor (and no rupture of the fetal membrane) and to 20% when labor ensued. When both labor and membrane rupture were present, the infection rate jumped to 43% (Gibbs, 1980). In our own experience amnionitis was observed in 41.6% of cases within 18 hours of ruptured membrane. The overall maternal infection rate was 22.4%: the infection rate between 12 and 24 hours of rupture membrane was 16%, and 34% after 24 hours. The incidence of infection increased as the time lag between the rupture of membrane and the onset of labor increased (Kochhar and Manjeet, 1978).

The increasing use of internal fetal monitoring has been accompanied by an increase in the intrauterine infection rate. In one study, intrauterine infections rose from 20.4% in unmonitored patients to 40.4% in the monitored women (Gasnner and Ledger, 1976). The retention of an intrauterine catheter for longer than 4 hours is also associated with maternal clinical infection (Bobitt and Ledger, 1978).

Women who had undergone more than seven vaginal examinations, and who had prolonged rupture of membrane, were found to have a greatly increased occurrence of postpartum infection (Lewis et al., 1976). Prolonged labor with ruptured membrane or an intrauterine fetal monitoring device in place, and cesarean section delivery are also high-risk factors.

THE PATHOLOGY OF PUERPERAL SEPSIS

Genital tract infection

Since puerperal infection is essentially a wound infection, the placental site is involved in most cases, with the exception of very mild infections.

Endometritis and metritis

Acute endometritis may be of two types: (1) septic endometritis, in which the uterus appears clean, a serous exudate is present, small uterine vessels contain infected thrombi, and bacteremia develops usually caused by hemolyticus streptococci; and (2) putrid endometritis, in which the uterine cavity contains placental tissue and blood clots, a foul-smelling discharge is present, the uterus remains subinvoluted with multiple abscesses. Putrid endometritis is caused by staphylococci and *E. coli*.

Lesions of the perineum, vulva, vagina, and cervix

Localized infections of repaired lacerations and episiotomies often occur. Wound edges become red and swollen, the surgical stitches cut through, and purulent discharge is present. Lacerations of vagina easily become infected and in neglected cases may result in atresia of the vagina, leading to subsequent dyspareunia and infertility. Cervical tears often extend to the base of the broad ligament and may be accompanied by lymphangitis, parametritis, and bacteremia.

Spread beyond the genital tract

Four types of pelvic lesions are encountered in puerperal sepsis:

(1) Pelvic cellulitis, usually stemming from an infected cervical injury, either directly or by way of the lymphatic system.
(2) Pelvic peritonitis with or without abscess formation; in severe cases, generalized peritonitis may follow.
(3) Acute salpingo-oophoritis leading to pyosalpingitis and ovarian abscess, and usually associated with perisalpingitis. The tubes are rarely subsequently occluded. Of interest is the fact that gonococcal salpingitis during the puerperium is rare.
(4) Pelvic thrombophlebitis with involvement of the uterine and broad ligament veins as a result of spread of infection. The ovarian veins are most commonly involved. The process may spread beyond the pelvis to the iliac and femoral veins and occasionally to the inferior vena cava (Dawn, 1982).

Extrapelvic lesions include those cases in which thrombosis of the infected vein suppurates and cause septicemia, pyemia, or thrombophlebitis of leg veins and the inferior vena cava. In some rare cases, extrapelvic lesions may lead to bacterial endocarditis, pericarditis, metastatic abscesses of the lungs, meningitis or arthritis. This kind of spread is rare, since the advent of antibiotics; in neglected cases, however, especially in developing countries, these conditions still occur and mortality due to septic endotoxic shock still occurs.

THE BACTERIOLOGY OF PUERPERAL SEPSIS

Pathogenic organisms may be introduced from exogenous sources or may originate in the resident flora of the cervix and lower genital tract.

Streptococci

Group A and B hemolytic streptococci were once the leading cause of puerperal infection but now are only rarely implicated. If present, however, the virulence of these organisms demands prompt treatment. Puerperal staphylococcal infections are especially difficult to treat, because penicillin-resistant organisms have now emerged. When *Clostridium perfringens* is the causative agent gas gangrene, hemolysis, septic shock, and even death are possible.

Anaerobic bacteroides species, *Clostridium perfringens*, and *C. tetani* are seldom pathogenic under normal circumstances, but can cause severe infections when necrotic tissue and blood clots are present. The presence of anaerobes in the genitourinary tract decreases during pregnancy but increases once again after delivery. By the third day after delivery (in uncomplicated cases) cultures reveal the presence of a moderate to heavy growth of at least one pathogen; 70–80% of the time, it is an anaerobic cocci (Gibbs *et al.*, 1975).

The type of organisms and the frequency of their occurrence is presented in

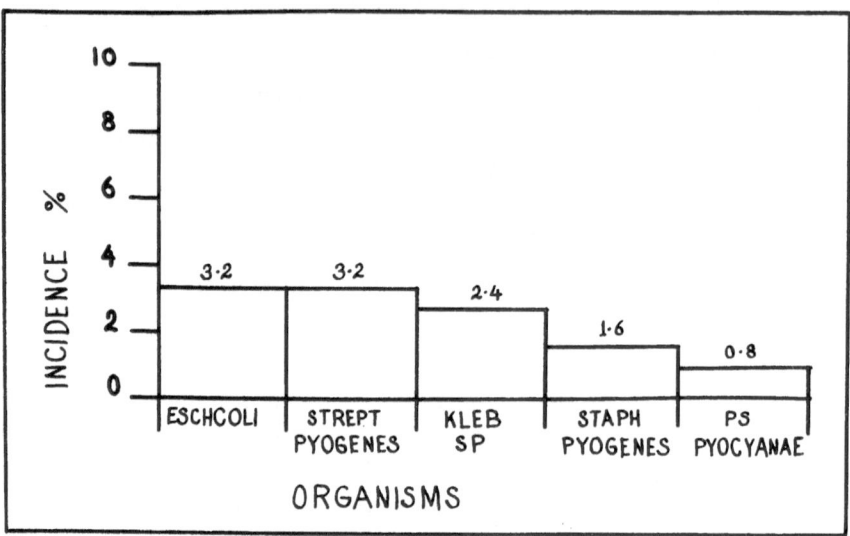

Fig. 1 Incidence of various organisms in high vaginal swab positive cases

Fig. 1. Anaerobic streptococci were not isolated, probably due to the lack of sensitivity of the analytical equipment. *Chlamydia trachomatis* was not cultured. The number of high vaginal swab positive cases had no significant association with time; however, there was a slight increase (10%) in the incidence of infection from 6 to 36 hours. The incidence of clinical maternal infection in the high vaginal swab positive cases was independent of the presence or absence of organisms in the vaginal canal: 64.2% of high vaginal swab positive cases developed infection, while 51.4% of high vaginal swab negative cases also showed infection ($p = 1.02$). There was no significant correlation between placenta-positive cases and the time after membrane rupture (Fig. 2).

Infection developed in 37.2% of the positive cases in contrast to the 12.3% of negative cases in whom infection developed. The incidence of maternal infection in placenta-positive cases without antibiotics was significantly lower (50%) at 12 hours and 24 hours (30%) (Kochhar and Manjeet, 1978).

There was a significant difference between the groups that had prophylactic antibiotics and those that did not. The incidence of maternal infection decreased over time in the groups that had no antibiotics while there was an increased incidence of infection with increasing time in the antibiotics groups (Fig. 3).

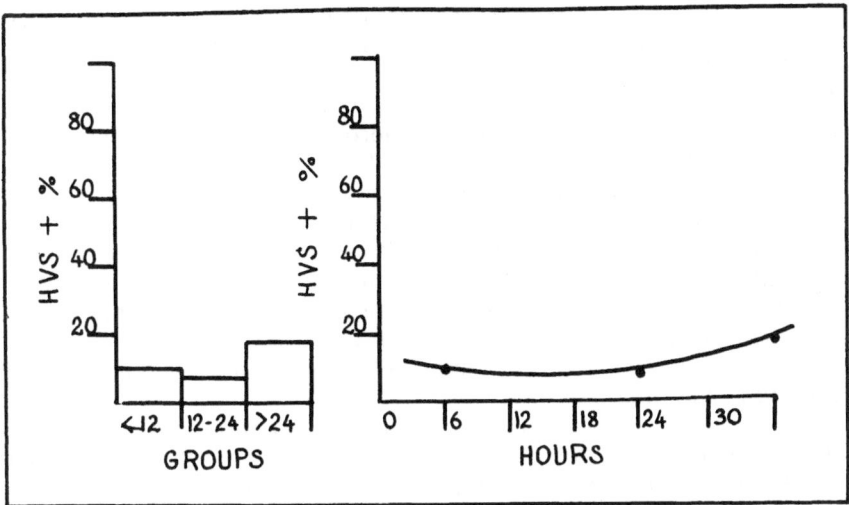

Fig. 2. Incidence of placenta-positive versus time

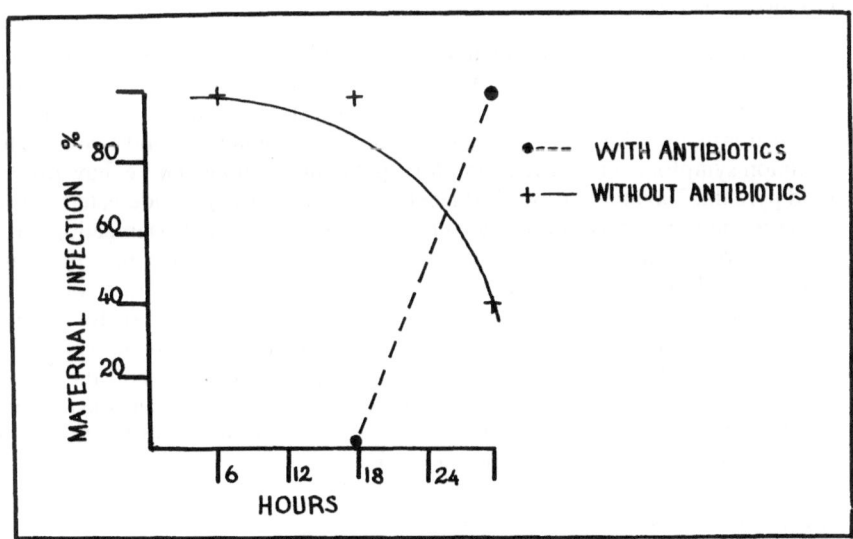

Fig. 3 Incidence of maternal infection in high vaginal swab positive cases with and without antibiotics

The fact that anaerobic streptococci were not isolated may be due to the lack of sensitivity of our analytical equipment. In clinical practice, sepsis caused by cross-infection of penicillin-resistant staphylococci remains a problem. It has been observed that the use of antibiotics may have led to more severe infection due to hemolytic streptococci and pneumococci; anaerobic and nonhemolytic streptococci, *Proteus*, enterococci, and coliform bacilli are resistant to antibiotics and often seem to acquire new and dangerous virulence.

The role of anaerobic organisms in such infections has only recently been recognized. Anaerobic streptococci and *Bacteroides* in perinatal and maternal mortality have been associated with amnionitis and puerperal sepsis respectively (Townsend *et al.*, 1966). *Bacteroides* organisms were isolated in 1.8/1000 live births (Pearson and Anderson, 1967). In 15 cases of newborn anaerobic streptococci, 14 *Veillonella* organisms and one *Clostridium* organism were isolated (Chow *et al.*, 1974).

The incidence of puerperal sepsis endometritis was 3.8% after vaginal delivery and 13–27% following cesarean section. Anaerobic bacteria were isolated in 55% of cases. *E. coli*, *Peptostreptococcus*, *Bacteroides*, and *Streptococcus* were the predominant organisms (Sweet and Ledger, 1973).

THE CLINICAL PRESENTATION OF PUERPERAL SEPSIS

The clinical features of puerperal infection vary greatly with the type and virulence of the organism, the primary site of infection, and the extent of its spread. The clinical picture, however, may be broken down into the two general types: localized and diffused infections.

Localized wound infection

Local infection of perineal, vaginal or cervical lacerations is not uncommon. The placenta is also a potential site for localized uterine sepsis. The abdominal incision made during cesarean section may also become infected, locally. In perineal infection the infected area becomes red, edematous and tender. The common symptoms are local discomfort, pain and burning. There may also be mild pyrexia. Vaginal and cervical lacerations sometimes go undetected unless a tear in the upper part of the vagina or cervix gets infected; this infection gives rise to sepsis and a purulent foul-smelling discharge. Uterine infection and mild cases of endometritis may show only elevation of temperature for 2 or 3 days. In more severe cases the temperature rises on the third or fourth day postpartum, sometimes to as high as 38–40 °C with accompanying chills and rigors. In most cases the pulse rate increases proportionally, and the lochia usually is profuse and foul-smelling. In some cases, however, the lochia remains scanty and the uterus is subinvoluted and soft due to drainage obstruction. The condition gradually improves over a week.

Diffuse infection

Pelvic cellulitis may be suspected if, by the end of the first week, there is a sharp rise in the temperature, tenderness of the lower abdomen, and tenderness and induration of fornices and uterosacral ligament on vaginal examination. Induration may extend to the lateral pelvic wall and above the inguinal ligament. Resolution takes place gradually and forms scarring in the parametrium. Suppuration and abscess formation in the posterior fornix also may occur.

Salpingo-oophoritis and pelvic peritonitis present a clinically similar picture to cellulitis. Pelvic peritonitis may result in pelvic abscess. High fever, diarrhea, and tenesmus are the important diagnostic features. There is also a tender, soft swelling in the Pouch of Douglas, which may burst into the vagina or rectum if not treated early. In severe cases there may also be generalized peritonitis with the signs and symptoms of severe infection: higher fever, rapid pulse, vomiting, and pain, tenderness, distension and rigidity of the abdomen. The patient looks ill and is dehydrated; diarrhea or signs of obstruction may be present. This condition is not common, but instances stemming from neglect are still seen in India and other developing countries.

Thrombosis of the pelvic veins may remain localized or may extend to the ovarian iliac veins and even infect the vena cava. Clinically, there is fever with rigors at the end of the second week of the puerperium. Tenderness of the calf muscles and edema of the lower limbs is also present. Septic emboli to other organs, especially the lungs, may prove fatal.

PROPHYLAXIS OF PUERPERAL SEPSIS

Antenatal prophylaxis

During pregnancy the general health of the mother should be considered and anemia treated; special care should also be taken regarding the diet. Any septic foci in the body should be treated, and coitus during the last weeks of pregnancy is not advised. All vaginal discharge should be treated, and unnecessary vaginal douches or examination should be avoided.

In developing countries, where the majority of deliveries are conducted at home, immunization against tetanus is becoming a routine, especially in our Maternal and Child Health Centers and hospitals (Devi, 1980).

During labor

Aseptic techniques should be employed in the delivery room. The vulva should be shaved and washed, and the patient may be given a shower and provided with a hospital gown. Vaginal examination should be restricted and performed only under strict aseptic conditions. The attendant must wear a clean mask, gloves, and gown, and delivery should be conducted with all aseptic precautions. Any attendant suffering from a septic focus, sore throat, common cold, or any other infection should be barred from entering the delivery room.

All lacerations or tears should be properly stitched. The placenta should be carefully examined to ensure that no membranes or pieces of placenta are retained, as these may cause uterine infection.

Prophylactic antibiotics are given in high-risk cases, such as in premature rupture of the membrane or in cases of prolonged labor or when patients are referred to hospitals after being handled by untrained midwives. It is better to take swabs for culture and sensitivity and later give antibiotic according to sensitivity. By giving antibiotics indiscriminately, significant differences in morbidity have been found between the groups with and without antibiotics. Incidence of maternal infection was decreased by 10 to 20% in mothers who were not receiving antibiotics and 20 to 50% in the neonates not receiving antibiotics (Kochhar and Manjeet, 1978).

It is true that antibiotics have made treatment of puerperal sepsis simple, but the general principles of asepsis and treatment of infection must still be applied.

Postpartum prophylaxis

All aseptic techniques must be maintained and care of the perineum and wound is necessary: sterile sanitary pads should be used. This practice is not effected in developing countries when delivery is conducted at home. Midwives should be given training in aseptic techniques.

In cases of pyrexia or infection the patient should be isolated; preferably, isolation wards should be separate from clean obstetrical units, although in many rural hospitals this is not feasible. At least barrier nursing should be provided and adequate measures taken to avoid cross-infection. The rules laid down by the Medical Research Council (1951) still hold true.

In short, the prevention of puerperal infection depends on the practice of good obstetric and nursing techniques in a suitable environment on women whose health is brought to a level of high local and general resistance (Bender, 1959).

DIAGNOSIS

Pyrexia after childbirth is usually caused by genital tract infection, but other causes must be ruled out, including cystitis, pyelonephritis, mastitis, wound sepsis (in the case of cesarean section), respiratory tract infection, malaria, and tuberculosis. This is especially true in developing countries. In Kasturba Hospital, fever during puerperium in 79 cases was due to malaria.

TREATMENT

The treatment of puerperal sepsis has undergone a revolution in recent years since the introduction of antibiotics. Good nursing care, diet and other forms of treatment still play important roles in the patient's ultimate recovery.

The principles of management of puerperal sepsis are:

(a) careful selection of cases for prophylactic antibiotic therapy;
(b) assessment of the nature, type and extent of infection;
(c) good supportive therapy including correction of anemia etc.,

(d) surgical intervention limited to drainage of abscesses or measures to prevent embolization.

Refractory fevers in the puerperium require careful search for specific foci, since flare-ups of old tuberculosis are not uncommon and tetanus is still prevalent in India and other developing countries. In one study (Saxena *et al.*, 1966) puerperal tetanus constituted 8.1% of 5550 cases of tetanus with a mortality of 27.7%. In India the incidence of tetanus presently has decreased due to routine immunization with tetanus toxoid during pregnancy.

General treatment

Bed rest, sedation and adequate diet are required. In mild cases an ordinary diet is sufficient, but in severe cases intravenous fluids are advised along with high levels of proteins and vitamins. If the patient is vomiting or in septic shock, more comprehensive measures need to be administered as well. Heavy doses of steroids can be given in cases of septic shock. Anemia is treated in severe cases by blood transfusion.

Approach to therapy

Antibiotic therapy should be determined by the results of sensitivity tests. In the absence of such data, however, antibiotics selected should be effective against both aerobic and anaerobic bacteria. The majority of anaerobic organisms, except *Bacteroides fragilis*, are sensitive to penicillin or tetracycline. Doxycycline is more effective than plain tetracycline; chloramphenicol is active against a wide range of anaerobic bacteria.

Metronidazole is active against anaerobic bacteria with a minimum of side-effects. Gentamycin and kenamycin, neomycin and streptomycin have little activity against anaerobes, while clindamycin and metronidazole are not effective against *E. coli*. Either clindamycin or chloramphenicol, in combination with gentamycin or kenamycin, should be used.

Treatment of infection with non-spore-forming anaerobes should follow general surgical principles (Seligman and Villi, 1980). There is widespread resistance of *B. fragilis* to penicillin and cephalosporins due to the production of *B. lactamase* (Tally *et al.*, 1979). Aminoglycosides are not active due to failure of active transport into anaerobic cells (Bryan *et al.*, 1979).

Chloramphenicol is not active against *B. fragilis*, probably because of rapid inactivation (Thadepalli *et al.*, 1977). The choice of chemotherapy lies between metronidazole, clindamycin and cefotaxime. Metronidazole is extremely effective and has no known side-effects. The incidence of wound sepsis following cesarean section has been reduced from 26% to 5%, and overall sepsis from 40% to 17% with the use of metronidazole as prophylaxis (Vaughan, 1979). Clindamycin is highly effective (Salaki *et al.*, 1976), but can cause colitis. Cefotaxime is a cefamycin with a wide spectrum against aerobes and anaerobes. It appears to be safe, but can be given only by injection and local reactions are troublesome. Moreover, this medication is still not available in India and other developing countries.

Symptomatic treatment

If pyrexia is present, hydrotherapy and antipyretic drugs should be given along with analgesics, sedatives, and mild tranquillizers for pain and sleeplessness.

If patients have diarrhea and abdominal distension due to pelvic or generalized peritonitis, treatment should include doses of antibiotics, parenteral fluids and nasogastric suction.

Local treatment

In the presence of infected local wounds, stitches should be removed and hot fomentation applied; analgesic should be given for pain and the infection treated by suitable antibiotics.

Uterine infection, if due to retained pieces of placenta or membrane, should be treated by very gentle removal or curettage under antibiotic coverage.

Pelvic cellulitis should be treated by anti-inflammatory drugs and specific antibiotics. If pelvic abscesses have formed, they should be drained by colpotomy.

In cases of generalized peritonitis, if improvement does not ensue after treatment with broad-spectrum antibiotics, intravenous drip and suction or if there are signs of pus collection in the peritoneal cavity, then laparotomy must be performed and a drainage tube left in place for 24–48 hours. In rare cases hysterectomy may be required to control the infection, especially in neglected cases with anaerobic organisms or *Clostridium perfringens*.

Specific treatment of complications

In pelvic thrombophlebitis and deep vein thrombosis, the treatment is the same as for pelvic cellulitis. Anticoagulants with proper monitoring should be started whenever deep vein thrombosis is diagnosed in order to prevent embolism. Dosages of anticoagulants should be regulated by repeated prothrombin times.

Ligation of the inferior vena cava and ovarian veins can be life-saving in cases of repeated septic emboli.

Pulmonary embolism

An important cause of maternal mortality may follow venous thrombosis of the lower limbs or pelvis, especially after cesarean section; 5.1% of the deaths (Rao *et al.* 1977) were due to pulmonary embolism.

Cerebral venous thrombosis

This condition has a particularly high incidence in the puerperium and may be accompanied by severe headache, disorientation, delirium or sudden convulsions. The maximum incidence of thrombosis occurs between 4 and 7 days after delivery. Anemia and dehydration are etiological factors.

Treatment is supportive with symptomatic anticoagulants used cautiously.

CONCLUSIONS

Before the advent of antibiotics, puerperal sepsis was one of the leading causes of maternal mortality. Thanks to the use of antibiotics that incidence, however, has decreased dramatically even in the rural areas of India where minimally trained or even untrained midwives are conducting deliveries. It should be emphasized, however, that although antibiotic usage has simplified the management of puerperal sepsis, the general principles underlying the prevention and treatment of this disease remains. Good midwifery is of primary importance. Prophylaxis, rather than treatment, is most important in minimizing the ill effects of puerperal sepsis and its sequelae.

Developing countries such as India have not yet organized their midwifery services to the point where they can assure that minimum standards of care are applied in all cases. Training midwives in aseptic techniques, improving the nutrition of the mother, and providing a mechanism for the early referral of patients with complications will go a long way in reducing puerperal sepsis.

More advanced countries are facing the growing problems of infection with gonococci, *Chlamydia* and other sexually transmitted organisms. Proper diagnosis and management of these diseases is essential to reduce their ill effects.

The role of anaerobes in venereal infections has only recently been recognized. Therapy should be determined by cultures and antibiotic susceptibility; in the absence of such data broad-spectrum antibiotics with activity against both aerobes and anaerobes of vaginal origin should be employed. Metronidazole is active against anaerobic bacteria and has minimal side-effects.

Although mortality due to puerperal sepsis has been all but eliminated in developed nations, morbidity after cesarean section and delivery is not uncommon. Therefore, the unwarranted use of cesarean section should be avoided.

References

Bender, S. (1959). The abnormal puerperium. *British Obstetrics and Gynaecological Practice*, 2nd edn., p. 892. The White Friars Press Ltd

Bobbit, J. R. and Ledger, W. J. (1978). Amniotic fluid analysis, its role in maternal and neonatal infection. *Obstet. Gynecol.*, **51**, 56

Bryan, L. E., Koward, S. K. and Van Den Elzen, H. M. (1979). Mechanism of aminologycoside antibiotic resistance in anaerobic bacteria clostridium perfringens and bacteroides. *Antimicrob. Agents Chemother.*, **15**, 7

Chi, I. C., Agoestina, T., Harbin, J. (1980). *Maternal Mortality at Twelve Teaching Hospitals in Indonesia: An Epidemiological Analysis*, p. 23. (New Delhi: New Roxy Press)

Chow, A. M., Leake, R. D. (1974). The significance of anaerobes in neonatal bacteremia: analysis of 23 cases and review of the literature. *Pediatrics*, **54**, 736

Chowdhary, N. N. R. (1980). *Factors Influencing Maternal Mortality*. 3rd International Seminar on Maternal and Perinatal Mortality: Termination and Sterilization, New Delhi

Cunningham, F. G., Hauth, J. C. (1978). Infections morbidity following C. section: comparison of two treatment regimens. *Obstet. Gynecol.*, **152**, 656

Dawn, C. S. (1982). The abnormal puerperium. In *Textbook of Obstetrics*, 8th edn., p. 475. (Calcutta: Sreemoti Aarti Dawn Publisher)

Devi, M., Rao, C. M., Devi, K. K. *et al.* (1975). *A 15-year Review of Maternal Mortality at*

Government Hospital, Hyderabad. 2nd international seminar on Maternal and Perinatal Mortality: Termination and Sterilization, Bombay

Devi, P. K. (1980). Pathology of the Puerperium. *Postgraduate Obstetrics and Gynaecology,* p. 153–4. (Madras, India: Orient Longman Ltd)

Donald, I. (1979). *Puerperal Infection,* 5th edn., p. 877. (London: Lloyd Luke (Medical Books) Ltd)

Engineer, A. D. and Lakshmi, M. S. (1975). Maternal mortality. *J. Obstet. Gynaecol. India,* **27**, 187

Gasnner, G. D. and Ledger, W. J. (1976). The relationship of hospital acquired maternal infection to invasive intra partum technique. *Am. J. Obstet. Gynecol.,* **126**, 33

Gibbs, R. S. (1980). Clinical risk factors for puerperal infection. *Obstet. Gynecol. Suppl.,* **55**, 175

Gibbs, R. S., O'Dell, T. N., MacGregor, R. R., Schwarz, R. H. and Morton, H. (1975). Puerperal endometritis: a prospective microbiologic study. *Am. J. Obstet. Gynecol.,* **121**, 919–25

Hingorani, V., Gupta, U., Oumochigui, A., Sarin, U., Verma, N. and Kumar, S. (1981). A study of bacterial flora in pre and post operative patients and in post partum and post abortal infections with special reference to anaerobic infection. 1st All India Symposium on Anaerobic Infection, New Delhi, p. 8

Holland, E. and Bourne, A. (1959). The abnormal puerperium. In 2nd edn. *British Obstetrics & Gynaecological Practice,* p. 877. (London: The White Friars Press Ltd)

Kochhar, M. (1982). *Kasturba Hospital Statistics.* New Delhi

Kochhar, M. and Manjeet, K. (1978). *Maternal and Neonatal Infection Following Premature Rupture of Membrane and the Role of Prophylactic Antibiotics.* Thesis. (University of Delhi)

Lewis, J. F., Johnson, P., Miller, P. (1976). Evaluation of amniotic fluid for aerobic and anaerobic bacteria. *Am. J. Clin. Pathol.,* **65**, 58

Maternal and Perinatal Mortality Committee, Department of Public Health, New South Wales (1969). Caesarean section in New South Wales 1966-7: a mortality and morbidity study. *Med. J. Aust.,* **1**, 319–23

Medical Research Council Memorandum (1951). The control of cross infection in hospital. (London: H.M.S.O.)

Mukherjee, S. and Kotwani, B. G. (1980). *Maternal Mortality at Maulana Azad Medical College, Delhi: A 17-year Survey.* 3rd International Seminar on Maternal and Perinatal Mortality: Termination and Sterilization, New Delhi

Narone, R., Narone, J. N., Chatterjee, T. K. (1980). *Maternal Mortality at University Teaching Hospital, Lusaka, Zambia.* 2nd International Seminar on Maternal and Perinatal Mortality: Termination and Sterilization, New Delhi

Ojo, O. A. and Sauage, V. Y. (1980). *Maternal Mortality: A 10-year Review at the University of College Hospital, Ibadan, Nigeria.* 2nd International Seminar on Maternal and Perinatal Mortality: Termination and Sterilization, Bombay

Pearson, H. E. and Anderson, G. V. (1967). Perinatal deaths associated with bacteroides infection. *Obstet. Gynecol.,* **30**, 486

Rao, K. B. and Malika, P. E. (1977). The study of maternal mortality in Madras City. *J. Obstet. Gynecol. India,* **27**, 877

Rao, K. B. (1980). *Maternal Mortality in India: A FOGSI Study.* 3rd International Seminar on Maternal and Perinatal Mortality: Termination and Sterilization, New Delhi

Richard, H. and Schwarz, M. D. (1980). Clinical risk factors for puerperal infection. *Discussion. Obstet. Gynecol. Suppl.* **55**, p. 183

Salaki, J. S., Black, R., Tally, F. P. and Kislak, J. W. *et al.* (1976). Bacteroides fragilis resistant to the administration of clindamycin. *Am. J. Med.,* **60**, 426

Saxena, O., Pareek, N. K., Hussain, S. A. (1966). Puerperal tetanus. *J. Obstet. Gynecol. India,* **16**, 181

Seligman, S. A. and Villi, S. T. (1980). Infection with non-sporing anaerobes. *Br. J. Obstet. Gynecol.,* **87**, 846

Shingawa, S. and Katagri, S. (1980). *Maternal Mortality and Its Background in Recent Japan.* 3rd International Seminar on Maternal and Perinatal Mortality: Termination and Sterilization, New Delhi

Stevenson, C. S., Behney, C. A. and Miller, N. F. (1966). Maternal death from puerperal sepsis: A 17-year study in Michigan. *Obstet. Gynecol.,* **29**, 181

Sweet, R. L. and Ledger, W. H. (1973). Puerperal infection morbidity: A 2-year review. *Am. J. Obstet. Gynecol.*, **117**, 1093

Tally, F. P., Snydman, D. R., Shimell, M. J. and Golden, B. R. (1979). Mechanics of antimicrobial resistance of bacteroides fragilis. *Roy. Med. ICS*, **18**, 19

Thadepalli, H. (1979). Anaerobic infection of the female genital tract. *Scand. J. Infect. Dis. Suppl.*, 1980

Thadepalli, H., Appleman, M. D., Maidman, J. E., Aroe, J. J. and Davidson, E. C. (1977). Antimicrobial effect of amniotic fluid against anaerobic bacteria. *Am. J. Obstet. Gynecol.*, **127**, 250

Tomkinson, J., Turnbull, A., Robson, G., Cloake, E. Adelestein, A. M. and Weatherall, J. (1979). Report on confidential enquiries into maternal deaths in England and Wales 1973-75. p. 103. (London: H.M.S.O.)

Townsend, L. (1966). Spontaneous premature rupture of membrane. *J. Obstet. Gynecol. Aust. N.Z.*, **6**, 227

Vaughan, J. E. (1979). Comparison of metronidazole and cephardine in the prevention of wound sepsis following C. section. *Roy. Med. ICS*, **18**, 203

Vohra, S., Jain, S., Rai, U., Kumari, S. (1982). *A Changing Trend in Cesarean Births: A Survey.* 5th annual scientific conference of Joint Symposium on Recent Advances in MTP, Delhi

William, J. W. (1979). Puerperal infection. In 16th edn. *Pnstetrocs*, p. 893. (New York: Pritchard MacDonald)

7
Autoimmune deficiency syndrome

M. D. BENSON, E. R. CASAS and M. W. METHOD

The public awareness of AIDS far exceeds present scientific understanding of this illness. Indeed, the layman's fear of this condition is far out of proportion to its incidence. For example, hospitalized patients repeatedly express their concerns about receiving blood transfusions as this therapy has been associated with transmission of AIDS. In contrast, the issue of hepatitis is rarely mentioned, although it is a much greater risk following blood transfusion than AIDS in terms of total morbidity and mortality. The attitude of the general public and, for that matter, the medical profession, stems from the mystery shrouding the manner of transmitting AIDS, the slow lingering death that often accompanies it, and medical science's present inability to explain or consistently provide a cure for this condition.

AIDS is an acronym for 'acquired immunodeficiency syndrome' – a descriptive title of an illness in which each word bears examination. The term 'acquired' separates AIDS from a variety of congenital immunodeficiency syndromes that are frequently genetically transmitted and are quite rare. The term 'immunodeficiency' suggests a fundamental derangment of the body's immune system and its ability to resist proliferation of common environmental microbes and even tumors. Finally, the term 'syndrome' refers to a variety of clinical presentations and pathologic conditions that may not at first glance appear to be related. These include systemic candidiasis, *Pneumocystis carinii* pneumonia, and Kaposi's sarcoma. All are different illnesses with different manifestations and etiologic agents but they share a single common factor – the impairment of the host's defenses. The history of AIDS, its epidemiology, and its clinical presentation will be reviewed in this chapter.

HISTORY

On 3 July 1981, the Centers for Disease Control reported in *Morbidity and Mortality Weekly Report* the clustering in California and New York during the previous 30 months of 26 homosexual men with the diagnosis of Kaposi's sarcoma (CDC, 1981). Eight of these patients died although Kaposi's sarcoma is usually an indolent cancer. The significance of this report was underscored by the past; only three cases were reported at the New York University Hospital during a 20-year period and no cases were treated at Bellvue during a recent 10-year period. Coexisting opportunistic infections were observed in the patients reported by the CDC as well. While initially only observed in homosexual adult males, the syndrome later was identified in drug abusers, Haitian refugees, hemophiliacs, and to a far lesser extent, women and infants. By December of 1983, 3000 cases of AIDS had been reported in 42 states and a variety of foreign countries (Gore and Machol, 1984).

The CDC defines AIDS as 'a disease, at least moderately predictive of a defect in cell-mediated immunity, occurring in a person with no known cause for diminished resistance to that disease'. Specifically the CDC states that:

> These infections include pneumonia, meningitis, or encephalitis due to one or more of the following; aspergillosis, candidiasis, cryptococcosis, cytomegalovirus, nocardiosis, strongyloidosis, toxoplasmosis, zygomycosis, or atypical mycobacteriosis; esophagitis due to candidiasis, cytomegalovirus, or herpes simplex virus; progressive multifocal leukoencephalopathy; chronic enterocolitis (more than four weeks) due to cryptosporidiosis; or unusually extensive mucocutaneous herpes simplex of more than five weeks duration (CDC, 1982a).

It has been suggested that only 10% of AIDS victims have been reported, since the CDC definition may omit patients with the early and chronic, low-grade forms of the syndrome (Gore and Machol, 1984).

EPIDEMIOLOGY

The epidemiological investigations of AIDS have provided most of the information available about this illness and, indeed, first made doctors aware that the increased incidence of rare illnesses within segments of the population was a new phenomenon. The individuals in the largest group afflicted by AIDS are homosexual men, comprising approximately 70% of all reported cases (CDC, 1983a). A study of 20 homosexual men with AIDS and 40 controls suggested that exposure to amyl nitrate, sexual promiscuity, and history of mononucleosis or sexually transmitted disease were all correlated with increased risk (Marmor et al., 1982). While increasing risk associated with promiscuity is generally accepted, the role of inhaled nitrates, widely used by homosexuals as sexual stimulants, is much less clear. Inhaled nitrates have been suggested to be mutagenic or immunosuppressive, but the data are not convincing (Jorgenson and Lawesson, 1982; Goedert et al., 1982). In one report, 87% of homosexual men were noted to have used nitrate inhalants versus 15% for heterosexual men within the previous 5 years (CDC, 1982b); however, the report also noted that its use was closely correlated with the number of sexual partners reported during the previous month, thus confounding the issue. The observation that AIDS seems to be sexually transmitted among homosexuals has led the CDC to issue warnings that the risk of acquiring AIDS is correlated with the number of sexual partners among homosexuals.

Those in the second major population at high risk for AIDS are the intravenous drug abusers. Twelve percent of AIDS victims are heterosexual males, the majority (63%) of whom have a history of i.v. drug abuse (CDC, 1982c). The high proportion of drug abusers in this group suggests that this may be a separate risk factor for acquiring AIDS.

Another group at increased risk of contracting AIDS comprises Haitian refugees. In July of 1982, the CDC reported 34 Haitians with AIDS (CDC, 1982d). By September 1982, Haitians accounted for 6% of all cases and 50% of cases in which homosexuality and i.v. drug abuse were denied (CDC, 1982a). The increased risk for AIDS among Haitians is even less well understood than for homosexual men and i.v. drug abusers in whom an obvious means of infection could be postulated.

Hemophiliacs also appear to have a high risk of contracting AIDS. While they account for only 0.3% of reported cases, their risk of contracting AIDS may force a change in the way they are treated for their hemophilia (CDC, 1982a). Currently, the 20,000 hemophiliacs in the US can treat themselves at home with Factor VIII concentrate, prepared from a pool of 200 to 1000 donors. This concentrate is easier to handle and more reliable in terms of dosage than its alternative, Factor VIII cryoprecipitate, which is prepared from one donor at a time. Some authorities have suggested returning to the use of cryoprecipitate if the concentrate increases the risk for AIDS transmission to hemophiliacs as is suspected by some (Desforges, 1982; CDC, 1982c). The fact that this blood product is a possible vector for the AIDS agent bolsters the notion that AIDS may be spread through contaminated blood.

While the press has given much attention to these specific four groups presently recognized to be at high risk for AIDS, two other groups of people may be afflicted – women and children. By December 1983, women comprised 7% of the 3000 AIDS cases reported to the CDC. While some of these women were prostitutes or i.v. drug abusers, many others were the monogamous sexual partners of men afflicted with AIDS or with subclinical immune deficiencies demonstrated by T-cell deficiencies on testing (Harris et al., 1983; CDC, 1983b). This finding provides further evidence for sexual transmission of the AIDS agent. A more controversial and potentially significant finding, however, is the description of AIDS in neonates and infants. The development of AIDS in children suggests alternative routes of transmission other than through sexual contact or contaminated blood. A report that appeared in J. Am. Med. Assoc., May 1983, described eight children from New Jersey who appeared to develop AIDS. Each of these children was in contact with a household member at high risk of contracting AIDS but not necessarily exhibiting the syndrome. The authors of this report suggest that normal hosts may develop AIDS and that the condition may be transmitted through ordinary household contact (Oleske et al., 1983). Another group of investigators reported an AIDS-like syndrome in seven children in the New York area. Symptoms and laboratory findings were similar to the adult syndrome. Six of the seven children were small for gestational age at birth, and they all subsequently demonstrated failure to thrive, lymphadenopathy, hepatosplenomegaly, and recurrent infections. The small size at birth of these infants and their poor course early in infancy suggested that AIDS may be transmitted *in utero* (Rubinstein *et al.*, 1983).

Finally, there are instances of AIDS transmission which seem to implicate blood transfusions or products. An infant in San Francisco who received a variety of blood products at birth for erythroblastosis fetalis developed evidence of immunodeficiency at 7 months with persistent oral candidiasis; subsequently, neutropenia and a variety of opportunistic infections developed (Amman *et al.*, 1983). One of the 19 blood donors to this infant subsequently developed AIDS and died. This account, together with the experiences of hemophiliacs and i.v. drug abusers, strongly suggests that AIDS can be transmitted through blood products.

There is no evidence of transmission through casual contact with affected individuals or by airborne spread, and there are no cases of AIDS among health-care workers that can definitely be ascribed to specific occupational exposures. The risk of AIDS transmission to health-care workers through percutaneous or mucosal inoculation of blood or body fluids from AIDS patients remains undefined, although currently available epidemiologic data suggest that the risk of transmission, if any, is small (MMWR, 1984).

CLINICAL PRESENTATION AND COURSE OF ILLNESS

How do patients with AIDS present? In one study of 14 of the sufferers, all had fever and either oral or esophageal candidiasis. Ninety-three percent also exhibited weight loss, and the majority had malaise and a cough. Fifty percent had lymphadenopathy. The average duration of symptoms was 9.5 months before medical help was sought. Basic laboratory findings included the averages

Table 1

	AIDS values	*Normal values*
HB	11.2	mean = 16
WBC	5.9	7.8±3.0
ESR	96+	less than 20
Lymphocytes	984	nl = 1500+
Albumin	3.2	more than 3.5
IgG, IgA	both elevated	—

shown in Table 1. All of the patients had decreased lymphocyte counts, increased sedimentation rates and increased serum IgG. In this particular study, seven of the 14 men went on to develop *Pneumocystis carinii* pneumonia, and one man developed disseminated mycobacterium intracellular infection, histoplasmosis, cryptococcosis, and cytomegalovirus infection. Twelve of the 14 patients had evidence of an associated viral infection as well, including Epstein–Barr virus (in nine), cytomegalovirus (in five), and herpes simplex type 2 (in two). At the time this report was prepared in March 1983, five of the 14 men had died from their illness (Small *et al.*, 1983)

This investigation corresponds well with other accounts of AIDS except for the conspicuous lack of Kaposi's sarcoma. By mid-1983, approximately 50% of AIDS patients had *Pneumocystis carinii* pneumonia, 25% had Kaposi's sarcoma and 8% had both. Only 15% did not have either disease but presented with another opportunistic infection as the primary diagnosis (CDC, 1983a). The overall mortality rate was 39%. Among those with Kaposi's sarcoma, 20% had died by the time of the report while the corresponding mortality rate for opportunistic infections was 50%. It should be noted that these death rates should not be considered complete as many of the patients are still ill and a variable time elapses from diagnosis to death.

Although the literature has focused on those patients meeting the CDC's criterion of a severe unexpected opportunistic infection in an individual without known predisposing factors, it also makes oblique references to those individuals with 'prodromal' AIDS – patients with weight loss, lymphadenopathy and lab. values suggesting immune depression but without florid opportunistic infections. As this group is not critically ill and their clinical presentation is highly variable it is difficult to discuss these prodromal cases. Very little is known about their long-term risk for acquiring the full-blown AIDS picture. It is also not known if there is a 'carrier' state or even a chronic, mild form of AIDS.

Pneumocystis carinii pneumonia, the chief killer in AIDS, was virtually unheard of in previously healthy young adults prior to 1981. It was first reported in the United States in 1955 as a parasitic infection resulting in an interstitial plasma cell pneumonia. Prior to 1981, the disease had been reported in three groups of individuals (Follansbee *et al.*, 1982). The most common form is a self-limited, clinically silent infection in children, which is accompanied by IgG seroconversion in 90% of cases.

The condition can also occur as a diffuse, fatal pneumonitis in malnourished infants. Finally, *P. carinii* occurred in adults, but only with immunosuppressive therapy, advanced malignancies or other serious underlying disorders. With the outbreak of AIDS however, the disease is now seen in previously healthy adults and is associated with a 50% mortality rate. In a study of 12 men who ultimately had *P. carinii* pneumonia, all had coughs, progressive shortness of breath, and dyspnea on exertion for 2–4 weeks prior to their admission to hospital (Gamsu *et al.*, 1982). Most of the patients also had a 1–7-month history of malaise, weight loss, diarrhea, fever, rash, joint pain, abdominal pain, and lymphadenopathy. All the men in this study were homosexuals, and they also had a history of prior infections including CMV, syphilis, gonorrhea, amebiasis, giardiasis, hepatitis, and herpes. On examination, the group had fever, increased respiratory rate, and most patients had rales. 'Cotton wool' exudates were frequently noted. Consistently abnormal studies included arterial blood gases with low Po_2 and a low Pco_2 (attributed to hyperventilation). PFTs revealed restrictive lung disease. Ten of the 12 patients had abnormal chest X-rays, although two of these were minimal change. The abnormal patterns include a diffuse, coarse ground-glass pattern or lymphadenopathy. The diagnosis in each case was made by methenamine silver stain of tissue obtained by transbronchial or open lung biopsy. Cytomegalovirus also was cultured from most of the lung specimens. All of the patients were initially treated with intravenous trimethoprim-sulfamethoxazole. If improvement occurred, the antibiotics were continued for 2–6 weeks. If no change occurred after 3–5 days, therapy was changed to intramuscular pentamidine (distributed solely by the CDC). Six of the patients in this study had progressive disease despite treatment and died from respiratory failure – in close agreement with national mortality statistics of 50%. Significantly, many of the patients experienced relapses after initial improvement.

The most common illness in AIDS after *P. carinii* pneumonia is Kaposi's sarcoma (KS), occurring in 25% of patients alone and in an additional 8% with *P. carinii* pneumonia. This cancer is a malignant vascular skin tumor that first appears as reddish-purple-to-dark-blue cutaneous lesions on the lower extremities. Prior to the outbreak of AIDS, KS was known to occur in three groups of individuals (Taff *et al.*, 1982). The first group is made up of elderly white males of either Jewish or Italian origin. In this population the tumor is not only extremely rare (0.021/100,000) but is indolent, with a mean survival of 8–13 years. Death usually results from a second malignancy, typically a lymphoreticular neoplasm, or from other diseases of the aged. KS is also common among a second group of people – central African blacks; it accounts for 9% of all malignancies in Uganda. Four types are seen; nodular, florid, infiltrative, and lympadenopathic (the most aggressive). Finally, the third group, renal transplant recipients on immunosuppressive therapy are also at high risk for this tumor.

KS in AIDS victims closely resembles the most aggressive African type. In one study of 19 homosexual KS patients, the mean duration of symptoms was 6 months and most of the patients had a fever for more than 3 weeks (Friedman-Kien *et al.*, 1982). Fifteen of the 19 patients had skin lesions widely distributed over the body; one patient had a single lesion on his forearm, and three patients had generalized lympadenopathy without skin lesions. In more than half of these patients, gastrointestinal lesions were ultimately found by endoscopy including three patients with oral lesions. Death from KS in AIDS victims occurs from visceral involvement and, according to previously noted CDC figures, runs approximately at 20%. Vinblastine, doxorubicin, and bleomycin have been used for chemotherapy, although the number of cases is too small to determine the most effective regimen.

SCIENTIFIC INVESTIGATION OF AIDS

An infectious agent has been postulated for AIDS, but the nature of this agent and its mechanism for causing the observed changes in AIDS victims is entirely unknown. Research into AIDS currently consists of collecting more observations in terms of etiology and clinical course. Investigators are also looking into host immune status and modifications that result from AIDS, the genetic make-up of AIDS victims, the possible role of specific viruses as infectious agents, and animal models for the syndrome.

The pattern of opportunistic infections in AIDS patients suggests a defect in the cell-mediated immune response. In most studies, AIDS patients are anergic;

that is, they fail to react to common antigens injected subcutaneously, a finding consistent with T-lymphocyte deficiencies. Homosexuals with KS had a ratio of T 'helper' cells to T 'suppressor' cells of 0.5, whereas healthy heterosexuals had a ratio of 1.75 (Stahl *et al.*, 1982). This finding may be significant, as T 'suppressor' cells are thought to block the immune response to foreign antigens while the 'helper' cells aid the response. Significantly, healthy homosexuals also had a decreased ratio of helper to suppressor cells (though not as low as in AIDS patients), and heterosexuals with KS had normal ratios (Stahl *et al.*, 1982).

Findings such as these bolster the notion that the homosexual lifestyle and repeated exposure to infectious agents may somehow alter the immune system, with the extreme alterations leading to AIDS. The previously cited study showed decreased T-lymphocyte proliferation in response to mitogens (growth factors); which also suggests a derangement among T-cells as a basic mechanism in the development of AIDS. Another study performed a functional assay on suppressor activity in 21 homosexual patients with the prodromal symptoms of AIDS (Hersh *et al.* 1983). As expected, the ability of these patients' lymphocytes to prevent normal lymphocytes from proliferating in response to mitogens was abnormally high and correlated well with the AIDS patients' decreased helper/suppressor cell ratio. Increased suppressor T-cell activity has been theoretically and experimentally linked with accelerated tumor growth in the general population. It should be noted that the T-cell impairment does not extend to B-cells since, as observed earlier, elevated levels of immunoglobulins (secreted by B-cells) have been widely reported in AIDS victims. Cytomegalovirus, epidemic among homosexuals, has been associated with lymphocyte suppression, but proof of a cause and effect relation in AIDS is lacking (Drew *et al.*, 1981, 1982). The causes for the increased activity of T-suppressor cells and the B-cells are still poorly understood.

A genetic predisposition to KS among AIDS patients has been suggested by a study in which HLA typing of patients with AIDS KS and classic KS revealed an equal 63% incidence of HLA allele DR5 (one of a group of specific cell surface proteins allowing the body to identify self from non-self (Friedman-Kien, 1982). This represented a 5.5 times increased incidence of this allele in those with KS over the general population, and suggests a genetic susceptibility to this malignancy.

The considerable expansion of evidence for the oncogene theory (that viral infections can transform normal cells into neoplastic ones) has carried over to the research on AIDS. A new retrovirus belonging to the human T-cell leukemia virus family has been isolated from a homosexual male with the prodromal symptoms of AIDS (Gallo *et al.*, 1983). Researchers found elevated levels of circulating antibodies to this virus as well. They concluded that this viral infection of T-cells may somehow impair the patient's response to repeated infections and thus lead to the immune deficiencies that seem to result in AIDS.

Finally, an AIDS-like syndrome has been noted in monkeys in two separate colonies – one in Boston and one on the West Coast. The symptoms of these monkeys, their laboratory findings, the presence of overwhelming opportunistic infections and death rate in the apparently infected colonies were remarkably similar to those same characteristics associated with human AIDS (Macek,

1983; Herrickson *et al.*, 1983; Letvin *et al.*, 1983). Significant differences from human AIDS include the facts that most of the animals were afflicted before reaching sexual maturity and an equal incidence was observed among sexes. Researchers have suggested using these monkey colonies as animal models for AIDS.

CONCLUSION

AIDS, 'acquired immunodeficiency syndrome', is a disease state characterized by the development of a severe opportunistic infection or Kaposi's sarcoma (KS) in an individual who has no obvious predisposing risk factor such as prior malignancy or medical treatment for severe, debilitating illness. Homosexuals and intravenous drug abusers are at particularly high risk to contract AIDS. Other high-risk groups include Haitian refugees, hemophiliacs, prostitutes, and female sexual partners of AIDS victims. The syndrome has also been reported in children with exposure to household members belonging to one of the 'high-risk' groups. The clinical syndrome consists of weight loss, malaise, and lymphadenopathy associated with lab. values indicative of an impaired immune system followed by the onset of a severe opportunistic infection or KS. The development of *P. carinii* pneumonia is the single event associated with the highest mortality rate, approaching 50%. The identification of an infectious agent, the precise route of transmission, and the possibility of carrier, or mild chronic, states are all pressing issues currently being investigated.

ACKNOWLEDGMENT

We wish to acknowledge review of this manuscript by Professor L. G. Keith of the Department of Obstetrics and Gynecology, Northwestern University Medical School.

References

Ammann, A. J., Wara, D. W., Dritz, S. *et al.* (1983). Acquired immunodeficiency in an infant: Possible transmission by means of blood products. *Lancet*, 956

Centers for Disease Control (1981). Kaposi's sarcoma and pneumocystis pneumonia among homosexual men – New York City and California. *Morb. Mort. Wkly. Rep.*, **30**, 305

Centers for Disease Control (1982a). Update on acquired immune deficiency syndrome (AIDS) – United States. *Morb. Mort. Wkly. Rep.*, **31**, 507

Centers for Disease Control (1982b). Epidemiologic aspects of the current outbreak of Kaposi's sarcoma and opportunistic infections. Report of the CDC, Task Force on Kaposi's sarcoma and opportunistic infections. *N. Engl. J. Med.*, 248

Centers for Disease Control (1982c). Update on Kaposi's sarcoma and opportunistic infections in previously health persons – United States. *Morb. Mort. Wkly. Rep.*, **31**, 294

Centers for Disease Control (1982d). Opportunistic infections and Kaposi's sarcoma among Haitians in the United States. *Morb. Mort. Wkly. Rep.*, **31**, 353

Centers for Disease Control (1982e). *Pneumocystis carinii* pneumonia among persons with hemophilia A. *Morb. Mort. Wkly. Rep.*, **31**, 365

Centers for Disease Control (1983a). Acquired immunodeficiency syndrome (AIDS) update – United States. *Morb. Mort. Wkly. Rep.*, **32**, 309

Centers for Disease Control (1983b). Immunodeficiency among female sexual partners of males with acquired immune deficiency syndrome (AIDS) – New York. *Morb. Mort. Wkly. Rep.*, **31**, 697

Desforges, J. F. (1982). AIDS and preventive treatment in hemophilia. *N. Engl. J. Med..*, **308**, 94

Drew, W. L., Lintz, L., Miner, R. C. *et al.* (1981). Prevalence of cytomegalovirus infection in homosexual men. *J. Infect. Dis.*, **143**, 188

Drew, W. L., Miner, R. C. and Ziegler, J. L. *et al.* (1982). Cytomegalovirus and Kaposi's sarcoma in young homosexual men. *Lancet*, **2**, 125

Follansbee, S. E., Busch, D. F. and Wofsy, C. B. *et al.* (1982). An outbreak of *Pneumocystis carinii* pneumonia in homosexual men. *Ann. Intern. Med.*, **96**, 705

Friedman-Kien, A. E., Laubenstein, L. J., Rubinstein, P. *et al.* (1982). Disseminated Kaposi's sarcoma in homosexual men. *Ann. Intern. Med.*, **96**, 693

Gallo, R. C., Sarin, P. S. and Gelmann, E. P. *et al.* (1983). Isolation of a T-lymphotropic retrovirus from a patient at risk for acquired immune deficiency syndrome (AIDS). *Science*, **220**, 868

Gamsu, G., Hecht, S. T., Birnberg, F. A. *et al.* (1982). *Pneumocystis carinii* pneumonia in homosexual men. *AJR*, **139**, 647

Goedert, J., Wallen, W. C., Mann, D. L. *et al.* (1982). Amyl nitrite may alter T lymphocytes in homosexual men. *Lancet*, **1**, 412

Gore, M. J. and Machol, L. (1984). Can AIDS be a threat to your patients? *Contemp. Obstet. Gynecol.*, **23**, 163

Harris, C., Small, C. B., Klein, R. S. *et al.* (1983). Immunodeficiency in female sexual partners of men with the acquired immunodeficiency syndrome. *N. Engl. J. Med.*, **308**, 1181

Henrickson, R. V., Osborn, K. G., Madden D. L. *et al.* (1983). Epidemic of acquired immunodeficiency in Rhesus monkeys. *Lancet*, **1**, 388

Hersh, E. M., Mansell, P. W. A., Reuben, J. M. *et al.* (1983). Suppressor cell activity among the peripheral blood leukocytes of selected homosexual subjects. *Cancer Res.*, **43**, 1905

Jorgenson, K. A. and Lawesson, S-O. (1982). Amyl nitrite and Kaposi's sarcoma in homosexual men. *N. Engl. J. Med.*, **307**, 893

Letvin, N. L., Eaton, K. A. and Aldrich, W. R. *et al.* (1983). Acquired immunodeficiency syndrome in a colony of Macaque monkeys. *Proc. Nat. Acad. Sci., USA*, **80**, 2718

Macek, C. (1983). Do these primates have AIDS? *J. Am. Med. Assoc.*, **249**, 1696

Marmor, M., Laubenstein, L., William, D. C. *et al.* (1982). Risk factors for Kaposi's sarcoma in homosexual men. *Lancet*, **1**, 1083

MMWR, leads from (1984). Prospective evaluation of health-care workers exposed via parenteral or mucous membrane routes to blood and body fluids of patients with AIDS. *J. Am. Med. Assoc.*, **251**, 2071

Oleske, J., Minnefor, An., Cooper, R. *et al.* (1983). Immune deficiency syndrome in children. *J. Am. Med. Assoc.*, **249**, 2345.

Rubinstein, A., Sicklick, M., Gupta, A. *et al.* (1983). Acquired immunodeficiency with reversed T_4T_8 ratios in infants born to promiscuous and drug-addicted mothers. *J. Am. Med. Assoc.*, **249**, 2350.

Small, C. B., Klein, R. S., Friedland, H. H. *et al.* (1983). Community-acquired opportunistic infections and defective cellular immunity in heterosexual drug abusers and homosexual men. *Am. J. Med.*, **74**, 433

Stahl, R. E., Friedman-Kien, A., Dubin, R. *et al.* (1982). Immunologic abnormalities in homosexual men. *Am. J. Med.*, **73**, 171.

Taff, M. L., Siegal, F. P. and Geller, S. A. (1982). Outbreak of an acquired immunodeficiency syndrome associated with opportunistic infections and Kaposi's sarcoma in male homosexuals. *Am J. Forensic Med. Pathol.*, **3**, 259

8
Sexually transmitted diseases in prepubertal boys

P. J. RETTIG

INTRODUCTION

During the past two decades, belated and inadequate attention has been given to the incidence and presentations of STDs in children (Bell, 1983). The two classic major venereal diseases, gonorrhea and syphilis, have in fact been diagnosed with increasing frequency among children, paralleling the trends

Table 1 Sexually transmitted and transmissible pathogens

Neisseria gonorrhoeae[a]	Herpes simplex virus (HSV)[a]
Chlamydia trachomatis[a]	Cytomegalovirus
Oculogenital strains	Hepatitis A virus
LGV strains	Hepatitis B virus
Genital mycoplasmas	Human papillomavirus (HPV)[a]
Mycoplasma hominis	Virus of molluscum contagiosum
Ureaplasma urealyticum	*Candida albicans*
Treponema pallidum[a]	*Trichomonas vaginalis*
Gardnerella vaginalis	*Phthirus pubis* (pubic louse)
Haemophilus ducreyi	*Sarcoptes scabiei* (scabies mite)
Calymmatobacterium granulomatis	
Enteropathogens	
Salmonella species	
Shigella species	
Campylobacter jejuni	
Entamoeba histolytica	
Giardia lamblia	

[a] Pathogens for which venereal transmission in childhood is documented

observed in adults. Moreover, a number of the 'new' STDs, particularly those for which the major or only mode of transmission is venereal, have also been recognized in prepubertal children (Table 1). Other infections on the list are best considered sexually transmissible, rather than transmitted, in the context of childhood infection. These include the variety of enteric infections commonly associated with 'the gay bowel syndrome', hepatitis A and B, and cutaneous infestations and infections such as scabies and molluscum contagiosum. All of these diseases occur commonly in children, but they are contracted most frequently through traditional, nonsexual modes of transmission.

This chapter will review the epidemiology, clinical manifestations, differential diagnosis, and therapy of sexually transmitted infections in prepubertal boys. The epidemiology and clinical pictures of STDs in sexually active adolescents are essentially identical to those in adults. Congenital and perinatal infections with these organisms and STDs in prepubertal girls are covered in chapter 9 in this volume.

GENERAL CONSIDERATIONS OF STDs IN PREPUBERTAL BOYS

Clinicians who treat male children presenting with a penile discharge are frequently unwilling to consider a diagnosis of gonorrhea or another STD. When the diagnosis has been established, however, the physician often remains reluctant to acknowledge that the infection may have been acquired venereally. This reluctance may account in part for the lower reported incidences of these infections in prepubertal boys. Clearly, once the diagnosis has been made, epidemiologic, anatomical, and physiologic evidence unique to the male all suggest that transmission is almost certainly via sexual contact.

In the prepubertal male the testes, prostate, and ejaculatory ducts are infantile, but these tissues lack specific anatomical or physiologic characteristics that would predispose the child to nonvenereal acquisition of infection with the gonococcus or other mucosal pathogens. Although Beilin (1931) has hypothesized that 'younger children are more susceptible to gonorrheal urethritis, perhaps due to the greater vulnerability of their urethral mucosae', there is no physiologic basis for this statement. Moreover, there is no evidence that the relatively protected prepubertal penile urethra is infected other than by direct contact with other infected mucosal surfaces.

The diagnosis in a prepubertal boy, of a disease that has almost certainly been transmitted sexually necessitates a thorough investigation into the mode of sexual exposure. Although heterosexual or homosexual exploratory behavior with peers may have occurred, the clinician has a clear responsibility to rule out sexual abuse by an older adolescent or adult. Evidence or suspicion of the latter requires that the appropriate child welfare authorities be notified.

GONORRHEA IN PREPUBERTAL BOYS

Epidemiology

The incidence of reported gonorrhea in children under age 10 increased from 1632 cases in 1960 to 3084 cases in 1979. The age-specific rates increased from

4.2/100 000 to 9.6/100 000 (Centers for Disease Control (CDC), 1981). During the same two decades the incidence of gonorrhea in 10–14-year-old adolescents increased 262%, to 50.4 cases per 100 000 in 1979. The female-to-male ratio of nationally reported cases in children less than 10 years of age in 1979 was 2.46 to 1. A review (Rettig, unpublished data, 1983) of 553 cases of childhood gonorrhea reported in the English literature from 1965 to 1983 revealed a female-to-male ratio of 4.7 to 1. This review comprised 21 reports of prepubertal gonorrhea in 553 patients of both sexes. All patients were less than 10 years of age or, if older, specifically defined as prepubertal. The reason for the discrepancy between the female-to-male ratios in these two databases is unclear, although it is probably due to reporting biases in the published series. In this review, the average age of the 60 male patients whose age was noted was 7.6 years, compared to 5.2 years for 222 female subjects. In most series the average age of male subjects has been 2 to 3 years greater than that of females.

The mode of transmission of prepubertal gonorrhea is controversial. Reports from the preantibiotic era commonly postulated that gonococcal infection, particularly vulvovaginitis, was transmitted by close nonsexual personal contact, by direct or manual contact with infected secretions or by infected fomites. Although gonococci in urethral secretions artificially implanted on fomites may remain viable for 2–3 hours (Gilbaugh and Fuchs, 1979), the role of contaminated toilet seats, toilet paper, or bedclothes in transmission remains unproven and highly unlikely.

A report of prepubertal gonorrhea in an Eskimo population (Shore and Winkelstein, 1971) has been widely cited in support of a theory of nonvenereal transmission. Seven children, aged 1–11 years, had 'indirect contact', consisting of sleeping with parent(s) who had concurrent or recent genital gonorrhea. Although it is theoretically possible that crowded sleeping arrangements and poor hygiene *may* permit nonvenereal infection of conjunctival or vulvar mucosa, this is a rare occurrence. In this study, each of three boys had acquired gonococcal urethritis through an 'unknown' mode of transmission.

Beilin (1931) spoke forcefully to this point over 50 years ago:

> While it is possible that a male child, sleeping with an actively infected mother or other person, may come in intimate contact with the discharge sufficiently soon to permit the transmission of infection, we believe this is a relatively infrequent occurrence. A careful inquiry into the prevailing social and environmental conditions will lead one to the conclusions that in young boys and often in girls a usual mode of infection is *per vias naturales*.

Recent comprehensive social and microbiologic investigations support this conclusion (Table 2; Branch and Paxton, 1965; Folland *et al.*, 1977; Sgroi, 1979; Meek *et al.*, 1979; Farrell *et al.*, 1981). Multiple family members (siblings and parents) are often found to have positive cultures for the gonococcus. Sexual contacts may be siblings or similarly aged playmates with whom the child participates in sex play and exploration. More commonly, however, the contact is with older family members or acquaintances, usually male, who have sexually abused the child. Comprehensive culturing of all household members will sometimes reveal asymptomatically infected siblings and adults (Folland *et al.*, 1977; Sgroi, 1979; Farrell *et al.*, 1981; Patamasucon *et al.*, 1981). These

Table 2 The role of sexual contact in the transmission of childhood gonorrhea

Study	Number of patients	Age range (years)	Number of patients with sexual contact		Number of contacts with gonorrheal/ Total number of contacts cultured	
Beilin (1931)	91	1–13	40	(44%)	Not done	
Branch and Paxton	45	1–9	42	(93%)	Not done	
(1965)	116	10–14	115	(99%)		
Folland et al. (1977)	53	1–9	18	(34%)	54/203	(27%)
Sgroi (1979)	15	4–12	8	(53%)	18/69	(26%)
Meek et al. (1979)	45	1–9	17	(38%)	13/45	(29%)
Farrell et al. (1981)	46	1–11	29	(63%)	28/83	(34%)

studies indicate that the usual mode of transmission of prepubertal gonorrhea is sexual.

Clinical characteristics

Gonorrhea in the prepubertal male most often manifests itself as a purulent urethral discharge. A yellow-green stain on the child's underpants may bring the condition to the mother's attention. The majority of boys experience dysuria and gross hematuria may occur (Beilin, 1931; Nelson et al., 1976; Rettig et al., 1980). Occasionally, a thin, watery urethral discharge is seen; asymptomatic urethral carriers may be detected among contacts who are screened microbiologically (Patamasucon et al., 1981). Balanitis and penile edema occur infrequently (Rettig et al., 1980; Patamasucon et al., 1981). Local complications such as epididymitis and periurethral abscess, previously reported by Beilin (1931), have been encountered only rarely in the antibiotic era. There are no contemporary reports of postgonococcal urethral stricture in boys.

Extragenital infection may be symptomatic or asymptomatic. Anal infection in girls may be due to 'spillover' of a contaminated vaginal discharge; in boys, however, this condition implies the direct inoculation of infected secretions, most likely via attempts at anal intercourse. Symptomatic proctitis has been described (Beilin, 1931), and asymptomatic anal carriers have been documented (Nelson et al., 1976). Anorectal infection appears to be less common in boys than in girls. Pharyngeal infection in the child may be due to autoinoculation of infected genital secretions but is more likely due to direct inoculation of organisms via fellatio. Although pharyngeal infection may be acutely symptomatic and produce tonsillopharyngitis (Wiesner et al., 1973), it is more commonly asymptomatic and may be found in as many as 18% of children with genital infection (Nelson et al., 1976; Silber and Controni, 1981; Groothuis et al., 1983). Any child in whom genital tract infection with Neisseria gonorrhoeae is documented should also have cultures of the oral and pharyngeal cavities performed on selective media.

Conjunctivitis due to N. gonorrhoeae has been reported in children beyond the neonatal period. The infection characteristically appears as an acute inflammatory process with intense conjunctivitis, marked chemosis, and large amounts of thick yellow or green purulent discharge. The eye may become infected by direct or indirect contact with the patient's or the index case's genital secretions. Three of six native Alaskan boys reported by Shore and Winkelstein (1971) had gonococcal conjunctivitis. Prompt antibiotic therapy is necessary to prevent the development of keratitis and subsequent perforation of the anterior chamber and endophthalmitis.

Gonococcal arthritis in childhood has been reported most frequently in young infants as a sequela of perinatal acquisition. The condition may also occur in older prepubertal children and has often been polyarticular (Fink, 1965). The arthritis–dermatitis syndrome or disseminated gonococcal infection syndrome is much more common in females and is very rare in children. This syndrome should be considered in the child who has migratory polyarthralgias and who displays characteristic distal skin lesions that progress from papular to pustular to necrotic stages.

Differential diagnosis

The differential diagnosis of a purulent urethral discharge in a prepubertal male is limited. *Chlamydia trachomatis* may cause a postgonococcal urethritis in boys (Rettig and Nelson, 1981). Poor hygiene and pyogenic infection under the foreskin may produce a purulent balanitis. Dysuria without frank urethral discharge occurs but is a poorly studied entity in boys (Williams and Mikhael, 1971). Cystitis (bacterial or viral), upper urinary tract infection, meatitis due to chemical or mechanical irritants, and urethral irritation due to external manipulation or to internal instrumentation (either iatrogenic or masturbatory) should be considered.

Diagnosis

The presence of intracellular Gram-negative diplococci in a urethral discharge is strong presumptive evidence of gonorrhea. Because of the psychosocial and medicolegal problems associated with this diagnosis, however, specimens from prepubertal children should be cultured to confirm the presence of *N. gonorrhoeae*. Anorectal and pharyngeal cultures should be obtained from all boys with urethral or extragenital infection. Pharyngeal and conjunctival isolates must be differentiated from *N. meningitidis* by carbohydrate fermentation or immunofluorescence.

Therapy

Recommended therapy for prepubertal gonococcal urethritis is outlined in Table 3 (Nelson *et al.*, 1976; Rettig *et al.*, 1980; Patamasucon *et al.*, 1981; Washington, 1982; CDC, 1982a). The oral route is preferable for young children, because it avoids the pain and fear associated with an injection, which would be an additional trauma to an already abused child. Complicated, extragenital infection should be treated as outlined for adults in the 1982 CDC

Table 3 Therapy of gonococcal infection in prepubertal children

Indication	Drug	Dosage	Maximum dose
Uncomplicated genital infection	(1) Amoxicillin + Probenicid *or*	50 mg/kg p.o. 25 mg/kg p.o.	3.0 g 1.0 g
	(2) Aqueous procaine penicillin G + probenicid	100 000 u/kg i.m. 25 mg/kg p.o.	4.8 million units 1.0 g
Penicillin allergy	Spectinomycin	40 mg/kg i.m.	2.0 g
Penicillinase-producing *N. gonorrhoeae* (PPNG)	(1) Spectinomycin *or*	40 mg/kg i.m.	2.0 g
	(2) Cefoxitin[a]+ probenicid *or*	40 mg/kg i.m. 25 mg/kg p.o.	2.0 g 1.0 g
	(3) Cefotaxime[a] *or*	25 mg/kg i.m.	1.0 g
	(4) Cefuroxime[b]	25 mg/kg i.m.	1.5 g

[a] Licensed in US but not evaluated in children as of June 1983
[b] Evaluated in children, but US licensure pending as of June 1983

recommendations, using scaled-down dosage schedules. In adults, amoxicillin has been less effective than procaine penicillin in treating anorectal infection (Washington, 1982), but in one study the oral regimen was effective in all children receiving this treatment (Nelson *et al.*, 1976). Similarly, spectinomycin and the oral penicillin regimens have had high failure rates in treating pharyngeal gonorrhea in adults (Washington, 1982). Groothuis *et al.* (1983) reported failure of procaine penicillin in three of seven children treated for pharyngeal gonorrhea. Successful therapy of infection at this site may require repeated doses of penicillin. The potential role of third-generation cephalosporins in treating pharyngeal infection has not yet been adequately examined. Tetracycline (40 mg/kg daily p.o. for 5 days; 2 g/day maximum dose) may be used for penicillin-allergic patients who are more than 8 years of age, but it should not be used to treat PPNG strains.

Patients with gonococcal conjunctivitis should receive parenteral penicillin G (200 000 u/kg per day). Topical antibiotics are not necessary, but copious saline irrigation of the affected eye is indicated until the purulent drainage has abated. Open drainage of gonococcal arthritis is appropriate only for bacteriologically confirmed infection of the hip, and antibiotic irrigations should not be used.

Antimicrobial therapy is only the first step in treating prepubertal gonococcal infection. Social investigation and microbiologic screening of all family members and other identified contacts must also be performed. Reporting of the case to child welfare authorities is mandatory. In certain situations, such as criminal assault, notification of the police is also necessary. Brief hospitalization may impress the parents with the gravity of the situation and appears to aid in investigations of the social milieu (Farrell *et al.*, 1981).

CHLAMYDIAL GENITAL INFECTIONS IN PREPUBERTAL BOYS

Epidemiology

The mode of transmission of chlamydial infection in adults is believed to be almost exclusively venereal. In adults hand-to-eye transmission of infected genital or ocular secretions and infected fomites may cause conjunctivitis due to oculogenital strains. Close, nonsexual interpersonal contact among young children is the primary mode of transmission of trachoma. Postnatal infection of infant's conjunctivae and nasopharynx is due to natal acquisition of chlamydiae from an infected maternal cervix. Although experiments have not tested the ability of *C. trachomatis* to survive on inanimate objects, the fact that it is an obligate intracellular parasite makes it unlikely that infectious forms could survive on fomites for prolonged periods. The mechanism of transmission of chlamydiae probably involves direct mucosal–mucosal contact or indirect contamination of mucosal surfaces with infected secretions.

Clinical characteristics

Urethral infection with *C. trachomatis* has been reported in prepubertal boys coincident with and subsequent to gonococcal infection (Rettig *et al.*, 1980; Rettig and Nelson, 1981; Patamasucon *et al.*, 1981). Urethral infection may be symptomatic, with a prolonged watery discharge that is less purulent than the yellow–green discharge typical of gonorrhea. Asymptomatic urethral infection of boys has also been documented. In the Dallas studies, 5 of 20 boys infected with gonorrhea had genital or anal chlamydial infection, as did 9 of 31 girls. (In adults, 11 to 34% of men and 24 to 62% of women have had dual chlamydial–gonococcal anogenital infection.) Concurrent infection with two sexually transmitted microorganisms in these children strongly argues for a venereal mode of acquisition, although we could not document this in all cases.

We have also documented chlamydial anal infection in children (Rettig *et al.*, 1980; Rettig and Nelson, 1981; Patamasucon *et al.*, 1981). Both male and female children have had asymptomatic infection at this site. One 14-year-old boy, who had participated in passive anal intercourse, had rectal bleeding and a purulent anal exudate that was positive for *C. trachomatis* and negative for *N. gonorrhoeae*. Of 11 patients with anal chlamydia, only three had concurrent or previous anorectal gonorrhea. The rectal presence of *C. trachomatis* has been noted in infected women and infants, and most commonly occurs in adult homosexual males (Quinn *et al.*, 1981). Infection in the former category of patients has been asymptomatic, while infection with oculogenital strains in homosexuals has produced mild proctitis or has been asymptomatic.

Examination of 12 prepubertal boys with nongonococcal urethritis (NGU), which is defined as dysuria and pyuria without bacteriuria, revealed that none were infected with *C. trachomatis* (Rettig and Nelson, 1981). Other studies of nonspecific urethritis in children have not included cultures for chlamydia (Williams and Mikhael, 1971). Given the frequency of *C. trachomatis* in NGU in adults, it is likely that future investigations of large numbers of children with urethritis will detect some who are infected with this organism. The etiology of epididymitis in prepubertal children is similar to that in older adults. Either classical urinary tract pathogens or no specific etiology are more commonly discovered than are STD pathogens (Doolittle *et al.*, 1966; Gierup *et al.*, 1975; Hermansen *et al.*, 1980; Berger *et al.*, 1979). In young, sexually active adults, chlamydial and gonococcal infection occur most frequently, having been found in 16 and 7 of 34 patients examined, respectively (Berger *et al.*, 1979). This finding is in contrast to studies in children, in which the largest number of cases are idiopathic and the next most common cause is urinary tract infection with coliform organisms. Gonococcal epididymitis occurs rarely in children (Beilin, 1931). A chlamydial etiology for childhood epididymitis has not been adequately investigated, but it is possible that *C. trachomatis* is responsible for some of those cases previously classified as idiopathic.

Conjunctivitis due to chlamydia has been demonstrated in children beyond infancy in association with chlamydial vulvovaginitis (Dunlop *et al.*, 1966). Conjunctivitis due to *C. trachomatis* has not been reported in prepubertal boys, but it should be considered in patients with follicular conjunctivitis who have chlamydial or gonococcal infection at other body sites or who are the victims of proved or suspected sexual abuse.

Lymphogranuloma venereum (LGV), one of the minor classic venereal diseases, is caused by L-1, L-2, and L-3 strains of *C. trachomatis*. It has rarely been reported in childhood. A recent review revealed only 20 case reports in the English literature from 1935 through 1979 (Wilfert and Gutman, 1981). Only five of these cases occurred in boys: three had matted inguinal nodes, one had rectal stricture, and one had cervical adenopathy. No venereal or other sources of infection were identified for any of these boys' infections. In none of the pediatric patients was a primary genital papule noted. Although inguinal adenopathy following a penile ulcer may be due to HSV, classic LGV is always and by definition caused by LGV strains of *C. trachomatis*. In most of these cases, the diagnosis was established through the Frei test (an intradermal test of delayed hypersensitivity to material prepared from LGV-infected lymphoid tissue) or by demonstration of complement-fixing serum antibodies. Both of these tests are nonspecific, and the diagnosis of LGV in several of the reported cases is suspect. The diagnosis of LGV should currently be made by the isolation of the organism from bubo pus, by the demonstration of typical histopathology, or by the detection of type-specific serum antibodies against LGV.

Differential diagnosis

Chlamydial urethritis in the male child should be considered in the differential diagnoses of purulent or mucoid urethral discharges and of dysuria and pyuria, in the manner outlined above for gonorrhea. A diagnosis of chlamydial urethritis should be carefully considered in the patient with gonorrhea who has a genital discharge persisting after the eradication of gonococcal infection (Patamasucon *et al.*, 1981).

C. trachomatis infection should also be considered in children with idiopathic epididymitis. Torsion of the testes or of the appendix testes or appendix epididymis, orchitis, tumor, and inguinal hernia must be ruled out in the boy who presents with unilateral scrotal swelling. Other causes of epididymitis to be investigated include tuberculosis, gonorrhea, urinary tract infection associated with structural anomalies, and systemic bacterial infection (Doolittle *et al.*, 1966; Gierup *et al.*, 1975; Hermanson *et al.*, 1982). Clinicians must be aware that epididymitis in the child can occasionally be the heralding sign of bacterial sepsis or meningitis due to the meningococcus or to *Haemophilus influenzae* type B (Davis and Scardino, 1972; Waldman *et al.*, 1977).

Diagnosis

The diagnosis of chlamydial genital infection in children depends on the isolation of *C. trachomatis* in tissue culture (Rettig and Nelson, 1981). Fourfold changes in serum titers are diagnostic but are rarely noted in uncomplicated genital tract infections (Rettig and Nelson, 1981). Traditional complement-fixation tests are relatively insensitive and are nonspecific because they detect antibody to chlamydial group antigens. Cytologic examination of conjunctival specimens can be a very sensitive and specific procedure for diagnosing ophthalmia neonatorum, although it is not very useful in older children. We have been unable to diagnose genital infection by examining Giemsa-stained smears of urethral scrapings or genital discharges.

Therapy

Pediatric genital infection with *C. trachomatis* should be treated with oral sulfonamides (120–150 mg/kg per day; maximum dose of 4 g/day) or erythromycin (40 mg/kg per day; maximum dose of 2 g/day) for a minimum of 10 days. Children aged 8 years or older may be treated with tetracycline (40 mg/kg per day; maximum dose of 2 g/day) or doxycycline (5 mg/kg per day; maximum dose of 200 mg/day). The diagnosis of chlamydial genital infection should prompt a search for coincident genital or extragenital gonococcal infection. A social and microbiologic investigation for presumed sexual abuse should be accomplished, as noted previously.

ACQUIRED SYPHILIS IN CHILDHOOD

Epidemiology

Although most pediatricians associate syphilis in children with congenital infection acquired from a syphilitic gravida, there has recently been an increased recognition of acquired syphilis in childhood (Ackerman *et al.*, 1972; Ginsburg, 1983). In 1981, 218 cases of primary or secondary syphilis in children 1–14 years of age were reported nationally, compared to 154 in 1979 (CDC, 1981, 1982b). These figures compare with 331 reported cases of congenital syphilis in 1979, and 287 in 1981. Several reviews of acquired syphilis in childhood from the preantibiotic era reported a congenital-to-acquired ratio of childhood syphilis of from 5.2:1 to 22.8:1 (Waugh, 1938; Smith, 1939). This suggests that the incidence of congenital syphilis has declined more markedly than that of acquired childhood infection, a phenomenon probably attributable to the almost universal practice of serologically screening pregnant women in the United States. [Ed.'s Note: see Vol. I, Chapter 13 for a discussion of congenital syphilis in Zambia.]

There are several modes of transmission of acquired syphilis in children. Because of the organism's poor survival outside the body, contagion via fomites is unusual. However, since primary or secondary lesions occur at extragenital sites and are highly infectious, chancre on the lip, face or fingertips, or mucous patches of the oral mucosa are as capable of transmitting infection as are genital lesions. In contrast to gonorrhea, syphilitic infection may be transmitted by nonvenereal, close interpersonal contact. Although detailed studies of the acquisition of pediatric acquired syphilis during the 1930s suggested that venereal transmission was rare it should nevertheless be suspected in cases where the primary lesion is genital and when the identified syphilitic contact is either the father or an adult, nonfamily member (Smith, 1939). Infected mothers have also been found frequently and thought to be responsible for nonvenereal transmission (Waugh, 1938). Recent reports have suggested that infection of prepubertal children continues to occur via venereal as well as nonvenereal routes of transmission (Ackerman et al., 1972; Ginsburg, 1983). The presence of a primary chancre on the genitals, in the perianal area, or in the pharynx is a strong indicator of sexual abuse.

More cases have been reported in prepubertal girls than in boys. Smith (1939) reported on 78 cases in females and 27 in males. In 1979, the female-to-male ratio was 2:1 in the 0–9 year age group and 3:1 in 10–14-year-olds (CDC, 1981). Whether this is due to increased venereal exposure or closer nonvenereal contact in girls has not been determined.

Clinical manifestations are essentially identical to those in adults (Ginsburg, 1983). The primary lesion is classically a single, indurated, and painless chancre. It may be absent in a quarter to a third of patients (Smith, 1939; Chapel, 1980). The cutaneous signs of secondary lues are protean. Generalized macular and papular rashes extending onto the palms and soles are seen most commonly. Lesions may develop a fine scale and become hyperkeratotic. Condyloma lata occur on the perineum, on the scrotum, and in the perianal area. Mucous patches may be seen on oral or genital mucosa. Prepubertal patients often have generalized lymphadenopathy, malaise, and pharyngitis. *The key to making the diagnosis on clinical grounds lies in recognizing the possibility of syphilitic infection.*

It is unlikely that latent acquired syphilis would be diagnosed in a prepubertal patient, because routine serologic testing is not indicated in pediatric populations. The fortuitous finding of a positive serology in a currently asymptomatic child necessitates a careful history and physical exam for historical evidence of previous acquired infection and for the subtle physical findings of congenital syphilis. The distinction between the two cannot be made solely on serologic grounds, but maternal history and serologic status may be enlightening.

Tertiary manifestations of late syphilis are not seen during childhood.

Differential diagnosis

A genital sore or ulcer in the prepubertal boy should suggest trauma (which may be due to insect bites, zipper injury, or injury from masturbatory activity), herpetic infection, impetigo, localized erythema multiforme, scabies or molluscum contagiosum. Other STDs that may cause a genital ulcer (chancroid, granuloma inguinale) have rarely been reported in children. Multiple painful penile or perianal ulcerative or vesicular lesions are characteristic of herpes infection.

The differential diagnosis of secondary syphilis in a child includes pityriasis rosea, psoriasis, tinea versicolor, drug eruptions (including erythema multiforme), and viral exanthems, especially those due to enteroviral infections or atypical measles. Perianal condyloma lata must be distinguished from condyloma acuminatum. Infectious mononucleosis with a macular-papular rash can mimic the constellation of generalized lymphadenopathy, pharyngitis, malaise, and rash seen in secondary syphilis.

Diagnosis

The definitive diagnosis of syphilis depends on either the demonstration of characteristic treponemes on darkfield examination of lesions or the detection of serum antibodies to nontreponemal and treponemal antigens. All suspicious primary genital and moist secondary lesions should be examined for spirochetes by darkfield examination. Oral and rectal lesions may be contaminated by saprophytic spirochetes and, therefore, are not suitable for such examination. Seroconversion, or a fourfold rise in antibodies against nontreponemal reagents (a Venereal Disease Research Laboratory (VDRL) test or a Rapid Plasma Reagin (RPR) test), is diagnostic of recent infection. These results should be confirmed by a treponemal-specific test, such as the FTA (fluorescent treponemal antibody-absorbed) test or the MHA-TP (micro-hemagglutination–*Treponema pallidum*) test. A patient with early primary syphilis may initially be seronegative, and repeat examinations at 1- and 4-week intervals are indicated. virtually all patients with secondary lues are seropositive by both treponemal and nontreponemal tests.

Therapy

Children with early acquired syphilis should receive 50 000 units/kg of benzathine penicillin i.m. in a single dose (maximum dose: 2.4 million units). Penicillin-allergic patients may be treated with erythromycin, 40 mg/kg per day p.o. (maximum dose: 2 g/day) for 15 days. Patients 8 years of age or older should receive tetracycline, 40 mg/kg per day p.o. (maximum dose: 2 g/day) for 15 days. Follow-up serologies should be checked 3, 6, and 12 months after therapy; almost all patients treated for early syphilis will become seronegative. The pediatric patient who does not become seronegative should receive a second course of therapy, especially if erythromycin has been used, to minimize the risk of sequelae decades later.

Both parents of a child with acquired syphilis must be examined for clinical and serologic evidence of lues. Other contacts and household members should be similarly evaluated. The child should be examined for evidence of other STDs and evidence of sexual abuse. A venereal mode of acquisition should be assumed unless disproven.

CONDYLOMA ACUMINATUM

Epidemiology

An increasing number of cases of condylomata acuminata in prepubertal children have been reported in the past decade (Mininberg and Rudick, 1976; Seidal et al., 1979; Stumpf, 1980). In reported childhood cases, there has been a 2 : 1 female-to-male ratio. On clinical and epidemiological grounds it appears that genital warts are transmitted venereally in most instances (Oriel, 1983). Young infants may contract human papilloma viruses (HPV) infection from maternal cervical or vulvar lesions at birth and subsequently develop perineal or perianal warts. Preliminary evidence indicates that laryngeal papillomas of infancy are caused by an HPV similar to that which causes maternal genital warts (Oriel, 1983). The mode of transmission of genital or anal warts to children beyond infancy is unclear, but venereal spread is most likely. Although the majority of reported pediatric cases have had no identified source of infection, five of six children in two recent reports were victims of sexual abuse (Mininberg and Rudick, 1976; Seidel et al., 1979).

Clinical characteristics

Condyloma acuminata in adult males most commonly occur on the glans or shaft of the penis, but may occur at the urethral meatus or intraurethrally. Perianal warts are commonly seen in homosexual males and are strongly associated with anal intercourse. Four of nine reported cases in boys were urethral, and five were perianal. The warts may be flat but are most often polymorphic and raised, pedunculated, or sessile. They frequently resemble a miniature head of cauliflower. Intraurethral lesions may be associated with a urethral discharge or urethral bleeding.

Differential diagnosis

Few cutaneous lesions mimic typical condylomata acuminata. Perianal skin tags are usually small and stalked. Hemorrhoidal tissue should not be confused with warts. Condylomata acuminata *must* be distinguished from condyloma lata. Warts are more raised and irregular, are darkfield-negative, and are not associated with rashes elsewhere on the body or with any constitutional symptoms.

Diagnosis

The diagnosis of genital or anal warts is made on clinical grounds. No laboratory tests are available, although biopsy reveals characteristic proliferation of the stratum spinosum and papillomatosis (Oriel, 1983).

Clinical and laboratory evidence of other STDs should be carefully sought in the child who has condylomata acuminata.

Therapy

There is no wholly satisfactory therapy for venereal warts (CDC, 1982a). Repeated topical application of 10% podophyllin is effective for most lesions occurring on cutaneous surfaces. This toxic resin should not be applied to mucosal surfaces. Intra-anal lesions can be managed by cryotherapy with liquid nitrogen or by electrocauterization. Meatal or intraurethral warts should be treated by an experienced urologist. Cryosurgery or surgical excision is often indicated for these warts. Anecdotal reports support the use of 5% 5-fluoro-uracil cream for intraurethral lesions.

GENITAL HERPES INFECTION IN CHILDREN

Epidemiology

Surprisingly few cases of genital herpes in prepubertal children have been reported in the past decade, despite the increased recognition of this condition in adults and the recent almost hysterical attention to genital herpes in the lay press. In the few reports available, this STD has been more commonly noted in girls than in boys (Nahmias *et al.*, 1968).

Genital herpes infection in adults is almost exclusively transmitted via genital–genital or orogenital contact (Corey *et al.*, 1983). Endogenous spread of infection may occur via the patient's hands to the conjunctivae or the pharynx. Despite a recent study indicating that this enveloped DNA virus may survive for as long as 18 hours on artificially infected fomites (Larson and Bryson, 1982), the role of inanimate objects in transmission of herpes remains unsubstantiated. Sufficient data on childhood infection are not available to allow conclusions concerning the mode of acquisition in this setting. Nahmias *et al.* (1968) suggested that auto-inoculation of type 1 HSV from the pharynx to the genitals may occur in children. Type 1 virus in adults is less likely to cause recurring genital lesions, although it may be found in 7–50% of primary genital episodes (Corey *et al.*, 1983). The type of virus isolated from a child's genital lesion may therefore have both clinical and epidemiologic implications; typing by a reference laboratory should be sought in pediatric cases. The traditional conclusion of 'type 1 above the waist, type 2 below' is no longer tenable with reference to adults. The increased incidence of isolation of type 1 virus from genital lesions in adults may be due to an increased frequency of orogenital sexual practices. The isolation of a type 2 virus from a child's genitalia, however, would increase the likelihood of a genital source of infection, and coincident isolation of type 1 viruses from both pharynx and genitalia would admit the possibility of nonvenereal autoinoculation.

Clinical characteristics

Primary genital herpes is commonly both a local and systemic disease. Multiple, painful grouped vesicles on an erythematous base occur on the glans or penile shaft in the male. Tender regional adenopathy is common, and the patient may have fever and systemic malaise. The total duration of illness is often 2–3

111

weeks. Recurrent lesions are few in number, and persist for less than a week; systemic signs and symptoms are infrequent. Extragenital manifestations of infection include perianal vesicles and proctitis in homosexual males, symptomatic pharyngitis, herpetic whitlow of a digit, and aseptic meningitis (Corey *et al.*, 1983). Asymptomatic oropharyngeal infection has been documented in a 3-year-old boy with genital vesicles due to type 1 HSV (Nahmias *et al.*, 1968). Transverse myelitis complicated vulvovaginitis due to type 1 HSV in an 8-year-old (Shturman-Ellstein *et al.*, 1976). The risk of genital recurrences in childhood infection is currently unknown.

Differential diagnosis

The lesions of primary herpetic genital infection are distinctive and not easily confused with other conditions. A contact dermatitis or drug eruption usually is less painful, of shorter duration, and not associated with systemic signs. Small numbers of recurrent lesions should be differentiated from scabies and molluscum contagiosum and from other STDs which cause genital ulceration. The history of previous herpetic lesions, the occurrence of prodromal pain or paresthesias, and a typical clinical course should all suggest the diagnosis of recurrent HSV infection.

Diagnosis

Although the diagnosis can be made on clinical grounds in most adults, virologic confirmation should be sought in all prepubertal cases. Typing of isolates from children may have epidemiologic importance, as noted above. Cytologic diagnosis is accurate in experienced hands but provides no information as to the type of HSV virus involved. Single or paired serologic tests for antibody to HSV are of limited diagnostic value. HSV is one of the more easily cultivated human viruses, and attempts to isolate it from all children with suspicious genital lesions are indicated.

Therapy

Acyclovir provides partially effective therapy for this infection. Several controlled studies support the efficacy of this antiviral compound in decreasing viral shedding and clinical symptoms during the initial genital episode (Corey and Holmes, 1983). The currently available 5% topical ointment should be used (four to six applications daily, for 7 days) to treat primary genital infections in adults as well as in children. Topical acyclovir does not appear to lessen the frequency of recurrences and offers no significant benefit in the therapy of recurrent disease. The multitude of other conventional and unconventional therapies for genital herpes are not effective and should be avoided.

OTHER STDs IN BOYS

Sexually transmitted pathogens not previously discussed in this chapter have not been shown to be venereally transmitted in childhood (see Table 1). As noted above, a number of agents which are often transmitted sexually in adults (particularly in homosexual males) are common pediatric pathogens. In children, however, these agents are acquired by traditional, nonvenereal modes of transmission. The potential for other sexually transmitted organisms to cause pediatric infection may be low because of the infrequent occurrence of these agents in the adult population. *Haemophilus ducreyi* and the etiologic agent of granuloma inguinale fall into this category. Finally, adequate laboratory and epidemiologic investigations of several STD agents in childhood genitourinary infections have not been performed. For example, previous investigations of NGU in prepubertal boys have not adequately cultured for *U. urealyticum*, an agent responsible for perhaps 40% of nongonococcal, nonchlamydial urethritis in adults (Williams and Mikhael, 1971; Rettig and Nelson, 1981). Similarly, the potential for urethral infection due to *Gardnerella vaginalis* or *Trichomonas vaginalis* has not been studied in boys.

None of these considerations should dissuade the clinician from entertaining the possibility of venereal transmission of an 'adult' STD in a prepubertal child. This is particularly true if the child has another STD known to be transmitted venereally to children or if there are clinical or epidemiologic features in the case consistent with a high risk of sexual abuse.

THE RELATION OF SEXUAL ABUSE TO CHILDHOOD STDs

No discussion of STDs in children can be complete without some discussion of the interrelationship between STDs and child sexual abuse. Two questions naturally arise: (1) What is the incidence of STDs in sexually abused children? and (2) To what degree is the discovery of an STD in a child evidence of sexual abuse?

Sexual abuse was brought into focus as a common manifestation of child abuse by Dr Henry Kempe, who defined such abuse as 'the involvement of dependent, developmentally immature children and adolescents in sexual activities that they do not fully comprehend, to which they are unable to give informed consent, or that violate the social taboos of family roles' (Kempe, 1977). It is currently estimated that 10–25% of all reported child abuse falls into this category, and that the total magnitude of this problem may be even greater, due to the reluctance of physicians to consider and to report this pediatric problem.

Reviews of 11 American studies of sexual abuse of children published from 1975 to 1983 revealed that 13.2% of 2618 cases occurred in male children. The proportion of male victims in individual reports ranged from 8.7% to 25.7%. The mean age of all patients for whom data were reported was 9.5 years. In several studies, male victims had an average age 1–3 years less than females (Ellerstein and Canavan, 1980; Rimsza and Niggemann, 1982; DeJong *et al.*, 1982).

Sexual abuse of children presents itself in several different guises (Kramer and Jason, 1982). A chief complaint of alleged abuse is made infrequently, and most commonly where a single episode of indecent exposure, fondling, or attempted intercourse by a stranger is claimed. Children may present with an

STD, in which case sexual abuse should always be suspected. Most frequently, the child presents with nonspecific genital or other physical, behavioral, or psychosomatic complaints. Contrary to popular belief, abuse by an unknown perpetrator outside of the home occurs infrequently. In seven series, the alleged victimizer was unknown to the child in only 7–53% of cases. A male family member or acquaintance is usually responsible for multiple episodes of abuse, which occur in the 'safe haven' of the victim's or the acquaintance's home. Male children may be more likely to be abused by a stranger, to be physically harmed, and to be victims of attempted anal or oral sodomy than females (Ellerstein and Canavan, 1980; DeJong et al., 1982).

The risk of STDs subsequent to sexual abuse has only been well evaluated for gonococcal infection (Kramer and Jason, 1982). From 0.7% to 19.7% of childhood victims of sexual abuse (male and female) who were cultured have been found to have gonorrhea. As many as 20% of such infections are asymptomatic (Rimsza and Niggemann, 1982). Epidemiologic or prophylactic therapy for gonorrhea is not indicated unless the perpetrator is known to be symptomatic or infected. However, all children should be cultured for *N. gonorrhoeae* at genital, anal, and pharyngeal sites. Our experience suggests that chlamydial cultures should also be obtained if possible. Cultures or serologic tests for additional STDs are not routinely indicated but may be necessary on a case-by-case basis after consideration of the assaulter's health status and the type of assault.

Epidemiologic considerations of childhood gonorrhea, as previously outlined in this chapter, lead to the following conclusion: 'Physicians should assume that children with gonorrhea have acquired it by sexual contact and that most such contacts are abusive' (American Academy of Pediatrics, 1983). The degree to which other STDs in children are also transmitted venereally remains a subject for further study; but, as previously indicated, the physician should consider that this is the most likely route of acquisition of these infections.

References

American Academy of Pediatrics Committee on Early Childhood, Adoption, and Dependent Care (1983). Gonorrhea in prepubertal children. *Pediatrics*, **71**, 553

Ackerman, A. B., Goldfaden, G. and Cosmides, J. C. (1972). Acquired syphilis in early childhood. *Arch. Dermatol.*, **106**, 92

Beilin, L. M. (1931). Gonorrheal urethritis in male children (with some observations on their sexual impulses). *J. Urol.*, **25**, 69

Bell, T. A. (1983). Major sexually transmitted diseases of children and adolescents. *Ped. Infect. Dis.*, **2**, 153

Berger, R. E., Alexander, E. R., Harnisch, J. P. *et al.* (1979). Etiology, manifestations and therapy of acute epididymitis: Prospective study of 50 cases. *J. Urol.*, **121**, 750

Branch, G. and Paxton, R. (1965). A study of gonococcal infections among infants and children. *Pub. Hlth. Rep.*, **80**, 347

CDC. (1981). *Sexually Transmitted Disease (STD) Statistical Letter for 1979.* No. 129. (Atlanta: Center for Disease Control)

CDC. (1982a). Sexually transmitted diseases: Treatment guidelines, 1982. *MMWR*, **31**, 415

CDC. (1982b). Annual summary, 1981. *MMWR*, **30**, 86

CDC. (1982c). Genital herpes infection: United States, 1966–79. *MMWR*, **31**, 137

CDC. (1983). Condyloma acuminatum: United States, 1966–81. *MMWR*, **32**, 306

Chapel, T. A. (1980). The signs and symptoms of secondary syphilis. *Sex. Transm. Dis.*, **7**, 161

Corey, L., Adams, H. G. and Brown, Z. A. et al. (1983). Genital herpes simplex virus infections: Clinical manifestations, course, and complications. Ann. Intern. Med., 98, 958

Corey, L. and Holmes, K. K. (1983). Genital herpes simplex virus infections: Current concepts in diagnosis, therapy, and prevention. Ann. Intern. Med., 98, 973

Davis, W. H. and Scardino, P. L. (1972). Meningitis presenting as epididymitis. S. Med. J., 65, 936

DeJong, A. R., Emmett, G. A. and Hervada, A. R. (1982). Sexual abuse of children. Am. J. Dis. Child., 136, 129

Doolittle, K. H., Smith, J. P. and Saylor, M. L. (1966). Epididymitis in the prepubertal boy. J. Urol., 96, 364

Dunlop, E. M. C., Al-Hussaini, M. K., Freedman, A. et al. (1966). Infection by Tric agent and other members of the Bedsonia group with a note on Reiter's Disease. III. Genital infection and disease of the eye. Trans. Ophthalmol. Soc. UK, 86, 313

Ellerstein, N. S. and Canavan, J. W. (1980). Sexual abuse of boys. Am. J. Dis. Child., 134, 255

Farrell, M. K., Billmire, M. E., Shamroy, J. A. et al. (1981). Prepubertal gonorrhea: A multidisciplinary approach. Pediatrics, 67, 151

Fink, C. W. (1965). Gonococcal arthritis in children. J. Am. Med. Assoc., 194, 123

Folland, D. S., Burke, R. E., Hinman, A. R. et al. (1977). Gonorrhea in preadolescent children: An inquiry into source of infection and mode of transmission. Pediatrics, 60, 153

Gierup, J., Hedenberg, C. V. and Osterman, A. (1975). Acute non-specific epididymitis in boys. Scand. J. Urol. Nephrol., 9, 5

Gilbaugh Jr., J. H. and Fuchs, P. C. (1979). The gonococcus and the toilet seat. N. Engl. J. Med., 301, 91

Ginsburg, C. M. (1983). Acquired syphilis in prepubertal children. Ped. Infect. Dis., 2, 232

Groothius, J. R., Vischoff, M. C. and Jauregui, L. E. (1983). Pharyngeal gonorrhea in young children. Ped. Infect. Dis., 2, 99

Hermansen, M. C., Chusid, M. J. and Sty, J. R. (1980). Bacterial epididymo-orchitis in children and adolescents. Clin. Pediatr., 19, 812

Kempe, C. H. (1978). Sexual abuse, another hidden pediatric problem: The 1977 C. Anderson Aldrich Lecture. Pediatrics, 62, 382

Kramer, D. G. and Jason, J. (1982). Sexually abused children and sexually transmitted diseases. Rev. Infect. Dis., 4, S883

Larson, T. and Bryson, Y. (1982). Fomites and herpes simplex virus: The toilet seat revisited. Pediatr. Res., 16, 244A

Meek, J. M., Askari, A. and Belman, A. B. (1979). Prepubertal gonorrhea. J. Urol., 122, 532

Minimberg, D. T. and Rudick, D. H. (1976). Urethral condyloma acuminata in male children. Pediatrics, 57, 571

Nahmias, A. J., Dowdle, W. R., Naib, Z. M. et al. (1968). Genital infection with herpes virus hominis types 1 and 2 in children. Pediatrics, 42, 659

Nelson, J. D., Mohs, E., Dajani, A. S. et al. (1976). Gonorrhea in preschool and school-age children: Report of the prepubertal gonorrhea cooperative study group. J. Am. Med. Assoc., 236, 1359

Oriel, J. D. (1983). Genital warts. In K. K. Holmes and P.-A. Mardh (eds.) International Perspectives on Neglected Sexually Transmitted Diseases: Impact on Venereology, Infertility, and Maternal and Infant Health, p. 125. (Washington: Hemisphere)

Patamasucon, P., Rettig, P. J. and Nelson, J. D. (1981). Cefuroxime therapy of gonorrhea and coinfection with Chlamydia trachomatis in children. Pediatrics, 68, 534

Quinn, T. C., Goodell, S. E., Mkrtichian, E. et al. (1981). Chlamydia trachomatis proctitis. N. Engl. J. Med., 305, 195

Rettig, P. J. and Nelson, J. D. (1981). Genital tract infection with Chlamydia trachomatis in prepubertal children. J. Pediatr., 99, 206

Rettig, P. J., Nelson, J. D. and Kusmiesz, H. (1980). Spectinomycin therapy for gonorrhea in prepubertal children. Am. J. Dis. Child., 134, 359

Rimsza, M. E. and Niggemann, E. H. (1982). Medical evaluation of sexually abused children: a review of 311 cases. Pediatrics, 69, 8

Seidel, J., Zonana, J. and Totten, E. (1979). Condyloma acuminata as a sign of sexual abuse in children. J. Pediatr., 95, 553

Sgroi, S. M. (1979). Pediatric gonorrhea beyond infancy. *Pediatr. Ann.*, **8**, 326

Shore, W. B. and Winkelstein, J. A. (1971). Nonvenereal transmission of gonococcal infections to children. *J. Pediatr.*, **79**, 661

Shturman-Ellstein, R., Borkowsky, W., Fish, I. *et al.* (1976). Myelitis associated with genital herpes in a child. *J. Pediatr.*, **88**, 523

Silber, T. J. and Controni, G. (1981). Pharyngeal gonorrhea. *Pediatrics*, **68**, 609

Smith Jr., F. R. (1939). Acquired syphilis in children: An epidemiology and clinical study. *Am. J. Syph. Gon. Vener. Dis.*, **23**, 165

Stumpf, P. G. (1980). Increasing occurrence of condylomata acuminata in premenarchal children. *Obstet. Gynecol.*, **56**, 262

Waldman, L. S., Kosloske, A. M. and Parsons, D. W. (1977). Acute epididymo-orchitis as the presenting manifestation of *Hemophilus influenzae* septicemia. *J. Pediatr.*, **90**, 87

Washington, A. E. (1982). Update on treatment recommendations for gonococcal infections. *Rev. Inf. Dis.*, **4**, S1758

Waugh, J. R. (1938). Acquired syphilis of infancy and childhood. *Am. J. Syph. Gon. Vener. Dis.*, **22**, 607

Wiesner, P. J., Tronca, E., Bonin, P. *et al.* (1973). Clinical spectrum of pharyngeal gonococcal infection. *N. Engl. J. Med.*, **288**, 181

Wilfert, C. and Gutman, L. (1981). Chlamydial infections. In: R. D. Feigin and J. D. Cherry (eds.) *Textbook of Pediatric Infectious Diseases*, p. 1431. (Philadelphia: W. B. Saunders)

Williams, D. I. and Mikhael, B. R. (1971). Urethritis in male children. *Proc. Roy. Soc. Med.*, **64**, 133

9
Sexually transmitted diseases in premenarchal girls

A. F. SINGLETON

INTRODUCTION

The incidence of sexually transmitted diseases (STDs) is increasing among children and assuming greater importance to physicians who treat children (Felman *et al.*, 1978). In some ways these diseases are similar in age groups, i.e. the simultaneous occurrence of gonococcal and chlamydial infections is common in both children (Rettig and Nelson, 1981; Fraser *et al.*, 1983) and adults (Karney *et al.*, 1977). There are, however, major differences in epidemiology, clinical manifestations, evaluation, and treatment. A pathophysiologic basis underlies many of these differences, an understanding of which is essential for rational management.

PATHOPHYSIOLOGY AND GENERAL THERAPEUTIC CONSIDERATIONS

The estrogenized adult female is relatively well protected against vulvovestibulovaginitis for at least three reasons: (1) the labia majora cover the subjacent structures; (2) the vaginal pH is acidic, largely due to the fact that lactobacilli predominate in the normal flora; and (3) the superficial epithelial layers of the exocervix, vagina, and vestibule are thick. Tissue trauma is less likely in the estrogenized female at any age because of the high content of elastic and collagen fiber in the vagina and vestibule and the apposition of the labia majora. On the other hand, the estrogenized female, in contrast to the pre-estrogenized female, is susceptible to pelvic inflammatory disease (PID) and glandular infections (endocervix, Bartholin's, Skene's, minor vestibular glands). These susceptibilities stem from the patency of the endocervical canal and the secretory activity of various glands, which become targets of infection.

In the pre-estrogenized female, the areas of greater resistance and vulnerability are exactly the opposite. Although vulnerable to vulvovestibulovaginitis and trauma, the young girl is relatively well protected against PID and glandular infections. A susceptibility to trauma results from the thinness of the superficial epithelial layers, the decreased content of elastic and collagen fiber in tissues of vagina and vestibule, and the non-apposition of the labia majora. In association with the 'benign mixed flora of childhood' (diphtheroids, enterococci, staphylococci and nonhemolytic coagulase-negative diplococci), the pH is 6.5–7.5, which is optimal for many organisms that cause vaginitis. Protection against PID is due to the absence of a patent endocervical canal; protection against glandular infections is due to the absence of secretory activity among the glands that are lined with simple cuboidal epithelium (Huffman *et al.*, 1981).

The major manifestations of genital infectious disease in the estrogenized female are endocervicitis, PID, and glandular infections. In the pre-estrogenized female, on the other hand, the primary problem is vulvovestibulovaginitis.

These physiologic differences dictate the approach that should be used in the physical examination. For example, the absence of glandular activity in the pre-estrogenized female results in a lack of lubrication of the genital mucosa. Thus, any instrument that is introduced into the pre-estrogenized vagina should first be lubricated with water or saline (not with bacteriostatic jellies) to diminish pain and abrasion. Even the most careful instrumentation may, however, result in tearing the nondistensible, collagen-poor tissues (Singleton, 1983; Figs 1 and 2).

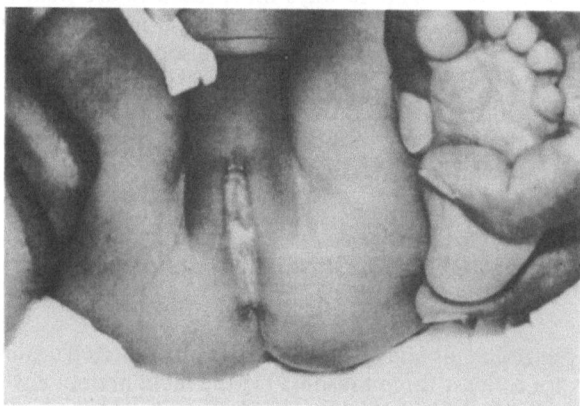

Fig. 1 The well estrogenized external genitalia of this neonate facilitate a successful, noninjurious examination. Tissues are distensible, thick, and well lubricated by endocervical secretions

In the adult, STDs associated with *Chlamydia trachomatis*, human papillomavirus, herpesvirus hominis, and granuloma inguinale may have a relationship to premalignant dysplasia (Handsfield, 1982; Davis, 1970). This relationship is, as yet, not clearly established in children. Instead, the major significance of STDs in childhood lies in their association with sexual abuse. STDs may be the only evidence that sexual abuse has occurred, since neither hymenal nor fourchette tears are necessarily present (Sgroi, 1982). Although a number of

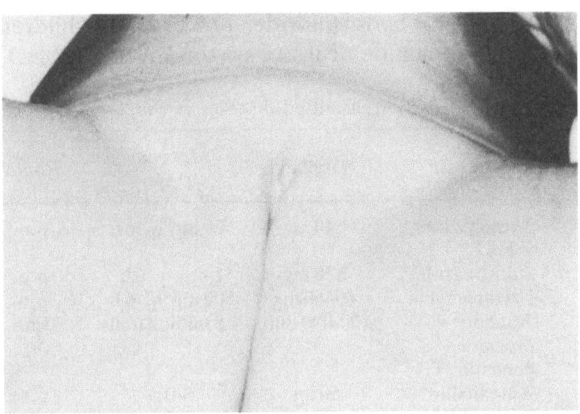

Fig. 2 The nonestrogenized external genitalia of this 18-month-old require lubrication of all instruments. Even with the greatest of care, injury of thin, nonlubricated tissues is possible

infectious agents (e.g. cytomegalovirus, *C. trachomatis*, genital mycoplasmas, *Gardnerella* species, Group B streptococci; human papillomavirus) may become established in the neonate's genital tract at the time of delivery and persist for variable lengths of time, sexual abuse must always be considered when these or other sexually transmissible agents are detected. In these instances all of the child's contacts should be evaluated. As in the adult, the finding of one STD should stimulate the search for others. The occurrence of STD in a child should also be reported to the appropriate authorities to enhance detection of sexual abuse.

SPECIFIC SEXUALLY TRANSMISSIBLE DISEASES

Disease due to *Chlamydia trachomatis*, A to K

The causative organism of chlamydial vulvovestibulovaginitis, *C. trachomatis*, may be found in the genital tract of the prepubertal child, though not necessarily as the result of sexual transmission. Symptoms appear 2–3 weeks following infectious contact and often include urinary frequency and pain, as well as genital pruritus and discharge. In most cases vaginal discharge and inflammation of the vulva, vestibule, and vagina are found, although some children are asymptomatic (Fraser *et al.*, 1983).

A vaginal wall scraping is a helpful diagnostic aid. The sample should be transferred immediately to an appropriate transport medium, such as the one available from Immunology Consultants, California (Schachter, 1978a-c). A Papanicolaou smear of the scraping may be positive for the organism (Saltz *et al.*, 1981). Culture of a swab from the anorectal canal may also be useful (Quinn *et al.*, 1981), but a throat culture is of questionable value (Schachter and Atwood, 1975; Bowie *et al.*, 1977). A clean catch urinalysis may reveal pyuria (Handsfield, 1982).

The treatment of choice for chlamydial infection in children 8 years of age and older is tetracycline hydrochloride. For younger children, the clinician may select either sulfonamide drugs or erythromycin (Table 1).

Table 1 Treatment of sexually transmitted diseases in childhood

Disease	Drug	Dose/kg	Maximal Dose	Route[a]	Duration
Chlamydia trachomatis	Tetracycline HCl	40 mg	500 mg q. 6 h	p.o.	10 days
	Sulfisoxazole	120 mg	1–2 g q. 6 h	p.o.	10 days
	Erythromycin	40–60 mg	500 mg q. 6 h	p.o.	10 days
Gonorrhea	Aqueous procaine penicillin G[b]	100,000 units	4.8 million units	i.m.	single dose
	Amoxicillin[b]	50 mg	3.0 g	p.o.	single dose
	Ampicillin[b]	100 mg	3.5 g	p.o.	single dose
	Spectinomycin	40 mg	2 g	i.m.	single dose
	Cefoxitin[b]	?	2 g	i.m.	single dose
	Cefuroxime	25 mg	2 g	i.m.	single dose
	Tetracycline HCl	40 mg	500 mg q. 6 h	p.o.	5 days
Herpes progenitalis	Acyclovir 5% ointment		q. 4–6 h	topical	10–14 days (primary) 5–7 days (recurrent)
Molluscum contagiosum	Cantharone			topical	1 application
Pubic lice	Kwell shampoo		one application	topical	4 min
	Synergized pyrethrins (RID)		one application	topical	10 min
Scabies	Kwell lotion or cream			topical	one application for 8–12 h; repeat in 1 week
	Crotamiton (Eurax)			topical	one application for 24 h; repeat in 24 h
Condyloma acuminatum	Podophyllin 25% ointment			topical	one application q. 2 weeks (6 h maximum per application)
Candida albicans	Nystatin			topical	q. h × 7 days
				intravaginal	q. h × 7 days
		400,000 units to 600,000 units q.i.d.		p.o.	48 h after symptoms or cultures have become negative
	Clotrimazole			topical	q. h × 7 days
				intravaginal	q. h × 7 days

Table 1 *cont.* Treatment of sexually transmitted diseases in childhood

Disease	Drug	Dose/kg	Maximal Dose	Route[a]	Duration
	Miconazole			topical	q. h × 7 days
				intravaginal	q. h × 7 days
Trichomonas vaginalis	Clotrimazole		100 mg h	p.o.	7–10 days
	Metronidazole		125 mg TID	p.o.	10 days
Acquired syphilis	Benzathine penicillin	50,000 units	2.4 million units	i.m.	once – incubating weekly intervals twice – early three times – late
	Tetracycline HCl	40 mg	500 mg q. 6 h	p.o.	15 days (early) 30 days (late)
	Erythromycin	40–60 mg	500 mg q. 6 h	p.o.	15 days (early) 30 days (late)

[a] i.m. = intramuscular; p.o. = orally (per os)
[b] With probenecid: 25 mg; 1 g; p.o.; single dose

Genital mycoplasmas

Mycoplasma hominis and *Ureaplasma urealyticum* have not been conclusively shown to be associated with clinical genital disease in either children or adults. Genital colonization may occur at the time of birth, and persist for variable durations in childhood, but sexual abuse might also introduce these organisms into the vaginal flora (Lee *et al.*, 1974). The organism may be cultured from the urine or the vagina, and serologic testing may reveal an acute rise in titer (Taylor-Robinson, 1980).

Gardnerella vaginalis (Hemophilus vaginalis; Corynebacterium vaginale)

Though generally transmitted venereally, *G. vaginalis* may also persist in the vagina following colonization at birth (Platt, 1971; Venkataramani and Rathbun, 1976). Symptomatic disease is rare before the menarche, but has been described in a series of girls 8–11 years of age, each of whom had a profuse mucopurulent discharge associated with vulvar irritation. A foul odor was not described (Huffman *et al.*, 1981).

Whether or not clue cells are present is, as yet, not clear. This morphology results from the organism's adherence to superficial vaginal epithelial cells, present only in a thin layer in the pre-estrogenized female. It may be that the characteristic pH and other factors do not provide the essential conditions for organism adherence. Whether or not the addition of 10% KOH to a specimen of discharge results in the production of a 'fishy' amine odor, as it does in the adult, is also not clear in children (Pheifer *et al.*, 1978). Cultures on blood agar plates at room temperature may elucidate the situation (Huffman *et al.*, 1981).

Treatment with ampicillin may be helpful in some cases (see Table 1). Resistant cases may respond to metronidazole, though pediatric doses for this condition have not been well established (Singleton, 1980). A positive response to intravaginal creams containing sulfonamides or tetracyclines has been reported (Huffman *et al.*, 1981).

Group B streptococcal disease

The etiologic agent of this disease may be transmitted venereally or may become established shortly after birth (Hammerschlag *et al.*, 1977). Though generally asymptomatic, earlier literature describes symptoms identical to those due to Group A streptococci, i.e. dysuria; discharge that is serous, bloody, or purulent; and inflammation of the genitalia (Powers and Boisvert, 1944; Boisvert and Walcher, 1948).

Gram stain or cultures on selective media may be positive. Serologic tests for antibody to capsular polysaccharides will reveal the organism's serotype (Baker *et al.*, 1976). Treatment with penicillin may eliminate symptoms, but the organism persists nonetheless (Siegel *et al.*, 1980).

Genital cytomegalovirus

Cytomegalovirus has not been well studied in the genital tract of postmenarchal girls (Caine *et al.*, 1981). Disease is asymptomatic after the menarche; cultures of cervix and specific antibody to cytomegalovirus can be used to establish its presence (Knox *et al.*, 1979)

Gonorrhea

Infection due to *Neisseria gonorrhoeae* involves the vagina, exocervix, vestibule, and vulva (vulvovestibulovaginitis). About 1 week after infectious contact, copious and mucopurulent discharge, genital pruritus, painful urination, and lower abdominal pain may be described by the patient. The physical examination reveals discharge, inflammation, and excoriation of the mucous membranes.

Gram stain of vaginal or urethral discharge may be positive for the organism and culture of discharge from these two sites, as well as from the pharynx and anorectal canal, should be obtained. Urine culture may also be positive for *N. gonorrhoeae*, and urinalysis may be consistent with urinary tract infection or with urethritis. The sensitivity and specificity of the Gram strain in the preestrogenized female have yet to be established.

Several treatment modalities are available. Single-dose therapy with probenecid plus penicillin or its derivatives is generally effective for genital, anorectal, and pharyngeal sites of gonococcal infection, as well as for incubating syphilis, which is present in combination in up to 3% of cases. Such therapy is not,

STDs IN PREMENARCHAL GIRLS

however, effective for *C. trachomatis*, which also coexists in a large percentage of cases.

For patients allergic to penicillin or those who have disease caused by penicillinase-producing *N. gonorrhoeae* (PPNG), single-dose therapy with spectinomycin may be administered. If the organism is resistant to this drug, cefoxitin may be used, although the pediatric dosage has not yet been established. These drugs have no effect on either incubating syphilis or *C. trachomatis*.

Tetracycline hydrochloride, which should be restricted to children 8 years of age and older, has the obvious advantage of being effective for gonorrhea, syphilis, and chlamydial infection, but has the major disadvantage of requiring multiple doses (see Table 1).

Patients treated with any regimen should have repeat cultures 3–7 days after the end of therapy (Singleton, 1981).

Herpes progenitalis

As in adults, this disease is caused by herpes simplex virus (herpesvirus hominis) types 1 or 2. Symptomatic disease is generally primary and may be characterized as follows: 3–7 days after exposure, the patient notes painful urination, genital or thigh pain, fever, vaginal discharge, irritability, and listlessness. Physical examination reveals inflammation of the external genitalia, inguinal nodes that are large and tender, and genital lesions, some of which are vesiculoulcerative with a grayish base, others of which are bullae, crusts, or pustules. Secondary infection of these lesions sometimes results in a foul odor (Hare and Mowla, 1977).

A Tzanck smear or a Papanicolaou stain may reveal multinucleated giant cells in material from scrapings of mucocutaneous lesions. Papanicolaou staining may also be useful in assessing vaginal scrapings for the presence of multinucleated giant cells with a ground-glass nuclear morphology. Acetone-fixed vaginal scrapings may be tested for the presence of fluorescent antibodies. Viral cultures of lesions or urine may be positive (Vesterinen *et al.*, 1977). The erythrocyte sedimentation rate may be elevated, and complement fixation titers may be increased in acute and convalescent sera.

Treatment with 5% acyclovir sodium (Zovirax) ointment is currently the choice for primary herpes simplex virus infections (Corey *et al.*, 1982). This drug is also available in oral and parenteral forms, though these routes have not yet been approved for use in the United States. Preliminary studies indicate that the drug is effective in reducing the duration of viral shedding and symptoms in primary disease, although it does not significantly decrease the recurrence rate. All secondary bacterial infections are treated with topical or systemic analgesics and nonsteroidal anti-inflammatory agents may be helpful.

Condyloma acuminatum

This granulomatous growth is caused by human papillomavirus type 6 (HPV-6) and manifests itself about 2–3 months following exposure. Transmission may be venereal, secondary to nonvenereal intimate contact, or the result of colonization at the time of delivery. The child presents with perineal pain, which may interfere with ambulation. Other symptoms include a perineal mass, burning on urination, genital discharge, or genital bleeding. A multiform mass, which generally involves the lower vagina, vestibule, labia minora, clitoris, fourchette or perineum may also be noted (Stumpf, 1980).

Biopsy of the mass is imperative in young girls, in order to distinguish it from other conditions, such as sarcoma botryoides. Papanicolaou smear of vaginal scrapings may reveal koilocytes, as in the adult (Purola and Savia, 1977; Fig. 3).

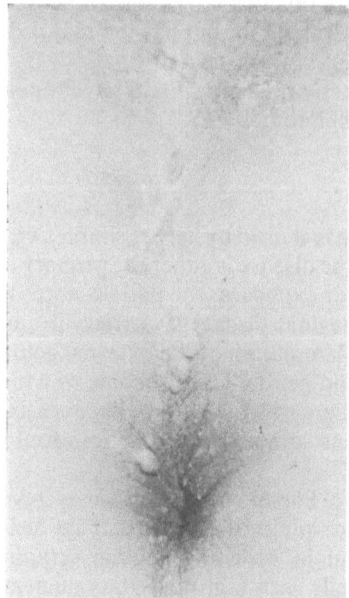

Fig. 3 Biopsy is essential whenever condyloma acuminatum is suspected. For example, in this case, biopsy showed unsuspected molluscum contagiosum infection

Podophyllin as a 25% ointment is recommended for older children; in younger children, cryotherapy is preferred, because podophyllin may accidentally spread to uninvolved areas, and damage normal tissues. The use of electrocautery and laser treatment is not well studied in children (Huffman *et al.*, 1981).

Candidiasis (moniliasis)

Candida albicans, a resident organism of the gut, may cause genital disease. Venereal transmission does occur, and should always be considered in the young child, but genital contact is not necessary for infection to occur. Symptoms include cheesy discharge, genital pruritus, and pain on urination. Vulvovestibulovaginitis and white plaques are noted.

A wet mount of vaginal fluid, to which 10% KOH has been added, is helpful in revealing the organism. Cultures on Sabouraud's or Nickerson's media may be positive. Since candidal infections are sometimes a clue to diabetes mellitus, a screening urine glucose determination should always be performed.

Antifungal creams (e.g. nystatin, clotrimazole, miconazole) should be instilled intravaginally, using the tip of a syringe (e.g. tuberculin; 2 cc or 5 cc) that is small enough for the child's introitus. The applicator that is provided with such medications is usually too large for pediatric use. These creams may also be applied topically to the vulva and vestibule. Oral nystatin may be essential to interrupt the pattern of recurrent candidiasis. The dose is 400,000–600,000 units q.i.d. for at least 48 h after the symptoms have disappeared or the cultures have returned to normal (Singleton, 1980).

Trichomoniasis

Though usually associated with venereal transmission, this infection sometimes may be contracted from swimming pools, or from intimate, nonvenereal contact. Symptoms include dysuria, genital pruritus, and pain, and a discharge that is foamy, grayish-yellow, and malodorous. Vulvovestibulovaginitis and excoriation are noted, however the 'strawberry cervix' is seen less commonly than in the post-menarchal group.

Wet mount of the discharge in saline permits observation of the motile *Trichomonas vaginalis* organism. Papanicolaou or Giemsa smears of the urinary sediment may also establish the diagnosis.

Multiple-dose treatment with clotrimazole or metronidazole may be effective (see Table 1). Single-dose metronidazole has not been sufficiently evaluated in the pediatric age group (Singleton, 1980).

Acquired syphilis

Infants and very young children may acquire infection with *Treponema pallidum* by feeding on a breast with a moist lesion or by other types of nonvenereal intimate contact with moist lesions. This infection is, however, often acquired venereally in even the youngest infant.

Symptoms appear 10–90 days after contact and follow the disease course described in the adult, i.e. a nonpainful, nontender primary stage with chancre and nodes and a secondary stage marked by a generalized rash, flu syndrome, and other systemic manifestations.

Among nonspecific tests, the Venereal Disease Research Laboratory (VDRL) and rapid plasma reagin (RPR) tests are most widely used in the United States. Specific antitreponemal tests include the micro-hemagglutination assay for *Treponema pallidum* (MHA-TP), the fluorescent treponemal antibody absorption test (FTA-ABS), and the *Treponema pallidum* inhibition test (TPI). The first two specific tests are generally available; the last is available in a few sites only.

The treatment of choice is benzathine penicillin, and the dose schedule depends upon whether the disease is incubating, early (present for less than 1 year), or late (present 1 year or longer). Tetracycline hydrochloride or erythromycin may be given to those who are allergic to penicillin, with duration of therapy changing according to duration of illness (see Table 1).

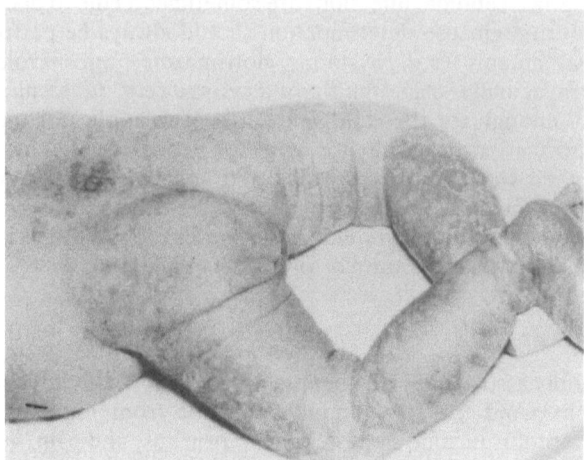

Fig. 4 At times it is not possible to distinguish between congenital and acquired syphilis. In this case the cutaneous pathology could represent either form of disease

It may be difficult to distinguish between acquired and congenital syphilis in some cases (Kelly and Singleton, 1980; Fig. 4).

Lymphogranuloma venereum

Though uncommon in childhood, this infection has been described in even the youngest of children. Caused by specific types (L1, L2, L3) of *C. trachomatis*, it is transmitted venereally or nonvenereally (fomites; laboratory accident; nonsexual contact; intrapartum transmission), with symptoms presenting up to 3 weeks after contact. In children it is generally of the purely inguinal type, unless there has been anal penetration, in which case rectal lesions may be seen (Levy, 1940).

Tender inguinal nodes (buboes), are symptomatic, with inflammation of the overlying skin. Anorexia, joint symptoms, and erythema nodosum may also be associated with this condition.

Diagnosis may be made by microbiologic (tissue-cell culture of aspirated bubo pus/tissue, or genital fluid), serologic (LGV complement fixation, microimmunofluorescence, counterimmunoelectrophoresis), immunologic (Frei skin test), or tissue (biopsy of involved tissue) methods. Eosinophilia and leukocytosis are commonly seen in childhood cases.

Available treatments include antibiotics (tetracycline hydrochloride; trimethoprim-sulfamethoxazole) and aspiration of fluctuant buboes, to prevent rupture and subsequent sinus tract formation (Holmes, 1977).

Granuloma inguinale (Donovanosis)

Although unusual in children this infection has been described following sexual and nonsexual intimate contact. Symptoms present an average of 30 days after inoculation, and ulcerative lesions generally involve the labia minora and fourchette. The ulcer is painless, and a pseudobubo is present (Ribeiro, 1972).

Puncture biopsy of the periphery of the lesion, with subsequent Giemsa-staining of an impression smear, is diagnostic. Treatment with tetracycline, streptomycin, chloramphenicol or gentamycin may be effective (Holmes, 1977).

Chancroid

The infection caused by *Hemophilus ducreyi* is rare in children, is transmitted venereally, and becomes symptomatic in 3–5 days. Painful lesions usually involve the labia minora and fourchette and present as papules, pustules, vesticulopustules, or ulcers. Lesions and nodes are painful. Malodorous discharge from the ulcer indicates secondary infection.

Though stained smear and biopsy of involved areas are suggestive of the diagnosis, isolation of *H. ducreyi* from the bubo confirms the diagnosis. An intradermal skin test is available (Holmes, 1977).

Treatment includes antibiotics (gantrisin, trimethoprim-sulfamethoxazole, cephalosporins, tetracycline; streptomycin, erythromycin, chloramphenicol) and aspiration of fluctuant nodes (Hart, 1979).

Molluscum contagiosum

This infection is caused by the *Pox viridae* virus and may be acquired by venereal and nonvenereal means. Breast feeding and fomites may be implicated.

Lesions appear 2 weeks to 2 months after contact, and may involve any skin surface, including the vulva.

Biopsy of involved skin reveals molluscum bodies. Serologic tests (e.g. fluorescent antibody, gel diffusion antibody) may be positive.

Treatment is by curettage, excision, or cantharidin collodion (Cantharone). Cryotherapy, trichloracetic acid and podophyllin have also been used (Postlethwaite, 1970).

Pubic lice (crabs)

The infestation caused by *Phthirus pubis* may be transmitted by fomites (e.g. undergarments), but is generally transmitted venereally. Reported cases involve pubic hair, axillary hair, eyelashes, and eyebrows; two cases have also been described in the scalp. Inflammation of the skin may occur, sometimes with crusting. Maculae caerulae may be present.

Low-power examination of a plucked hair often reveals nits. Treatment with 1% lindane shampoo (Kwell), or with synergized pyrethrin solution (e.g., RID) is effective. For eyelashes and eyebrows, yellow oxide of mercury with or without epilation may be required. Bed linen and towels should be treated with synergized pyrethrins (e.g. R & C Spray or Liban) (Epstein, 1975; Smith and Walsh, 1980).

Scabies

Infestation with *Sarcoptes scabiei* may follow venereal or nonvenereal contact, as well as contact with fomites. Itching appears 3–6 weeks later. Lesions may be present on any skin surface, including the vulva, breasts, umbilicus, buttocks and back. The burrow-like appearance of lesions is not essential.

Low-power light microscopic examination of scrapings of lesions often reveals mites. Treatment with 1% lindane (Kwell) lotion or cream for 12–24 hours, or with crotamiton (Eurax) lotion or cream for 24–48 hours is effective. Steroids may be helpful in alleviating the itching, which outlasts the infestation (Fiumara, 1982).

SUMMARY

The pediatrician should regard the presence of any STD as a possible indicator of sexual abuse. The presence of one STD should stimulate the search for others; genital, anorectal canal, and pharyngeal cultures, as well as eye cultures, should be obtained. Anoscopy is indicated in some cases. Since a child's consort may be unidentified, all contacts should be evaluated and treated appropriately. As in the adult, STD may be asymptomatic in children.

The proper management of the premenarchal child having STD requires an understanding of the pathophysiology of the pre-estrogenized genital tract. Thus, vulvovestibulovaginitis is the major manifestation of disease, and one must be able to distinguish it from the normal reddish-orange mucosa of the pre-estrogenized female genitalia. Dysuria may be one of the major symptons of STD in children as in adults.

The pediatrician should assure that all objects inserted into the non-estrogenized genital tract are lubricated with saline or water in order to maximize chances of obtaining an informative examination and evaluation. Specimens

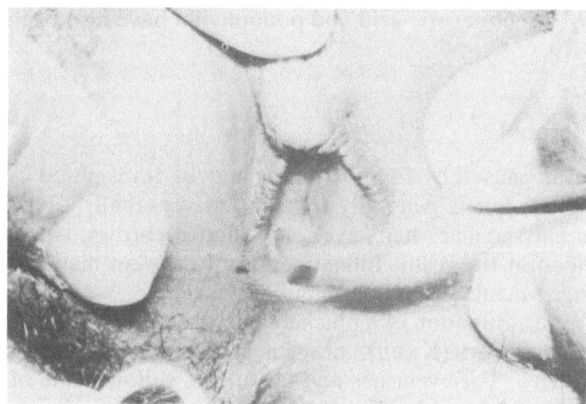

Fig. 5   Collection of vaginal contents is facilitated by introducing a lubricated No. 8 French feeding tube

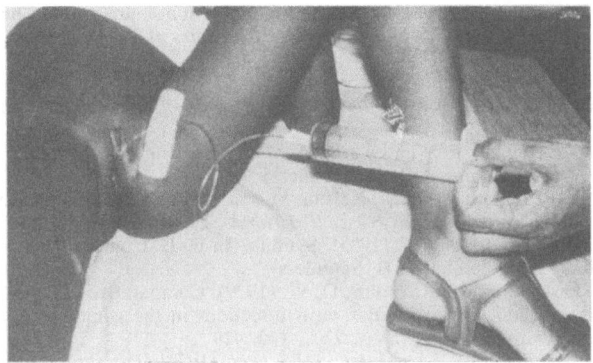

Fig. 6 Vaginal contents may be aspirated either with or without prior vaginal washing

may be collected with the aid of a No. 8 French feeding tube, with or without vaginal washing (Figs 5 and 6)

In treating STD in children, doses of systemic medications should be determined per unit of body weight. Topical vaginal medications should be instilled with the tip of a small syringe.

The knowledgeable pediatrician may effectively serve as a child's advocate, by knowing the hallmarks of sexual abuse, as well as by insisting that sexual relations, inflicted or voluntary, are nonphysiologic in the estrogen-deficient child.

References

Baker, C. J., Goroff, D. K., Albert, S. L. *et al.* (1976). Comparison of bacteriological methods for the isolation of Group B streptococcus from vaginal cultures. *J. Clin. Microbiol.*, **4**, 46

Boisvert, P. L. and Walcher, D. N. (1948). Hemolytic streptococcal vaginitis in children. *Pediatrics*, **2, 24**

Bowie, W. R., Alexander, E. R. and Holmes, K. K. (1977). Chlamydial pharyngitis? *Sex. Transm. Dis.*, **4**, 140

Caine, V. A., Handsfield, H. H., Chandler, S. C. *et al.* (1981). Sexual transmission of cytomegalovirus (Abstract). *Inter-Science Conf. on Antimicrobial Agents and Chemotherapy* (Chicago)

Corey, L., Nahmias, A. J. and Guinan, M. E. (1982). A trial of topical acyclovir in genital herpes simplex virus infections. *N. Engl. J. Med.*, **306**, 1313

Davis, C. M. (1970). Granuloma inguinale: a clinical, histological and ultrastructural study. *J. Am. Med. Assoc.*, **211**, 632

Epstein, E. (1975). Pediculosis pubis. *Med. Asp. Hum. Sexual.*, **9, 8**

Felman, Y. M., William, D. C. and Corsaro, M. C. (1978). Gonococcal infections in children 14 years and younger. *Clin Pediatr.*, **17**, 252

Fiumara, N. J. (1982). Scabies and genital herpes: a problem in management. *Am. Fam. Pract.*, **25**, 125

Fraser, J. J., Rettig, P. J. and Kaplan, D. W. (1983). Prevalence of cervical Chlamydia trachomatis and Neisseria gonorrhoeae in female adolescents. *Pediatrics*, **71**, 333

Hammerschlag, M. R., Baker, C. J., Alpert, S. *et al.* (1977). Colonization with group B streptococci in girls under 16 years of age. *Pediatrics*, **60**, 473

Handsfield, H. H. (1982). Sexually transmitted diseases. *Hosp. Pract.*, **17**, 99

Hare, M. J. and Mowla, A. (1977). Genital herpesvirus infection in a prepubertal girl. *Br. J. Obstet. Gynaecol.*, **84**, 141

Hart, G. (1979). Chancroid, Donovanosis and Lymphogranuloma venereum. U.S. Dept. HEW (CDC), **79**, 8302

Holmes, K. K. and Perine, P. T. (1977). Lymphogranuloma venereum. In Thorn, G., Adams, R. D., Braunwald, E. *et al.* (eds.). *Harrison's Principles of Internal Medicine*, p. 972 (New York: McGraw-Hill)

Holmes, K. K. (1977). Granuloma inguinale; chancroid; syphilis. In Thorn, G., Adams, R. D., Braunwald, E. *et al.* (eds.). *Harrison's Principles of Internal Medicine*, p. 872 (New York: McGraw-Hill)

Huffman, J. W., Dewhurst, J. and Capraro, V. (1981). *The Gynecology of Childhood and Adolescence*. (Philadelphia: W. B. Saunders)

Karney, W. W., Pederson, A. H. B., Nelson, M. *et al.* (1977). Spectinomycin vs. Tetracycline for the treatment of gonorrhea. *N. Engl. J. Med.*, **196**, 889

Kelly, A. P. and Singleton, A. F. (1983). Syphilis. In R. B. Conn (ed.). *Current Diagnosis: 1980*, p. 202 (Philadelphia: W. B. Saunders)

Knox, G. E., Pass, R. F. and Reynolds, D. W. (1979). Comparative prevalence of subclinical cytomegalovirus and herpes simplex virus infections in the genital and urinary tracts of low-income urban women, *J. Infect. Dis.*, **140**, 419

Lee, Y-H., McCormack, W. M., Marcy, S. M. *et al.* (1974). The genital mycoplasmas: their role in disorders of reproduction and in pediatric infections. *Pediatr. Clin. N. Am.*, **21**, 457

Levy, H. (1940). Lymphogranuloma venereum in childhood. *Arch. Pediatr.*, **57**, 441

Pheifer, T. A., Forsyth, P. S., Durfe, M. A. *et al.* (1978). Nonspecific vaginitis: role of Haemophilus vaginalis and treatment with metronidazole. *N. Engl. J. Med.*, **298**, 1429

Platt, M. S. (1971). Neonatal Hemophilus vaginalis (Corynebacterium vaginalis) infection. *Clin. Pediatr.*, **10**, 513

Postlethwaite, R. (1970). Molluscum contagiosum: a review. *Arch. Envir. Hlth.*, **21**, 432

Powers, G. F. and Boisvert, P. (1944). Age as a factor in streptococcosis. *J. Pediatr.*, **25**, 481

Purola, E. and Savia, E. (1977). Cytology of gynecologic Condyloma acuminatum. *Acta Cytol.*, **21**, 26

Quinn, T. C., Goodell, S. E. and Mkrtichian, E. (1981). Chlamydia trachomatis proctitis. *N. Engl. J. Med.*, **305**, 195

Rettig, P. J. and Nelson, J. D. (1981). Genital tract infection with Chlamydia trachomatis in prepubertal children. *J. Pediatr.*, **99**, 206

Ribeiro, J. (1972). Granuloma inguinale. *Practitioner*, **209**, 628

Saltz, G. R., Linnemann, C. C., Brookman, R. R. *et al.* (1981). Chlamydia trachomatis cervical infections in female adolescents. *J. Pediatr.*, **98**, 981

Schachter, J. (1978a). Chlamydial infections. I. *N. Engl. J. Med.*, **298**, 428

Schachter, J. (1978b). Chlamydial infections. II. *N. Engl. J. Med.*, **298**, 490

Schachter, J. (1978c). Chlamydial infections. III. *N. Engl. J. Med.*, **298**, 540

Schachter, J. and Atwood, G. (1975). Chlamydial pharyngitis? *J. Am. Vener. Dis. Assoc.*, **2**, 12

Sgroi, S. M. (1982). Pediatric gonorrhea and child sexual abuse: the venereal disease connection. *Sex Transm. Dis.*, **9**, 154

Siegel, J. D., McCracken, G. H., Threlkeld, N. *et al.* (1980). Single-dose penicillin prophylaxis against neonatal group B streptococcal infections. *N. Engl. J. Med.*, **303**, 769

Singleton, A. F. (1980). Vaginal discharge in children and adolescents: evolution and management – a review. *Clin. Pediatr.*, **19**, 799

Singleton, A. F. (1981). An approach to the management of gonorrhea in the pediatric age group. *J. Nat. Med. Assoc.*, **73**, 207

Singleton, A. F. (1983). Gynecology of the premenarchal child; a guide for the general pediatrician. In J. M. Mellinger and G. B. Stickler (eds.). *Critical Issues of Pediatrics*, p. 258 (Philadelphia: J. B. Lippincott)

Smith, D. E. and Walsh, J. (1980). Treatment of pubic lice infestation. *Cutis*, **26**, 618

Stumpf, P. G. (1980). Increasing occurrence of Condylomata acuminata in premenarchal children. *Obstet. Gynecol.*, **56**, 262

Taylor-Robinson, D. and McCormack, W. M. (1980). The genital mycoplasmas. II. *N. Engl. J. Med.*, **302**, 1063

Venkataramani, T. M. and Rathbun, H. K. (1976). *Corynebacterium vaginale (Hemophilus vaginalis)* bacteremia: clinical study of 29 cases. *The Johns Hopkins Med. J.*, **139**, 93

Vesterinen, E., Purola, E., Saksela, E. *et al.* (1977). Clinical and virological findings in patients with cytologically diagnosed gynecologic herpes simplex infections. *Acta Cytologica*, **21**, 199

2
Special Topics

10
Ureaplasma urealyticum infections in infertility and pregnancy

W. FOULON, A. NAESSENS, S. LAUWERS and J. J. AMY

INTRODUCTION

The organism *Ureaplasma urealyticum* was first isolated from a man with nongonococcal urethritis (Shepard, 1954). It formerly was known as *T. mycoplasma* or *T-strain mycoplasma* because of the very small size of its colonies (tiny form PPLO colonies). Since it has the unique ability to metabolize urea, this organism was placed in a new genus, and is now called *Ureaplasma urealyticum* (Shepard *et al.*, 1974). At least 10 serotypes are recognized.

Ureaplasma are commonly found in the genital tracts of both men and women. Infants generally become colonized during their passage through the birth canal, a phenomenon that occurs less frequently among those delivered by Cesarean section (Klein *et al.*, 1969). Neonatal colonization does not persist, however, and most infants are soon free of the organisms. Adults may acquire ureaplasma during sexual contact. The likelihood of harboring *U. urealyticum* increases with the number of sexual partners (McCormack *et al.*, 1972).

Other factors affecting the colonization rate are race and socioeconomic status. Ureaplasmas have been isolated more frequently from black than from white women (McCormack *et al.*, 1973; Braun *et al.*, 1971), the colonization rate is higher among patients from lower socioeconomic classes (McCormack *et al.*, 1973). The prevalence of genital ureaplasma infection decreases after the menopause (Mårdh and Westrøm, 1970).

UREAPLASMA UREALYTICUM IN INFERTILITY

Kundsin (1970) was the first to report a case in which a successful pregnancy was achieved following eradication of ureaplasma from the genital tracts of an infertile couple. The initial suggestion of an association between genital ureaplasma infestation and subfertility generated considerable interest. Gnarpe and Friberg (1972) isolated ureaplasma significantly more frequently ($p<0.001$) from the cervix (86% vs. 23%) or the semen (83% vs. 26%) in 36 couples with primary infertility of unknown origin of more than 5 years than in fertile subjects. Similar observations were made in 19 couples having serum antibodies agglutinating donor sperm. In these 55 couples doxycycline therapy for up to 5 months was followed by pregnancy in 15 cases (27%) (Friberg and Gnarpe, 1973). This study, however, did not include controls; furthermore, doxycycline could have eradicated other organisms implicated in the pathogenesis of subferti-lity.

A study investigating 120 infertile couples and 92 pregnant women was unable to find any differences in the isolation rates for *Ureaplasma urealyticum* (de Louvois *et al.*, 1974). In another study, subfertile subjects were treated with either doxycycline or a placebo, and no discernible difference was observed in terms of the pregnancy rate (Harrison *et al.*, 1975). These observations have since been confirmed by other authors (Matthews *et al.*, 1975, 1978).

Numerous other isolation studies, however, have shown divergent results (Tables 1 and 2). In a 1978 report, Stray-Pedersen *et al.* documented higher ureaplasma isolation rates from the cervix (83% vs. 49%) and from the endometrium (50% vs. 7%) in infertile than in fertile women. Only the difference in endometrial infestation rates reached statistical significance, how-ever. In a later study, Stray-Pedersen (1979) reported isolation of ureaplasma from the endometrium in 26% of 375 infertile patients as compared to only 8% in a control group. Similar differences in the isolation rates were found regardless of the cause of infertility (tubal occlusions, male infertility, other known cause of infertility, unexplained infertility). Eradication of ureaplasma from the endometrium did not result in an increased number of conceptions in the group with unexplained infertility. None of the women with a husband suffering from azoospermia harbored ureaplasma in the endometrium, even though five of the women harbored the organism in the cervix.

Table 1 Isolation studies of *Ureaplasma urealyticum* in infertile and fertile patients

Authors	Isolation in infertile patients			Isolation in fertile patients		
	N	Cervix/vagina (%)	Semen (%)	N	Cervix/vagina (%)	Semen (%)
Gnarpe *et al.* (1972)	36	86	83	40	23	—
	19	100	89	23	—	26
de Louvois *et al.* (1974)	120	52	—	92	55	—
	109	—	39	38	—	32
Matthews *et al.* (1975)	124	51	40	92	66	—
Rehewy *et al.* (1978)	21	47	—	17	35	—
Nagata *et al.* (1979)	40	63	—	80	65	—
Graber *et al.* (1979)	25	84	—	25	60	—
Stray-Pedersen *et al.* (1979)	379	57	—	40	48	—
Cassell *et al.* (1983)	133	42	—	61	34	—

Table 2 Pregnancy rate in infertile women after treatment for *Ureaplasma urealyticum* infection

Authors	Treatment group	N	Pregnancy rate (%)
Friberg and Gnarpe (1973)	Unexplained infertility		
	Treated doxycycline	55	27
Harrison *et al.* (1975)	Unexplained infertility		
	Treated doxycycline	30	17
	Treated placebo	28	14
Matthews *et al.* (1978)	Unexplained infertility		
	Ureaplasma pos. treated	51	20
	Ureaplasma pos. not treated	18	22
	Ureaplasma neg. treated	21	14
	Ureaplasma neg. not treated	24	25
Rehewy *et al.* (1978)	Infertility		
	Treated tetracycline	19	5
Stray-Pedersen *et al.* (1979)	Unexplained infertility		
	Pos. endometrium treated	46	26
	Pos. cervix not treated	56	22
	Neg. not treated	73	16

Toth *et al.* (1983) treated 161 couples in whom *U. urealyticum* was isolated in the male partner. Within 3 years of treatment, pregnancy was achieved in 60% of the couples who were successfully treated for the ureaplasma infection; in contrast, only 5% of those in whom the microorganism could not be eradicated were able to achieve pregnancy. Cassell *et al.* (1983) investigated 56 fertile couples and 194 couples with infertility of various origins. The rates of colonization by ureaplasma of the lower genital tract were comparable among women belonging to either the fertile (34%) or the subfertile group (42%). In women whose partners were considered the cause of infertility, the prevalence of ureaplasma infestation of the lower genital tract was significantly higher than in any other infertility subgroup ($p < 0.05$) and was more than twice as high as in all infertile women combined ($p < 0.005$). The endometrium was colonized in only 1% of the subjects having a positive cervical culture.

Numerous investigators have reported on the role of *U. urealyticum* in relation to the quality of the semen. Some studies suggest that ureaplasma may interfere with spermatogenesis. Semen samples containing ureaplasma had fewer spermatozoa, and those present were less motile and included more aberrant forms than ureaplasma-free samples (Fowlkes *et al.*, 1975). Ureaplasma has also been isolated from testicular biopsy specimens of infertile men (Engel and Baumann, 1979) and from prostatic tissue (Hofstetter, 1977). A return to normal semen quality may take as long as 6 months after spermatogenesis has been restored. The length of this interval may be one of the reasons why some authors failed to observe an improvement in the quality of the semen following eradication of *U. urealyticum* (Swenson *et al.*, 1979). Aparicco *et al.* (1980) and Toth and Lesser (1982) reported improved quality of the semen following treatment of men with genital ureaplasma infection and impaired sperm motility and vitality. Contradictory results were published by Desai *et al.* (1980) and Cintron *et al.* (1981). Valvo *et al.* (1982) found that genital infection by *U. urealyticum* resulted in a higher pH of the semen that reverted to normal following eradication of the microorganism.

The variable results obtained by different investigators may partly stem from the lack of uniformity in the definitions used as well as differences in study methodology. Nonetheless, it would presently seem that ureaplasma does not play an 'all-or-none' role in the etiology of human infertility. Since infertility frequently is multifactorial in origin, these microorganisms may play a contributory role. To elicit the latter, further investigation of the effects of *U. urealyticum* on specific aspects of human fertility is needed.

UREAPLASMA UREALYTICUM IN SPONTANEOUS ABORTION

Epidemiology

The frequency of recognized spontaneous abortion in the general population ranges between 15% and 20%. A recent study that used a radioimmunoassay technique for human chorionic gonadotropin (HCG) found an embryonic wastage rate of 43% (Thiller *et al.*, 1981). It generally has been estimated that the very early spontaneous abortion rate ranges from 30% to 50%. In view of this apparent high frequency of spontaneous abortion only patients with repeated early pregnancy wastage should be investigated. In about 50% of these cases no etiologic factor is found. Despite one decade of research, it remains unclear whether *U. urealyticum* can cause spontaneous and/or recurrent spontaneous miscarriage.

The recovery of *U. urealyticum* from the decidua, chorion, and amnion following spontaneous abortion at 17 weeks' gestation by Kundsin *et al.* (1967) has suggested a possible role for this microorganism in the causation of miscarriage. Support for this view is provided by the results of two prospective studies that demonstrated a higher incidence of genital tract colonization by *U. urealyticum* among women who eventually aborted spontaneously than among women who carried their pregnancies successfully to term (Kundsin *et al.*, 1970; Braun *et al.*, 1971). The demonstration of such an association is of great interest, since treatment of the infection with a tetracycline or another antibiotic is possible.

In 1969, Driscoll *et al.* reported on six women with a history of recurrent abortion. In five of them cervical cultures for *U. urealyticum* were performed and four yielded the microorganism. All six women were subsequently treated with Declomycin before and during their next pregnancy. Only one of these pregnancies ended in spontaneous abortion. Other workers also described successful pregnancies after antibiotic treatment (Kundsin, 1970; Stray-Pedersen, 1979; Quinn *et al.*, 1983). Unfortunately, these observations are inconclusive since a control group treated with a placebo was not studied as well.

Ureaplasmas were isolated more often from products of conception after spontaneous first and midtrimester abortions than after induced abortion (Caspi *et al.*, 1972; Sompolinsky *et al.*, 1975). However, it is not clear from these studies whether *U. urealyticum* is involved in the etiology of spontaneous abortion, or whether the microorganism only invades the uterine cavity after fetal death has occurred from some other cause.

Another possible role for *U. urealyticum* in recurrent abortion was suggested by Stray-Pedersen *et al.* (1979). These researchers studied the presence of *U. urealyticum* in the cervix and endometrium in a group of 46 habitual aborters and found that cervical colonization was more frequent in the recurrent abortion group (61%) than in a group of controls (49%). Moreover, endometrial colonization was significantly higher in the study group (28% vs. 7% for the control subjects). The post-treatment pregnancy rate showed an improved outcome in the group with positive endometrial colonization.

Colonization of the cervix and the endometrium by *U. urealyticum* in women with repeated fetal wastage was also investigated by Foulon *et al.* (1983), who isolated the organism in 71% of 31 patients with recurrent spontaneous abortion. This isolation rate was significantly higher than the 40% found in 205 normal pregnant women. Endometrial tissue obtained in patients with recurrent abortions was more often positive (35%) than that obtained in the control group of 34 normal fertile patients (12%). These results suggest an association between maternal colonization by *U. urealyticum* and pregnancy wastage. However, considering only patients with positive cervical cultures in the group of habitual aborters and in the fertile group, no significant difference in endometrial colonization would be shown. This is probably due to the small number of patients with positive cervical cultures studied. Subclinical endometrial infection with *U. urealyticum* was considered to be an important factor in recurrent miscarriage by the last two groups of investigators.

Quinn *et al.* (1983b) studied the antibody levels in eight serotypes of *U. urealyticum* in 14 women with a history of spontaneous abortion. In this small group the mean levels assessed at delivery showed a significant elevation for serotypes 4 and 8 and a smaller, nonsignificant elevation for serotype 6. Since these antibodies did not cross the placenta, they might be IgM-specific and indicate the mothers' immune response to the infection. Infants of mothers with previous pregnancy losses had elevated levels for serotypes 6 and 8, suggesting that the fetuses responded immunologically to an *U. urealyticum* infection *in utero*. These results support the idea that there may be a true maternal and fetal infection during pregnancy. Some serotypes such as 4, 6 and 8, may be more pathogenic than others.

Pathogenesis

It is not clear by what mechanisms *U. urealyticum* exerts its pathogenic effects. A direct fetal infection resulting in fetal death is one possible explanation. The recovery of ureaplasma from the lungs and viscera of spontaneously aborted fetuses suggests such a possibility. The microorganism was isolated from the placenta, heart and lungs of a fetus aborted in the 19th week of gestation (Romano *et al.*, 1971). Histologic examination showing an inflammatory process in the lungs suggested that an overwhelming acute infection had taken place before fetal death. Recovery of ureaplasma from placentas obtained during cesarean sections performed before rupture of the membranes confirms that these agents can gain access to the amniotic cavity even through intact membranes (Caspi *et al.*, 1976).

Chromosomal aberrations are found in the products of conception in approximately 50% of first trimester spontaneous abortions (Boué *et al.*, 1975). It is not known whether these abnormalities arise spontaneously from random errors in meiosis or mitosis, or whether they result from exposure to noxious agents. *In vitro* studies have revealed that *U. urealyticum* infection may damage chromosomes in cell cultures (Kundsin *et al.*, 1971). This finding suggests that *U. urealyticum* may induce chromosomal aberrations in the zygote with subsequent miscarriage.

The induction of a subclinical inflammation of the endometrium is a third possible mechanism by which ureaplasmas may exert pathogenic effects. Horne *et al.* (1973) found an association between positive ureaplasma cultures in the cervix and urine and histologic evidence of endometritis. The low pathogenicity of the microorganism may explain the absence of clinical signs of endometritis. Indeed, it is likely that *U. urealyticum* can colonize the uterine cavity in some specific pathologic conditions such as death *in utero*, an open cervical canal, or bleeding in pregnancy. It is more difficult to explain how ureaplasma gain access to the endometrium in the absence of any pathology. It is possible that spermatozoa may carry ureaplasma to the interior of the uterine cavity before pregnancy commences. Scanning electronmicroscopy of infected semen samples has revealed that ureaplasma can adhere to spermatozoa (Fowlkes *et al.*, 1975). In most cases they are localized at the junction between the spermhead and the midpiece (Hofstetter *et al.*, 1978). These findings could explain the endometrial colonization in some patients.

Management and therapy

Since the prevalence of *U. urealyticum* in the cervix of normal pregnant women is high, it is not advisable to perform routine prenatal cultures. Neither is it necessary to treat couples with a history of one spontaneous abortion. However, in patients with two or more spontaneous abortions it is reasonable to obtain a culture of the cervix, endometrium and sperm for *U. urealyticum*. If one of these cultures is positive, doxycycline should be given to both partners for 10 days. Contraception must be provided because of the known harmful effect of this antibiotic on the embryo. One month after therapy a repeat culture should be obtained. Treatment should be continued until the couple is clear of ureaplasma, although this is not always easy to achiéve (Gnarpe and Friberg, 1973). If cultures remain positive after 10 days of therapy, a sensitivity test should be performed; approximately 10% of *U. urealyticum* strains show *in vitro* resistance to tetracycline (Evans and Taylor-Robinson, 1978). Some alternative antibiotic therapy should be chosen in accordance with the sensitivity studies.

UREAPLASMA UREALYTICUM IN INTRAUTERINE GROWTH RETARDATION

In a double-blind study, Elder *et al.* (1968) reported that women who had been treated for 6 weeks with a tetracycline during pregnancy gave birth to fewer infants weighing less than 2500 g than those who had received no antibiotics. It is possible that tetracycline-sensitive organisms (which also include the ureaplasma) might have been responsible for the observed difference. The first direct evidence that *U. urealyticum* could retard intrauterine growth was reported by Klein *et al.* (1969). They found that newborns colonized by ureaplasma weighed significantly less (2605 g) than infants not colonized (2952 g; $p<0.01$). Similarly, Braun *et al.* (1971) stated that women with ureaplasma in either cervix or urine gave birth to infants weighing a mean of 202 g less than women of the same gestational age who were not colonized. ureaplasma was cultured from the nose or the throat of 28% of the newborns of 2500 g or less, but only in 5% of those with a birthweight of over 2500 g ($p<0.001$). According to Embree *et al.* (1980), placental colonization by *U. urealyticum* was found significantly more frequently in growth-retarded pregnancies (22.4%) than in a control group (9.3%; $p<0.01$).

In spite of these observations, no correlation was found in other studies between maternal genital colonization by *U. urealyticum* and intrauterine growth retardation (IUGR). Thus, Shurin *et al.* (1975) observed no increase in vaginal colonization by ureaplasma in women with growth-retarded pregnancies. Moreover, the mean birth weight of infants born to mothers colonized was 3169 g, whereas it was 3107 g in babies belonging to the control group. The isolation of ureaplasma from the newborn was significantly associated to the presence of chorioamnionitis. Ross *et al.* (1981) also found no relation between maternal cervical colonization by *Ureaplasma* and birth weight of the infant. In our own material (Naessens *et al.*, 1983), neither cervical (47% of the cases) nor placental colonization (24%) were associated with low birth weight or prematurity. Patients with positive cervical or placental cultures gave birth to infants weighing a mean of 111 g and 93 g less, respectively, than those of the control group; but these differences were not statistically significant.

It has been suggested that *U. urealyticum* could induce IUGR by causing chorioamnionitis, thereby interfering with fetomaternal exchanges. Indeed, chorioamnionitis was found significantly more frequently when ureaplasma were cultured from the newborn (Shurin *et al.*, 1975) and remained at a statistically significant level even when other factors causing chorioamnionitis were taken into consideration. Note, however, that the chorioamnionitis was only related to the isolation of ureaplasma from the newborn and not to genital colonization of the mother, suggesting that the isolation of ureaplasma from the newborn could merely be the consequence of membrane rupture. Chorioamnionitis was also related to positive placental cultures for ureaplasmas. Embree *et al.* (1980) found not only a correlation between chorioamnionitis and positive placental cultures, but also a correlation between a positive placental culture and the duration of membrane rupture. From the available data it cannot be ruled out that both the colonization of the fetus and the placenta and the chorioamnionitis merely resulted from the rupture of the membranes.

There are two explanations for the discrepancies among these observations. First, certain serotypes of *U. urealyticum*, perhaps more pathogenic than others, might be more prevalent in certain geographic areas. This question needs further investigation. Second, patients of lower socioeconomic status might be more susceptible to develop infection by ureaplasma and/or complica-

INFECTIONS IN REPRODUCTIVE HEALTH

tions. Tafari *et al.* (1976) isolated *U. urealyticum* as the sole microorganism from the lungs of 21 stillborn infants. Autopsy revealed signs of congenital pneumonitis, indicating that infection had taken place prior to fetal death. This study was done in Addis Ababa, Ethiopia, where the socioeconomic level is low. Braun *et al.* (1971) and Shurin *et al.* (1975), studying populations of low socioeconomic status and with a high percentage of blacks, reported isolation rates of ureaplasmas from the lower genital tract of 79% and 75% respectively. In contrast, Ross *et al.* (1981) and Naessens *et al.* (1983) found genital colonization by ureaplasma in only 43% and 41%, respectively, in women belonging to a higher socioeconomic class.

In the study by Braun *et al.* (1971), infection by ureaplasma was associated with lower birth weights only in black patients, strongly suggesting that socioeconomic status plays a role in the causation of IUGR, in the presence of the microorganism.

Table 3 *Ureaplasma urealyticum* isolation in relation to infant birth weight

			Birth weight in g		p value
Authors	N	Site cultured	Pos. cultures	Neg. cultures	
Klein *et al.* (1969)	221	Newborn	2605	2952	p<0.01
Braun *et al.* (1971)	485	Cervix/urine	3099	3297	p<0.003
Shurin *et al.* (1975)	249	Vagina/newborn	3169	3107	NS
Embree *et al.* (1980)	446[a]	Placenta (high risk)	3248		p<0.001
	108	Placenta (control)		3526	
Ross *et al.* (1982)	134[b]	Cervix	3490	3260	p<0.025
Naessens *et al.* (1983)	128	Cervix	3190	3301	NS
		Placenta	3299	3392	NS

NS: not significant
[a] Only birth weights of infants with a gestational age of at least 38 weeks are recorded
[b] Only data on Caucasian women are recorded

References

Aparicco, N. J., Muchirik, G., Levalle, O. *et al.* (1980). The effect of a treatment with doxycycline on semen of asthenospermic patients with T-mycoplasma genital infection. *Andrologia*, **12**, 521

Boué, I., Boué, A. and Lazar, P. (1975). Retrospective and prospective epidemiologic studies of 1500 karyotyped spontaneous human abortions. *Teratology*, **12**, 11

Braun, P., Lee, Y. H., Klein, J. O. *et al.* (1971). Birth weight and genital mycoplasmas in pregnancy. *N. Engl. J. Med.*, **284**, 167

Caspi, E., Solomon, F. and Sompolinsky, D. (1972). Early abortion and mycoplasma infection. *Israel J. Med. Sci.*, **8**, 122

Caspi, E., Solomon, F., Langer, R. *et al.* (1976). Isolation of mycoplasmas from the placentas after cesarean section. *Obstet. Gynecol.*, **48**, 682

Cassell, G. H., Younger, J. B., Brown, M. B. *et al.* (1983). Microbiologic study of infertile women at the time of diagnostic laparoscopy. Association of *Ureaplasma urealyticum* with a defined subpopulation. *N. Engl. J. Med.*, **308**, 502

Cintron, R. D., Wortham, J. W. and Acosta, A. (1981). The association of semen factors with the recovery of *Ureaplasma urealyticum*. *Fertil Steril.*, **36**, 648

de Louvois, J., Blades, M., Harrison, R. F. *et al.* (1974). Frequency of mycoplasma in fertile and infertile couples. *Lancet*, **1**, 1073

Desai, S., Cohen, M. S., Khatamee, M. *et al.* (1980). Ureaplasma urealyticum (T-myco-plasma) infection: does it have a role in male infertility? *J. Urol.*, **124**, 469

Driscoll, S. G., Kundsin, R. B., Horne, H. W. *et al.* (1969). Infections and first trimester losses: possible role of mycoplasmas. *Fertil. Steril.*, **20**, 1017

Elder, H. A., Smith, R. and Kass, E. H. (1968). *Effects of Tetracycline on Outcome of Pregnancy in Nonbacteriuric Patients.* VIII interscience conference on Antimicrobial Agents and Chemotherapy. New York

Embree, J. E., Krause, V. W., Embil, J. A. *et al.* (1980). Placental infection with Mycoplasma hominis and Ureaplasma urealyticum: Clinical correlation. *Obstet. Gynecol.*, **56**, 475

Engel, S. and Baumann, B. (1979). Das Vorkommen von Mykoplasmen in Hoden gewebe. *Dermatol. Monatschr.*, **165**, 593

Evans, R. T. and Taylor-Robinson, D. (1978). The incidence of tetracycline resistant strains of ureaplasma urealyticum. *J. Antimicrob. Chemother.*, **4**, 57

Foulon, W., Naessens, A., Volckaert, M. *et al.* (1983). *Prevalence of Ureaplasma Urealyticum in Habitual Abortion.* XI World Congress on Fertility and Sterility, Dublin

Fowlkes, D. M., Dooher, G. B. and O'Leary, W. M. (1975). Evidence by scanning electron microscopy for an association between spermatozoa and T-mycoplasmas in men of infertile marriages. *Fertil. Steril.*, **26**, 1203.

Fowlkes, D. M., MacLeod, J. and O'Leary, W. M. (1975). T-mycoplasmas and human infertility: Correlation of infection with alterations in seminal parameters. *Fertil. Steril.*, **26**, 1212

Friberg, J. and Gnarpe, H. (1973). Mycoplasma and human reproductive failure. III. Pregnan-cies in 'infertile' couples treated with doxycycline for T-mycoplasmas. *Am. J. Obstet. Gynecol.*, **116**, 23

Gnarpe, H. and Friberg, J. (1972). Mycoplasma and human reproductive failure. I. The occurrence of different mycoplasmas in couples with reproductive failure. *Am. J. Obstet. Gynecol.*, **114**, 727

Gnarpe, H. and Friberg, J. (1973). T-mycoplasmas as a possible cause for reproductive failure. *Nature*, **242**, 120

Graber, C. D., Creticos, P., Valicenti, J. *et al.* (1979). T-mycoplasma in human reproductive failure. *Obstet. Gynecol.*, **54**, 558

Harrison, R. F., Blades, M., de Louvois, J. *et al.* (1975). Doxycycline treatment and human infertility. *Lancet*, **1**, 605

Hofstetter, A. (1977). Mycoplasmen Infektion des Urogenital Traktes. *Hautarzt*, **28**, 295

Hofstetter, A., Schmeidt, E., Schill, W. B. *et al.* (1978). Genital Mykoplasmen Stämme als Ursache der männlichen Infertilität. *Helv. Chir. Acta*, **45**, 329

Horne, H. W., Hertig, H. T., Kundsin, R. B. *et al.* (1973). Subclinical endometrial inflamma-tion and T-mycoplasma: A possible cause of human reproductive failure. *Int. J. Fertil.*, **18**, 226

Klein, J. O., Buckland, D. and Finland, M. (1969). Colonization of newborn infants by mycoplasmas. *N. Engl. J. Med.*, **280**, 1025

Kundsin, R. B. (1970). Mycoplasma in genitourinary tract infection and reproductive failure. In: S. H. Sturgis and M. Taymor (eds.) *Progress in Gynecology*, vol. 5, p. 275. (New York: Grune & Stratton)

Kundsin, R. B., Ampola, M., Streeter, S. *et al.* (1971). Chromosomal aberrations induced by T-strain mycoplasmas. *J. Med. Genet.*, **8**, 181

Kundsin, R. B., Driscoll, S. G. and Ming, P. L. (1967). Strain of mycoplasma associated with human reproductive failure. *Science*, **157**, 1573

Mårdh, P.-A. and Westrøm, L. (1970). Mycoplasmas in the genito-urinary tract of the female. *Acta Pathol. Microbiol. Scand.*, **78**, 367B

Matthews, C. D., Clapp, K. H., Tansing, J. A. *et al.* (1978). T-mycoplasma genital infection: The effect of doxycycline therapy on human unexplained infertility. *Fertil. Steril.*, **30**, 98

Matthews, C. D., Elmslie, R. G., Clapp, K. H. *et al.* (1975). The frequency of genital mycoplasma infection in human fertility. *Fertil. Steril.*, **26**, 988

McCormack, W. M., Almeida, P. C., Bailey, P. E. *et al.* (1972). Sexual activity and vaginal colonization with genital mycoplasmas. *J. Am. Med. Assoc.*, **221**, 1375

McCormack, W. M., Rosner, B. and Lee, Y. H. (1973). Colonization with genital mycoplas-mas in women. *Am. J. Epidemiol.*, **97**, 240

Miller, J. F., Williamson, E. M., Glu, J. *et al.* (1981). Fetal loss after implantation: prospective study. *Lancet*, **2**, 554

Naessens, A., Foulon, W., Volckaert, M. *et al.* (1983). Cervical and placental colonization with Ureaplasma urealyticum and fetal outcome. *J. Infect. Dis.*, **148**, 333

Nagata, Y., Iwasaka, T. and Wada, T. (1979). Mycoplasma infection and infertility. *Fertil. Steril.*, **31**, 392

Quin, P. A., Shewchuk, A. B., Shuber, J. *et al.* (1983). Efficacy of antibiotic therapy in preventing spontaneous pregnancy loss among couples colonized with genital mycoplasmas. *Am. J. Obstet. Gynecol.*, **145**, 239

Quin, P. A., Shewchuk, A. B., Shuber, J. *et al.* (1983b). Serologic evidence of Ureaplasma urealyticum infection in women with spontaneous pregnancy loss. *Am. J. Obstet. Gynecol.*, **145**, 245

Rehewy, M. S. E., Jasczak, C., Hafez, E. S. E. *et al.* (1978). *Ureaplasma urealyticum* (T-mycoplasma) in vaginal fluid and cervical mucus from fertile and infertile women. *Fertil. Steril.*, **30**, 297

Romano, N., Romano, F. and Carollo, F. (1971). T-strains of mycoplasma in bronchopneumonic lungs of an aborted fetus. *N. Engl. Med. J.*, **285**, 950

Ross, J. M., Furr, P. M., Taylor-Robinson, D. *et al.* (1981). The effect of genital mycoplasmas on human fetal growth. *Br. J. Obstet. Gynaecol.*, **88**, 749

Shepard, M. C. (1954). The recovery of pleuropneumonia-like organisms from Negro men with and without non-gonococcal urethritis. *Am. J. Syph. Gon. Vener. Dis.*, **38**, 113

Shepard, M. C., Lunceford, C. D., Ford, D. K. *et al.* (1974). *Ureaplasma urealyticum* gen. nov., sp. nov.: proposed nomenclature for the human T (T-strain) mycoplasma. *Int. J. Sys. Bacteriol.*, **24**, 160

Shurin, R. P., Alpert, S., Rosner, B. *et al.* (1975). Chorioamnionitis and colonization of the newborn infant with genital mycoplasmas. *N. Engl. J. Med.*, **293**, 5

Sompolinsky, D., Solomon, F., Ellkina, L. *et al.* (1975). Infections with mycoplasmas and bacteria in induced mid-trimester abortion and fetal loss. *Am. J. Obstet. Gynecol.*, **121**, 610

Stray-Pedersen, B. (1979). Female genital colonization with Ureaplasma urealyticum and reproductive failure. *Curr. Ther. Res.*, **26**, 771

Stray-Pedersen, B., Eng, Y. and Reikvam, T. M. (1978). Uterine T-mycoplasma colonization in reproductive failure. *Am. J. Obstet. Gynecol.*, **130**, 307

Swenson, C. E., Toth, A. and O'Leary, W. M. (1979). Ureaplasma urealyticum and human infertility: The effect of antibiotic therapy on semen quality. *Fertil. Steril.*, **31**, 660

Tafari, N., Ross, S., Naege, R. L. *et al.* (1976). Mycoplasma T-strain and perinatal death. *Lancet*, **1**, 108

Toth, A. and Lesser, M. L. (1982). Ureaplasma urealyticum and infertility: the effect of different antibiotic regimens on the semen quality. *J. Urol.*, **128**, 705

Toth, A., Lesser, M. L., Brooks, C. *et al.* (1983). Subsequent pregnancies among 161 couples treated for T-mycoplasma genital tract infection. *N. Engl. J. Med.*, **208**, 505

Valvo, J. R., Caldamone, A. A., Hipp, S. *et al.* (1982). Elevated seminal pH and *Ureaplasma urealyticum*. *J. Androl.*, **3**, 144

11
The bacteriology, pathogenesis and treatment of *Ureaplasma urealyticum* in human infertility

A. TOTH

INTRODUCTION

Since mycoplasma was first isolated from a genital tract abscess in 1937 (Dienes and Edsall, 1937), the role of this organism in reproductive failure has been controversial. Studies performed during the last several decades have associated mycoplasma with other conditions, such as reproductive failure and relative or absolute infertility. Several investigators have demonstrated that the relative frequency of T-mycoplasma (*Ureaplasma urealyticum*) colonization of the genital tract depends on the number of sexual partners (Horne *et al.*, 1973; Rehewy *et al.*, 1978) and that infertile couples tend to have higher colonization rates than fertile controls (Graber *et al.*, 1979). Nonetheless, epidemiological studies of patients with *Ureaplasma urealyticum* genital tract infections have provided conflicting results regarding its role in infertility and other disorders of the reproductive tract (Shepard *et al.*, 1974).

Ureaplasma has been isolated from tubo-ovarian abscesses (Braun and Besdine, 1973) and in cultures from patients with nonspecific urethritis (Shepard, 1970). Lesions found in certain endometrial biopsy specimens have been attributed to *U. urealyticum* infection (Horne *et al.*, 1973). The organism has also been implicated with spontaneous abortion (Kundsin *et al.*, 1967), chorioamnionitis (Shurin *et al.*, 1975), low birth weight of infants (Braun *et al.*, 1971), and unexplained infertility (Gnarpe and Friberg, 1972; O'Leary and Frick, 1975). The organism can attach itself to spermatozoa and adversely affect spermatozoal motility and morphology (Taylor-Robinson and Manchee, 1967b; Swenson and O'Leary, 1980). However, it is presently not clear whether the organism itself or its metabolic products interfere with sperm function and motility, germ cell migration, and early embryonic development. It remains possible that the organism may simply cause local inflammatory processes in the genital tract which then lead to direct pelvic inflammatory disease or chorioamnionitis. Table 1 lists the chronology of associations of *Ureaplasma* to reproductive failure.

Table 1 Chronology of significant studies relating ureaplasma to reproductive failure

Author	Year	Comment
Taylor-Robinson and Manchee	1967	First demonstration of spermadsorption
Kundsin *et al.*	1967	Recovery of 'T'-mycoplasma from women with reproductive failure
Braun *et al.*	1971	Low birth weight associated with T-mycoplasma infection
Gnarpe and Friberg	1972	High frequency of T-mycoplasma in infertile couples
Friberg and Gnarpe	1973	27% conception rate among unexplained infertile couples after doxycycline therapy
Horn *et al.*	1973	T-mycoplasma-associated endometrial lesion described
deLouvois *et al.*	1974	Same incidence of infection for both fertile and infertile couples
Shurin *et al.*	1975	Mycoplasma isolated from chorioamnionitis
O'Leary and Frick	1975	High frequency of T-mycoplasma in idiopathic infertility cases
Fowlkes *et al.*	1975	Scanning electron microscopic demonstration of ureaplasma and sperm attachment
Matthews *et al.*	1975	Same pregnancy rates with or without ureaplasma among unexplained infertile women treated with antibiotics
Toth *et al.*	1978	Light microscopic predicting factors described in seminal fluid
Swenson *et al.*	1979	Improved semen quality after antibiotic therapy
Cassell	1983	Higher colonization rate in women whose infertility was associated with a male factor
Toth *et al.*	1983	Three-year follow-up of treated patients showing significantly higher pregnancy rates among ureaplasma negative couples, compared with couples colonized with doxycycline-resistant strains

MICROBIOLOGICAL CONSIDERATIONS

Mycoplasmas are the smallest self-replicating procaryotes; they stand between bacteria and viruses and possess RNA as well as DNA components which enable them to reproduce without the host DNA. Because mycoplasmas do not have cell walls, antibiotics that interfere with cell wall synthesis do not affect their replication. Information about the mycoplasma family has significantly increased during the last decade, and there are now over 60 different species described in this group (Tully and Razin, 1977).

Recently, mycoplasma-like organisms have been isolated from insects, plants, rumens of cattle and sheep, and coal refuse. Human mycoplasmas have been isolated frequently from the oral, pharyngeal and genital mucous membranes. *M. pneumoniae* (the Eaton agent) causes atypical pneumonia

(Chanock *et al.*, 1962). *M. salivarium, M. oralae, M. buccale, M. faucium, M. lipophilum,* and *Acholeplasma ladlawii,* all are part of the normal oropharyngeal flora. *M. fermentans* and *M. primatum* have been recovered only occasionally from the human genital tract and have not been implicated convincingly with disease processes (Taylor-Robinson and McCormack, 1979). Two members of the mycoplasma family, the *M. hominis* and the T-mycoplasma (*U. urealyticum*) can frequently be isolated from the genitourinary tract of both males and females. Henceforth, every allusion in this chapter to generic mycoplasma, unless otherwise stated, refers to T-mycoplasma (*U. urealyticum*) or to *M. hominis.*

ISOLATION AND CULTIVATION OF *MYCOPLASMA*

The use of a culture medium which is rich in the basic ingredients (fatty acids, cholesterol) necessary for cell membrane synthesis aids in the isolation and identification of individual *Mycoplasma* species. The addition of horse serum to the media supplies all the essential components and results in a better growth rate. The ureaplasma group differs significantly from the rest of the mycoplasmas because of its ability to hydrolyze urea. This organism fails to grow in conventional mycoplasma media to a titer higher than 10^7 colony units per ml.

Culture specimens for *M. hominis* or for *U. urealyticum* can be obtained from the urogenital tract of both sexes. From the male a urethral swab, urine specimen or semen specimen can be used. From the female vaginal discharge from the posterior fornix, a swab from the cervical canal, a secretion of the periurethral glands, or urine specimen will serve. Cervical cultures tend to give lower yields than vaginal pool specimens. While urine specimens are more convenient to obtain for culture studies, the yield is significantly less than either direct culture of seminal fluid or cervical and vaginal pool aspirations (Tarr *et al.*, 1976; Braun, *et al.*, 1970; Mårdh and Westrøm, 1970; Lee *et al.*, 1972; Toth *et al.* 1978). In our laboratory we use fresh semen specimens (0.2 ml) or a freshly obtained specimen from the endocervical canal or the posterior fornix of the vagina and immediately inoculate it into 5 ml of U-9 broth (Shepard and Lunceford, 1970), modified by the addition of 2.5μ/ml of amphotericin B (E. R. Squibb & Sons, Princeton, NJ) and 30μ/ml of lincomycin hydrochloride (Grand Island Biological Company, Grand Island, NY). The hydrolysis of urea to ammonia and carbon dioxide by the urease system of *U. urealyticum* results in a rise of pH and a visible change in the fenol red indicator from yellow to red. *M. hominis* similarly metabolizes arginin to ammonia in an arginin-containing medium; the pH rises and the fenol red indicator signals the presence of mycoplasma. When a positive change occurs, a sample is subcultured to a second broth and onto an A7 differential agar (Shepard and Lunceford, 1976). This agar medium contains manganese sulfate; urease-positive colonies turn brown to black as a result of the formation of particles of manganese dioxide.

In a laboratory testing on the average of 5–10 specimens daily, fresh media should be prepared biweekly. A specimen is considered positive only when the

145

secondary broth changes color and brown to black accretion colonies of typical size and morphology are noted on the differential agar. Colonies of *M. hominis* are about 200–300 μm in diameter and, as classically described, exhibit a fried-egg appearance. The *Ureaplasma* was originally termed as T strain because of the tiny colony sizes (15–30 μm in diameter). This organism fails to grow beyond the titer; that is, higher than the 10^7 colony units per ml. It has been speculated that the exhaustion of essential nutrients or accumulation of certain metabolic products in the immediate vicinity of the colony acts as a growth-limiting factor. Adding a continuous supply of urea or applying exchange resins to remove ammonia or carbon dioxide produced by the urea hydrolysis still does not change the colony size (Masover *et al.*, 1977; Windsor and Trigwell, 1976). It has also been hypothesized that a slowly dialyzable thermostable and catalase-resistant substance accumulates in ureaplasma cultures and is responsible for limiting the colonies' growth (Furness, 1973).

PATHOGENICITY OF *MYCOPLASMA* INFECTIONS

Toxic cell products such as peroxide, an end-product of respiration, are suspected to be cytotoxic for the host (Razin, 1969). In order for peroxide to exert its deleterious effect on the cell membrane, close adherence by the mycoplasma colony is needed. Lipid peroxidation will damage the cell wall if peroxidase activity is not high enough for a steady, high concentration of peroxide to be produced locally by the mycoplasmas (Cohen and Somerson, 1969). *M. hominis* uses arginin as a substrate and metabolizes it into ammonia and carbon dioxide. *U. urealyticum*, while splitting urea through its urease system, produces the same end-products. A concentration of ammonia can be toxic for the host. In the case of *M. hominis*, however, it is speculated that the depletion of the host's arginin supply is responsible for the toxic effect rather than the accumulated ammonia which is rapidly cleared as an end-product (Barile, 1973; Schneider and Stanbridge, 1975). Unlike other mycoplasma strains, such as *M. neurolyticum* which has a neurotoxin (Tully, 1974), or *M. fermentans* that can be lethal to laboratory animals when a homogenate is injected intravenously (Gabridge *et al.*, 1972), neither *M. hominis* nor *U. urealyticum* has been shown to produce exo- or endotoxins.

SURFACE ADHERENCE

Although it has been shown (Harwick *et al.*, 1970) that *M. hominis* can invade the blood stream in febrile women undergoing elective abortion, this organism generally adheres to and colonizes the epithelial lining surfaces of the respiratory and urogenital tract and is regarded as a surface parasite. Beside spermatozoal attachment (Taylor-Robinson and Manchee, 1967b), mycoplasmas attach to erythrocytes (Manchee and Taylor-Robinson, 1968), fibroblasts in monolayers (Brown *et al.*, 1974), HeLa cells (Boatman *et al.*, 1977), macrophages (Sobeslavsky *et al.*, 1968), tracheal epithelium (Manchee and Taylor-Robinson, 1969), and glass and plastic surfaces (Taylor-Robinson and Manchee,

1967a). Intimate attachment of mycoplasmas to the host cell wall provides a favorable milieu for the colonies to take up host nutrients; at the same time, the colonies exert a toxic effect on the host cell walls by continuously producing metabolic products. It is possible that mycoplasmas utilize host cell wall components such as cholesterol and fatty acids for structural purposes. Although the details of the binding sites are uncertain, when mycoplasma is bound to bronchial epithelial or urethral epithelial cells, the binding seems to be strong enough to resist ciliary activity or wash off by urine flow. Electron microscopic photographs demonstrate that a distinct space exists between the host cell wall and the mycoplasma cell membrane; thus no direct fusion occurs between the host and the parasite (Gnarpe and Friberg, 1973).

The specific role of *U. urealyticum* in the genital tract has been investigated in detail by several authors. In the case of spermatozoa, membrane adherence can be of especial significance. The first study showing a correlation between spermatozoa of inferior quality and mycoplasma attachment surface was reported in 1967 (Taylor-Robinson and Manchee, 1967b). Further studies, using scanning electron microscopy, have shown mycoplasmas adhering to human spermatozoa of patients with low fertility (Gnarpe and Friberg, 1973; Fowlkes *et al.*, 1975). The granular deposition of mycoplasma colonies over the tail and head segment of the spermatozoa and the coiling of spermatozoal tails as seen on scanning electron microscopy have been confirmed through light microscopic examinations (Toth *et al.*, 1978; Swenson *et al.*, 1979). Two distinct abnormalities were described in association with mycoplasma contamination of the seminal fluid: coiling of the sperm tails and a greenish, fuzzy appearance of the tail segments when using the standard Papanicolaou stains (Fig. 1). This cytologic feature allowed the authors to predict in 70% of the cases the presence of ureaplasma in a given seminal fluid. Subsequent studies convincingly documented the finding that seminal fluid specimens infected with *U. urealyticum* have a significantly improved motility rating after successful antibiotic therapy (Toth and Lesser, 1981). Other studies not only showed that ureaplasma-infected specimens exhibited inferior quality in terms of motility and tail morphology, but a lower percentage of oval forms and a relatively increased number of the small forms. Moreover, increased viscosity of the seminal fluid is present when ureaplasma infection exists (Toth and Lesser, 1982). The sum of these studies document that ureaplasma infection interferes with overall semen quality and that therapy can significantly improve the individual parameters. Because it possesses a viscous surface, the ureaplasma colony, by coating spermatozoal heads, tails, or midpiece sections, could serve as an adhesive for bacteria to use the spermatozoa as vehicles to gain access to higher genital tract structures. Recent studies have shown, however, that bacterial attachment can occur even without the presence of ureaplasma (Toth *et al.*, 1982).

The literature is not clear on what damage ureaplasma may exert on the female internal genital tract. Although many investigators have isolated *M. hominis* and *U. urealyticum* from patients with vaginitis and cervicitis, it is difficult to say whether this organism or other associated pathogens such as *Trichomonas vaginalis*, *Neisseria gonorrhoeae*, *Haemophilus vaginalis* or *Candida albicans* are the cause of direct cervical infection resulting in a poor postcoital test (McCormack *et al.*, 1973; Taylor-Robinson and McCormack, 1979).

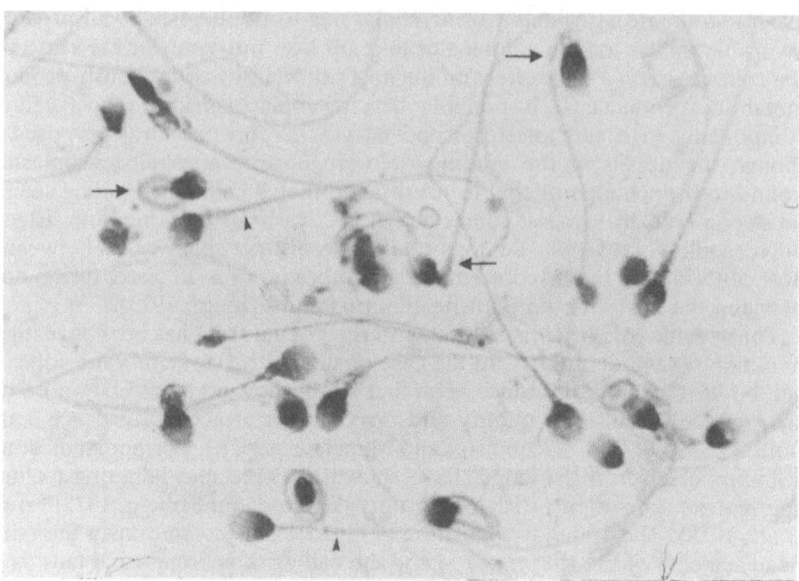

Fig 1. Typical features of seminal fluid infected with ureaplasma. Note: different degree of coiling (large arrows) and fuzzy appearance of tail segments (small arrows). Papanicolaou stained smear, original magnification ×1000

Tissue cultures from respiratory and oviduct epithelium help to explain the possible pathogenic effects of genital mycoplasma in the female (Collier *et al.*, 1969; Mårdh *et al.*, 1976). After adherence of mycoplasma to ciliary epithelium, a slowing of ciliary activity is observed; this is followed by complete ciliostasis. When the infection progressed, complete destruction of the ciliary epithelium was noted and the desquamation of the superficial epithelial cells took place in the presence of ureaplasma (Stalheim *et al.*, 1976). Although the exact nature of the toxic factors is not known, it is postulated that ammonia and/or hydrogen peroxide could be at least partially responsible for local tissue damage. Toxic substances or breakdown products of the lipid membrane of the mycoplasma colonies are postulated to be toxic to the host as well.

If laboratory results observed on oviductal epithelial culture cells were extrapolated to the human, they would show that mycoplasma colonization of the fallopian tubes could severely interfere with egg transport by reducing or completely blocking ciliary activity. Local destruction of the ciliary epithelium could also cause entrapment of the traveling ova and facilitate the development of an ectopic pregnancy.

The effect of ureaplasma on the endometrial lining is less certain. Studies correlating endometrial lesions with ureaplasma infection describe a subclinical endometrial inflammation with microgranuloma formation (Horne *et al.*, 1973). Whether ureaplasma directly affects ovulation and other ovarian functions, or whether the presence of ureaplasma can lead to pelvic inflammatory disease and become a mechanical component in infertility through tubal blockage, is less certain. Mycoplasmas, especially *M. hominis*, have been isolated from a large percentage of patients with pelvic inflammatory disease. It is possible that this organism, alone or in combination with *U. urealyticum*, has a primary pathogenic role in some cases of acute pelvic inflammatory disease. Since this entity is a complex disorder with additional micro-organisms involved, future studies are needed.

CLINICAL STUDIES

In evaluating the numerous papers dealing with genital infection by ureaplasma, it is useful to keep in mind that mycoplasmas occur with such high frequency in the lower genitourinary tract of sexually active healthy men and women that some authorities regard them as part of the normal bacterial flora. It is also important to remember that there are at least 11 different serotypes of ureaplasmas, and that each probably possesses a different pathogenicity. The prevalence of *U. urealyticum* infection in both males and females depends on a great variety of factors including age, race, socioeconomic status, sexual activity, the use of oral contraceptives and pregnancy.

Congenital infection is possible during passage through the birth canal, since infants delivered by cesarean section have a lower colonization rate than those delivered vaginally (Klein *et al.*, 1969). After puberty, however, colonization primarily occurs through sexual intercourse (McCormack *et al.*, 1972). The isolation of ureaplasma from the chorion and from the fetus of a patient with spontaneous mid-trimester abortion has given impetus to much mycoplasma research and to studies evaluating the role of this organism in reproductive failure (Kundsin *et al.*, 1967). A correlation has also been reported (Braun *et al.*, 1971) between the occurrence of ureaplasma in the urine and in cervical cultures and pregnancies which result in low birth-weight infants.

A higher recovery rate of *U. urealyticum* has been reported from the genital tracts of infertile couples than from fertile controls (Gnarpe and Friberg, 1972). Moreover, when doxycycline was used to eradicate these infections a higher pregnancy rate ensued (Friberg and Gnarpe, 1973, 1974). Other investigators have failed, however, to demonstrate a significant difference in the isolation rates of *U. urealyticum* among fertile as opposed to infertile couples, or a significant difference between the pregnancy rates after antibiotic therapy. In addition, there were no significant differences in isolation rates between women with unexplained infertility and women in whom the cause of infertility was known (de Louvois *et al.*, 1974; Matthews *et al.*, 1975; André *et al.*, 1978; Khatamee and Decker, 1978; Nagata *et al.*, 1979). Unfortunately, many papers concerning the relationship between ureaplasma and infertility do not contain controls. Other studies involved so few patients that a small but significant difference could easily have been missed.

After reviewing the literature, it seemed clear to us that the role of urea-plasma in human infertility could best be determined through a double-blind, prospective study that evaluated clearly defined cases of infertility considered as two distinct groups: antibiotic-treated and a placebo control. A long-term follow-up of these two groups might provide concrete answers about ureaplasma's role in infertility.

It also became apparent five years ago, when our laboratory became interested in ureaplasma, that such a study could not be carried out because so many publications supported the beneficial effects of antibiotic therapy. Any clinician who deals with apprehensive, infertile couples knows that it would be impossible and unfair to administer placebos to them not to mention requesting a 2-year follow-up period, when time was of such importance to these patients.

Our approach, therefore, was different. For 3 years our clinic systematically cultured semen specimens and recommended doxycycline therapy for both husband and wife when the husband was found to have a ureaplasma infection of the genital tract. We proposed to compare the 3-year follow-up of pregnancy rates in women whose husbands' infections were successfully eradicated (demonstrated by a negative post-therapy culture) in contrast to that of women whose husbands' infections were not eradicated. After the therapy, the rate of successful pregnancies was 60% for the group in which ureaplasma was eradicated and 5% for the group in which it was not.

We are not certain whether this difference was due solely to the successful eradication of ureaplasma or to the eradication of other aerobic and anaerobic bacteria and chlamydia for which doxycycline is also an effective antibiotic. We examined a series of variables, and none was directly correlated with success or failure in eradicating ureaplasma. It is our opinion that after therapy, positive cultures for ureaplasma represented doxycycline-resistant strains. Whether this organism represents a more pathogenic serotype is uncertain, but the emergence of this group of ureaplasmas is a growing concern (Toth and Lesser, 1982). The median time to achieve pregnancy after obtaining a negative mycoplasma culture was 10.6 months. The majority of women became pregnant without any additional fertility test or drug.

Multivariate statistical analysis selected the negative post-therapy mycoplasma status as the most important factor in predicting a couple's chance to achieve a pregnancy within the ensuing 3 years (Toth et al., 1983). We believe, therefore, that for couples who have no obviously detectable cause for infertility but in whom a positive ureaplasma isolate is found, either in the seminal fluid or in the cervical mucus, doxycycline therapy is indicated. Our laboratory recommends a full month doxycycline therapy course for both husband and wife, 100 mg twice daily. Two weeks following the completion of this therapy course, a repeat culture should be obtained. If either partner has a positive culture for ureaplasma, erythromycin is chosen as the second therapy at a dose of 500 mg four times daily for 2 weeks.

The drug regimen described above eradicates approximately 98% of all genital tract ureaplasma infections. For the remaining 1–2% of patients, we recommend a cyclic antibiotic therapy. Starting on the first day of the woman's cycle, the couple resumes the best-tolerated antibiotic, either doxycycline 100 mg twice daily or erythromycin 500 mg four times daily for 15 days. Unless the woman's period resumes, no further antibiotic therapy is given. If pregnancy ensues and the ureaplasma culture is still positive, erythromycin therapy is continued for an additional 2 weeks. If pregnancy does not occur, the couple repeats the cyclic antibiotic therapy course for 6 months. For women who habitually abort, and who present with a missed menstrual period, 3 weeks of erythromycin, 500 mg four times daily for both partners are recommended. Clindomycin and spectinomycin have been reported effective against mycoplasma infections, but since our clinic rarely uses these drugs we cannot recommend the therapy (Table 2).

Table 2 Antibiotic therapy for *Ureaplasma urealyticum* genital tract infection for couples with infertility or poor reproductive history

Doxycycline 100 mg b.i.d. × 30 days for both husband and wife	
Repeat culture 2 weeks after completion of therapy course	Cure rate 81%, if positive
Erythromycin 500 mg q.i.d. × 2 weeks for both husband and wife	Cure rate 98%, if positive
Doxycycline or erythromycin cyclic therapy 1–15 days of the woman's cycle for 6 months	Cure rate close to 100%

PITFALLS IN THERAPY

Even in a well-established, routine working laboratory, slow-growing mycoplasma strains can be missed in 1–2% of cases. It is therefore advisable, especially after antibiotic therapy, that culture tubes be saved for at least 10 days. Normally, the culture can be read and reported within 3 days. Mycoplasmas exposed to tetracycline-type drugs tend to have a slower growth rate.

If the follow-up culture is performed too soon after therapy is concluded, a positive isolate can be missed. We have repeatedly seen cultures submitted too soon after the cessation of therapy reported as negative. A month later, however, a positive culture was again obtained. We recommend a 2–3-week waiting period after the last day of antibiotic therapy before the culture is repeated.

In our experience, the use of generic tetracycline is contraindicated due to the emergence of tetracycline-resistant mycoplasma strains; moreover, patients often comply poorly with the four-times-daily regimen. On the other hand, doxycycline is well tolerated once the patient learns to cope with the gastrointestinal side-effects and to prevent sun exposure; the twice-a-day dosage makes compliance easy.

There are three major categories of resistant mycoplasma strains among patients previously exposed to tetracycline-type drugs. First, strains from the Far East, where tetracycline-type drugs were widely available during the Vietnam War, need special attention (Toth and Lesser, 1982). Two extreme cases in our clinic required 6 months of intermittent vibramycin and erythromycin therapy courses before a negative ureaplasma culture was obtained and pregnancy occurred. Second, in patients who have received tetracycline in low doses for dermatological conditions, there is a potential cross-resistance to doxycycline. Third, in patients who have undergone infertility work-ups and received short courses of tetracycline without proper pre- or post-therapy testing, we found only a 50% cure rate after a 10-day tetracycline course for ureaplasma (Toth and Lesser, 1982).

If a pregnancy does not occur within 6 months after eradication of the ureaplasma, a repeat culture should be done. We have encountered several cases in which properly taken repeat post-therapy culture studies were reported as negative, and 6 months later a follow-up study revealed positive colonization once again. Whether these instances represent reinfection through extramarital relationships is uncertain. Another possibility is the presence of chronic prostatitis or cervicitis where isolated pockets of organisms can potentially remain for years. The futility of treating chronic infections in these two sites may be responsible for the recurrence of ureaplasma infection.

CONCLUSION

The available clinical data support the beneficial effect of antibiotic therapy directed against ureaplasma. This is especially true in cases of unexplained infertility or where borderline-to-poor semen quality is diagnosed (Toth *et al.*, 1983; Cassell *et al.*, 1983).

References

André, D., Sepetjian, M., Mikaelin, S. *et al.* (1978). Role des mycoplasmes dans la sterilite: Etude de 150 femmes sterile. *J. Gynecol. Obstet. Biol. Reprod.* (Paris). **7**, 51

Barile, M. F. (1973). Mycoplasmal contamination of cell cultures: Mycoplasma-virus-cell culture interactions. In Fogh, J. (ed.) *Contamination in Tissue Culture*, p. 131. (New York: Academic Press)

Boatman, E., Cartwright, F. and Kenny, G. (1977). Morphology, morphometry and electron-microscopy of HeLa cells infected with bovine mycoplasma. *Cell Tis. Res.*, **170**, 1

Braun, P. and Besdine, R. (1973). Tuboovarian abscess with recovery of T-mycoplasma. *Am. J. Obstet. Gynecol.*, **177**, 86

Braun, P., Klein, J. O., Lee, Y. H. *et al.* (1970). Methodologic investigations and prevalence of genital mycoplasmas in pregnancy. *J. Infect. Dis.*, **121**, 391

Braun, P., Lee, Y. H. and Klein, J. O. *et al.* (1971). Birth weight and genital mycoplasmas in pregnancy. *N. Engl. J. Med.*, **284**, 167

Brown, S., Teplits, M. and Revel, J.-P. (1974). Interaction of mycoplasmas with cell cultures, as visualized by electron microscopy. *Proc. Natl. Acad. Sci. USA*, **71**, 464

Cassell, G. H., Younger, B. J., Brown, M. B. *et al.* (1983). Microbiologic study of infertile women at the time of diagnostic laparoscopy: association of *Ureaplasma urealyticum* with a defined sub-population. *N. Engl. J. Med.*, **308**, 502

Chanock, R. M., Hayflick, L. and Barile, M. F. (1962). Growth on artificial medium of an agent associated with atypical pneumonia and its identification as a PPLO. *Proc. Natl. Acad. Sci. USA*, **48**, 41

Cohen, G. and Somerson, N. L. (1969). Glucose dependent secretion and destruction of hydrogen peroxide by *Mycoplasma pneumoniae*. *J. Bacteriol.*, **98**, 547

Collier, A. M., Clyde, W. A., Jr. and Demy, F. W. (1969). Biologic effects of Mycoplasma pneumoniae and other mycoplasmas from man on hamster tracheal organ culture. *Proc. Soc. Exp. Biol. Med.*, **132**, 1153

deLouvois, J., Blades, M., Harrison, R. F. *et al.* (1974). Frequency of mycoplasma in fertile and infertile couples. *Lancet*, **1**, 1073

Dienes, L. and Edsall, J. (1937). Observations on L-organisms of Klieneberger. *Proc. Soc. Exp. Biol. Med.*, **36**, 740

Fowlkes, D. M., Dooher, G. B. and O'Leary, W. M. (1975). Evidence by scanning electron microscopy for an association between spermatozoa and T-mycoplasmas in men of infertile marriage. *Fertil. Steril.*, **26**, 1203

Friberg, J. and Gnarpe, H. (1973). Mycoplasma and human reproductive failure. III. Pregnancy in infertile couples treated with doxycycline for T-mycoplasmas. *Am. J. Obstet. Gynecol.*, **116**, 23

Friberg, J. and Gnarpe, H. (1974). Mycoplasmas in semen from fertile and infertile men. *Andrologia*, **6**, 45

Furness, G. (1973). T-mycoplasmas: their growth and production of a toxic substance in broth. *J. Infect. Dis.*, **127**, 9

Gabridge, M. G., Abrams, G. D. and Murphy, W. H. (1972). Lethal toxicity of *Mycoplasma fermentans* for mice. *J. Infect. Dis.*, **125**, 153

Gnarpe, H. and Friberg, J. (1972). Mycoplasma and human reproductive failure. I. The occurrence of different mycoplasmas in couples with reproductive failure. *Am. J. Obstet. Gynecol.*, **114**, 727

Gnarpe, H. and Friberg, J. (1973). T-mycoplasmas on spermatozoa and infertility. *Nature* (London), **245**, 97

Graber, C. D., Creticos, P., Valicenti, J. *et al.* (1979). T-mycoplasma in human reproductive failure. *Obstet. Gynecol.*, **54**, 558

Harwick, H. J., Purcell, R. H., Iuppa, J. B. *et al.* (1970). *Mycoplasma hominis* and abortion. *J. Infect. Dis.*, **121**, 260

Horne, H. W., Hertig, A. T., Kundsin, R. B. *et al.* (1973). Sub-clinical endometrial inflammation and T-mycoplasma: a possible cause of human reproductive failure. *Int. J. Fertil.*, **18**, 226

Khatamee, M. A. and Decker, W. H. (1978). Recovery of genital mycoplasma from infertile couples using New York City medium. *Infertility*, **1**, 155

Klein, J. O., Buckland, D. and Finland, M. (1969). Colonization of newborn infants by mycoplasmas. *N. Engl. J. Med.*, **280**, 1025

Kundsin, R. B., Driscoll, S. G. and Ming, P. L. (1967). Strain of mycoplasma associated with human reproductive failure. *Science*, **157**, 1573

Lee, Y.-H., Bailey, P. E. and McCormack, W. M. (1972). T-mycoplasmas from urine and vaginal specimens: decreased rates of isolation and growth in the presence of thallium acetate. *J. Infect. Dis.*, **125**, 318

McCormack, W. M., Almeida, P. C., Bailey, P. E. *et al.* (1972). Sexual activity and vaginal colonization with genital mycoplasmas. *J. Am. Med. Assoc.*, **221**, 1375

McCormack, W. M., Braun, P., Lee, Y.-H. *et al.* (1973). The genital mycoplasmas. *N. Engl. J. Med.*, **288**, 78

Manchee, R. J. and Taylor-Robinson, D. (1968). Haemadsorption and haemagglutination by mycoplasmas. *J. Gen. Microbiol.*, **50**, 465

Manchee, R. J. and Taylor-Robinson, D. (1969). Studies on the nature of receptors involved in attachment of tissue culture cells to mycoplasmas. *Br. J. Exp. Pathol.*, **50**, 66

Mårdh, P.-A., Westrøm, L., von Mecklenburg, C. *et al.* (1976). Studies on ciliated epithelia of the human genital tract. *Br. J. Vener. Dis.*, **52**, 52

Masover, G. K., Razin, S. and Hayflick, L. (1977). Effects of carbon dioxide, urea and ammonia on growth of *Ureaplasma urealyticum* (T-strain mycoplasma). *J. Bacteriol.*, **130**, 292

Matthews, C. D., Elmslie, R. G., Clapp, C. H. *et al.* (1975). The frequency of genital mycoplasma infection in human fertility. *Fertil. Steril.*, **26**, 988

Nagata, Y., Iwasaka, T. and Wada, T. (1979). Mycoplasma infection and infertility. *Fertil. Steril.*, **31**, 392

O'Leary, W. M. and Frick, J. (1975). The correlation of human male infertility with the presence of mycoplasma T-strains. *Andrologia*, **7**, 309

Razin, S. (1969). Structure and function in mycoplasma. *Ann. Rev. Microbiol.*, **23**, 317

Rehewy, M. S. E., Jaszczak, S., Hafez, E. S. E. *et al.* (1978). *Ureaplasma urealyticum* (T-mycoplasma) in vaginal fluid and cervical mucus from fertile and infertile women. *Fertil. Steril.*, **30**, 297

Schneider, E. L. and Stanbridge, E. J. (1975). Comparison of methods for the detection of mycoplasma contamination of cell cultures: a review. *In Vitro.*, **11**, 20

Shepard, M. C. (1970). Nongonococcal urethritis associated with human strains of 'T' mycoplasmas. *J. Am. Med. Assoc.*, **211**, 1335

Shepard, M. C. and Lunceford, C. (1970). Urease color test medium U-9 for the detection and identification of 'T' mycoplasmas in clinical material. *Appl. Microbiol.*, **20**, 539

Shepard, M. C., Lunceford, C. (1976). Differential agar medium (A7) for identification of

Ureaplasma urealyticum (human T-mycoplasmas) in primary cultures of clinical material. *J. Clin. Microbiol.*, **3**, 613

Shepard, M. C., Lunceford, C. D., Ford, D. K. *et al.* (1974). Ureaplasma urealyticum: Proposed nomenclature for the human (T-strain) mycoplasmas. *Int. J. Sys. Bacteriol.*, **24**, 160

Shurin, P. A., Alpert, S., Rosner, B. *et al.* (1975). Chorioamnionitis and colonization of the newborn infant with genital mycoplasmas. *N. Engl. J. Med.*, **293**, 5

Sobeslavsky, O., Prescott, B. and Chanock, R. M. (1968). Adsorption of Mycoplasma pneumoniae to neuraminic acid receptors of various cells and possible role in virulence. *J. Bacteriol.*, **96**, 695

Stalheim, O. H. V., Proctor, S. J. and Gallagher, J. E. (1976). Growth and effect of ureaplasmas (T mycoplasmas) in bovine oviduct organ cultures. *Infect. Imm.*, **13**, 915

Swenson, C. E. and O'Leary, W. M. (1980). Examination of human semen infected with Ureaplasma urealyticum by fluorescence microscopy. *Arch. Androl.*, **5**, 373

Swenson, C. E., Toth, A. and O'Leary, W. M. (1979). Ureaplasma urealyticum and infertility: The effect of antibiotic therapy on semen quality. *Fertil. Steril.*, **31**, 660

Tarr, P. I., Lee, Y.-H., Albert, S. *et al.* (1976). Comparison of methods for the isolation of genital mycoplasmas from men. *J. Infect. Dis.*, **133**, 419

Taylor-Robinson, D. and Manchee, R. J. (1967a). Adherence of mycoplasmas to glass and plastic. *J. Bacteriol.*, **94**, 1781

Taylor-Robinson, D. and Manchee, R. J. (1967b). Spermadsorption and sperm agglutination by mycoplasmas. *Nature* (London), **215**, 484

Taylor-Robinson, D. and McCormack, W. M. (1979). Mycoplasmas in human genitourinary infections. In Tully, J. G. and Whitcomb, R. F. (Eds) *The Mycoplasmas: Human and Animal Mycoplasmas*, vol. 2, p. 307. (New York: Academic Press)

Toth, A., Ledger, W. and O'Leary, W. M. (1982). Evidence for microbial transfer by spermatozoa. *Obstet. Gynecol.*, **59**, 556

Toth, A. and Lesser, M. L. (1981). Ureaplasma urealyticum and infertility. A. The effect of different antibiotic regimens on semen quality. B. Two-year follow-up on pregnancy rate after antibiotic therapy. *INSERM*, **103**, 509

Toth, A. and Lesser, M. L. (1982). *Ureaplasma urealyticum* and infertility: the effect of different antibiotic regimens on the semen quality. *J. Urol.*, **128**, 705

Toth, A., Lesser, M. L., Brooks, C. *et al.* (1983). Subsequent pregnancies among 161 couples treated for T-mycoplasma genital tract infection. *N. Engl. J. Med.*, **308**, 505

Toth, A., Swenson, C. E. and O'Leary, W. M. (1978). Light microscopy as an aid in predicting ureaplasma infection in human semen. *Fertil. Steril.*, **30**, 586

Tully, J. G. (1974). Mycoplasma neurotoxins: Partial purification of the toxin from Mycoplasma neurolyticum. *INSERM*, **33**, 317

Tully, J. G. and Razin, S. (1977). The mollicutes (mycoplasmas). In Laskin, A. I. and Lechevalier, H. A. (Eds) *CRC Handbook of Microbiology*, 2nd edn., p. 405. (Cleveland: CRC Press)

Windsor, G. D. and Trigwell, J. A. (1976). Prolonged survival of *Ureaplasma urealyticum* in liquid culture. *J. Med. Microbiol.*, **9**, 101

12
Genital papillomavirus infections in the human

K. J. SYRJÄNEN

INTRODUCTION

Genital warts (condylomata acuminata) have a long history in the medical literature. They were a widespread condition in antiquity, particularly during the Roman–Hellenistic era, and were described by the ancient physicians as 'condylomas', which means 'figs' (Oriel, 1971). Through the centuries genital warts were associated with venereal diseases, first with syphilis and later with gonorrhea, and they were long thought to be transmitted by homosexual intercourse between men (Oriel, 1971, 1977, 1981). It was not until 1954, however, that the true venereal transmission of genital warts was affirmed in studies on returning servicemen who had acquired penile warts from heterosexual intercourse in Korea (Barrett et al., 1954). In these studies the incubation period of the vulvar and other genital warts in the wives of the returning servicemen appeared to be 4–6 weeks (Barrett et al., 1954).

Although identified in skin warts in 1949, viral particles were not discovered in genital warts until 1968 (Dunn and Ogilvie, 1968). The structures of these viral particles proved to be identical to those of common warts, which are now designated as human papillomavirus (HPV) (Rowson and Mahy, 1967). The hypothesis that common warts, juvenile flat warts, and genital warts are caused by the same papillomavirus (PV), and that the differences in their clinical and histologic appearances are due to their different anatomical locations, was espoused for many years by both clinicians and researchers (Rowson and Mahy, 1967). During the past few years, however, this concept has been subjected to a complete re-evaluation, following the discovery of many different PV types and subtypes in man (zur Hausen, 1977, 1980), as well as of significant differences in the epidemiology of the different HPVs. Other ideas regarding genital warts have also been recently re-evaluated because of the discovery in 1976 of two new morphological entities of HPV lesions, which have been named flat and inverted (endophytic) condylomas (Meisels and Fortin, 1976;

Purola and Savia, 1977). Subsequently, these lesions were reported to be frequently associated with concomitant intraepithelial neoplasia (CIN) and occasionally with invasive squamous cell carcinomas of the uterine cervix (Syrjänen, 1979). This finding and the data accumulated on the malignant transition of laryngeal papillomas, genital giant condylomas, and lesions of EV (epidermodysplasia verruciformis, an HPV lesion in the skin), as well as the emerging data on cervical cancer as a venereal disease, have raised HPV as a possible etiologic agent in human squamous cell carcinomas, especially those of the genital tract (Powell, 1978; zur Hausen, 1976, 1977; zur Hausen and Gissmann, 1980; Syrjänen, 1979, 1980).

CHARACTERIZATION OF HUMAN PAPILLOMAVIRUS

Physical characterization

PVs are icosahedral particles of approximately 45–55 nm in diameter and consist of 72 capsomers. They belong as a subgroup (A) to the family Papova viruses (Rowson and Mahy, 1967). PV particles do not contain lipids and are not inactivated by lipid solvent. When subjected to equilibrium centrifugation in cesium chloride gradient, the particles separate into two discernible bands at densities $1.34\,g/cm^3$ (full particles) and $1.29\,g/cm^3$ (empty particles) (zur Hausen and Gissmann, 1980). Tubular capsids are frequently discovered in the band with lower density and, occasionally, particles with increased density are found which differ slightly in their protein pattern from that of the full particles. The sedimentation coefficients for the full and empty particles are determined as 296S and 168S, respectively (zur Hausen and Gissmann, 1980).

Papillomavirus DNA

Detailed analysis of HPV DNA has become possible by cleaving it with a variety of restriction endonucleases and by analyzing the fragments via gel electrophoresis (zur Hausen et al., 1974). This method has allowed researchers to demonstrate the characteristic cleavage patterns of HPV DNA and to construct physical maps of cleavage sites for restriction endonucleases in the genomes of different PVs (zur Hausen, 1977; zur Hausen and Gissmann, 1980). The different types of HPVs discovered so far and their preferential sites of infection will be discussed in detail later (see below).

HPV particles contain a circular, double-stranded DNA molecule, that weighs approximately 5×10^6 daltons (zur Hausen, 1977; zur Hausen and Gissmann, 1980). When analyzed by velocity sedimentation, HPV DNA reveals three components: supercoiled circular DNA (22–23S), nicled circular DNA (17S), and linear viral DNA (16S) (zur Hausen, 1977; zur Hausen and Gissmann, 1980). The guanosine–cytosine content, as calculated from buoyant density determinations, is 41%, and HPV1 DNA, for example, is known to contain short palindromic sequences of about 180 nucleotides. This latter finding has been demonstrated by the self-annealing of individual strands (zur Hausen and Gissmann, 1980).

Proteins of human papillomavirus

It appears that the DNA of HPV is covered with histone-like proteins, which comigrate in the SDS–polyacrylamide electrophoretic gel with calf thymus histones H2a, H2b, H3, and H4. Further characterization of these proteins is forthcoming (zur Hausen and Gissman, 1980).

The structural proteins of HPV are poorly defined as yet, mainly due to technical difficulties. Most authors have used pooled wart tissues for virus particle extraction; this practice, however, carries a risk of obtaining mixtures of different HPV types, as has been pointed out by zur Hausen (1977). When individual isolates have been used, the protein patterns of some HPV and bovine PV types have been analyzed in SDS–polyacrylamide gel electrophoresis. Such analyses have revealed a major capsid protein in HPV1 with a molecular weight of 57 000 daltons and some minor differences in the molecular weight of major capsid proteins among individual HPV types (zur Hausen and Gissmann, 1980).

Very little is known about the virus-specific nuclear antigens in HPV-transformed cells. Two nonvirion antigens were described in wart tissue: one distributed throughout the nucleus and the other located exclusively on the cell surface. Whether these antigens originated from a fetal source remains to be determined. When specific antisera against purified HPV virions are used, viral capsid antigens specific for each HPV type can be visualized in the nuclei of wart tissues (Jablonska *et al.*, 1982). Thus, such antisera are type-specific with no cross-reactivity with other HPV types (Jenson *et al.*, 1980). When antisera are raised against the SDS-disrupted HPV virions, however, they cross-react with the capsid antigens of most, if not all, HPVs as well as with PVs of other animal species (Jenson *et al.*, 1980). Thus, there are amino acid sequences in the major capsid proteins of PVs that are responsible for this genus-specific antigenic cross-reactivity and that are not exposed on the surface of the virion particles, i.e. are not type-specific (Jenson *et al.*, 1980). Further studies are essential to characterize these nonvirion capsid antigens associated with HPV-transformed cells; such characterization would be especially pertinent to the attempts to define the events leading to rejection of these tumors by immunologic mechanisms.

Immunologic reactions against human papillomavirus

Since skin warts are rejected by immunologic mechanisms, it is clear that HPV infection in man elicits a specific humoral (Pyrhönen, 1978) and cell-mediated immunity (CMI) (Jablonska *et al.*, 1982). The assessment of these immune reactions has been skewed by the fact that pooled virus preparations were previously used as antigens, which has prevented the type-specific evaluation of the response evoked. Only gradually are data emerging on humoral and cell-mediated immune responses against specific HPV types.

Immunofluorescent techniques have revealed specific antibodies against HPV types 1, 2, 3, 5, 8, and 9, i.e. the viruses responsible for cutaneous disease (Table 1) (Jablonska *et al.*, 1982). Attempts to correlate the clinical course of these lesions with the immunologic findings have yielded inconclusive results

Table 1 HPV types and their clinical manifestations

HPV type	Clinical entity
HPV 1	Myrmecia type of deep plantar wart
HPV 2	Common wart and mosaic type of plantar wart
HPV 3	Flat warts and less severe types of epidermodysplasia verruciformis
HPV 4	Palmar and plantar warts of small hyperkeratotic type
HPV 5	Macular lesions of epidermodysplasia verruciformis
HPV 6	Genital warts
HPV 7	Common warts in butchers, papillomatous warts
HPV 8	Macular lesions of epidermodysplasia verruciformis
HPV 9	Macular lesions of epidermodysplasia verruciformis
HPV 10	Flat warts
HPV 11	Laryngeal papillomas
HPV 13	Focal epithelial hyperplasia, oral papillomas, oral condylomas
HPV 16, 18	Bowenoid papulosis of genitalia
HPV (?)	Esophageal papillomas (?)
HPV (?)	Nasal and paranasal sinus papillomas (?)

(Pyrhönen, 1978; Jablonska *et al.*, 1982). Since the specific antigens of the virions found in genital warts (HPV6) are not available, studies completed so far have utilized pooled HPVs and/or condyloma extracts, thereby obviating type-specific assays.

As is the case with studies of humoral immunity, the most intensely studied CMI responses are in the cutaneous HPV lesions (warts and EV) (Jablonska *et al.*, 1982). In these studies, nonspecific CMI has been evaluated *in vivo* using DNCB sensitization, and *in vitro* with tests of mitogen stimulation and E-rosette formation. The results have disclosed a varying degree of impairment in CMI in patients with different types of warts (Jablonska *et al.*, 1982); this finding suggests that susceptibility to infection with a particular HPV type is related to the magnitude of the CMI defect. Data on genital warts and CMI are extremely scanty. In a series of 16 women with impaired CMI, widespread *in situ* carcinomas were found in the genital tract, suggesting that inability to reject these tumors might be partially due to impairment of CMI (Jablonska *et al.*, 1982). Only recently have analyses been made on the cellular infiltrates in the lesions of genital HPV infection (Syrjänen, 1983). In these lesions, B lymphocytes far outnumber T lymphocytes and macrophages; no significant differences have been observed between the three condyloma types (flat, inverted, papillomatous). Work is under way to analyze the phenotypic differentiation of the immunocompetent cells in these HPV lesions and to correlate the data with the clinical course of the disease. These analyses may lead to an insight in the mechanisms involved in rejection and progression of HPV infection in the genital tract.

INFECTIONS CAUSED BY HUMAN PAPILLOMAVIRUS

Nongenital HPV infections

Since the discovery of HPV particles in cutaneous and genital warts, characteristic viral particles have regularly been demonstrated in a variety of human squamous cell papillomas at many sites within the body (zur Hausen, 1977; zur Hausen and Gissmann, 1980; Howley, 1982; Jablonska *et al.*, 1982). Following the application of modern immunohistochemical and molecular biological techniques, an increasing number of tumors have been suspected of having HPV origins. These techniques have enabled the assessment of the various HPV types with distinct cleavage pattern for restriction endonucleases; and, at this time, 26 different HPV types are recognized (Jablonska *et al.*, 1982). Most of these types seem to have a predilection for a particular site of infection and are responsible for a typical clinical manifestation (see Table 1). Recently, some successful attempts have been made to characterize the HPV type on the basis of the lesion morphology (Gross *et al.*, 1982; Jablonska *et al.*, 1982). It is quite apparent, however, that many new HPV types and their clinical manifestations will be discovered in the near future.

HPV infections in the genital tract

Penile HPV infections (Buschke–Loewenstein)

In 1896, Buschke and, later, Loewenstein described huge penile condylomas, which have subsequently become known as giant condylomas or Buschke–Loewenstein (B-L) tumors. These authors emphasized the close similarities between these lesions and the squamous cell carcinomas arising in the genital tract. This relationship has been emphasized repeatedly, and B-L tumors have been called 'carcinoma-like condylomas' or 'condyloma-like carcinomas' to underline the difficulty in distinguishing between these two entities. It later was suggested (Kraus and Perez-Mesa, 1966) that B-L tumor was a variant of verrucous carcinoma, characterized by slow growth, fungus-like appearance, and ulceration. The viral (HPV) etiology of B-L tumor has been repeatedly documented; however, its eventual clinical course is quite distinct from that of the usual genital wart, even though the early stages are identical. Nodular areas of induration soon develop that gradually lead to fistulas exuding putrid-smelling purulent fluid. The genitalia may eventually become overgrown with luxuriant condylomatous masses that are extraordinarily difficult to eradicate (Boxer and Skinner, 1977). The literature of B-L tumors has grown rapidly, and by 1977 a total of 65 cases in which a B-L tumor had undergone a malignant transition into a squamous cell carcinoma had been reported (Boxer and Skinner, 1977). Since the ultrastructure of B-L tumor and carcinoma appear identical, this finding lends further support to the concept that this HPV lesion has a neoplastic nature.

Another type of lesion recently observed in the penis of young adults and attributed to HPV is called Bowenoid papulosis (Berger and Hori, 1978; Wade *et al.*, 1979). These lesions reportedly undergo spontaneous regression; they also show features of *in situ* squamous carcinoma, as their name implies. Viral particles identical to those of HPV have been identified in Bowenoid papulosis (Kimura *et al.*, 1978), lending further support to the hypothesis of an HPV etiology. Although the biologic behavior of most cases reported so far has been entirely benign, it may be unpredictable, and clinicians should recognize this entity as distinct from the usual condyloma, lichen planus, or psoriasis (Berger and Hori, 1978; Wade *et al.*, 1979). The type of HPV involved seems to be 16 or 18 in most cases (see Table 1).

Urethral HPV infections

Codyloma acuminatum confined to the urethra of adult male was first described in 1891. In the large, recent series of Debenedictis *et al.* (1977), as well as in many other reports, the symptoms, diagnosis, and management of the urethral condylomas have been well outlined; the etiologic aspects, however, have not been discussed as thoroughly (Debenedictis *et al.*, 1977). It is generally agreed, however, that urethral condylomas are tumors of HPV origin; HPV antigens have also been demonstrated recently in a flat type urethral condyloma by immunoperoxidase–PAP (IP-PAP) technique (Syrjänen and Pyrhönen, 1983). Although condylomas involve the urethra in only 5% of cases and the bladder only rarely (Debenedictis *et al.*, 1977), they usually pose serious treatment problems. Due to their luxuriant growth, huge size, ulceration, extension, and penetration into the deeper tissues the gross similarities of urethral condylomas to carcinoma have been emphasized by a number of authors. Whether the HPV type responsible for urethral condylomas is identical to that of genital warts has not been determined.

Vulvar HPV infections

The literature of vulvar HPV lesions and their possible role in premalignant (*in situ*) and malignant lesions is vast and beyond the scope of this chapter. Case reports are continuously appearing on malignant transformation of vulvar condyloma and B-L tumors into squamous cell carcinomas. Thus, as in the penis, evidence suggests that HPV-induced tumors possess the potential to become malignant in some patients (Rhatigan and Saffos, 1977; Schmauz *et al.*, 1978). Of special interest in this context is verrucous squamous cell carcinoma, which has recently been discussed in terms of the problems in its differential diagnosis vs. condylomas, B-L tumors, and squamous cell papillomas (Väyrynen *et al.*, 1981).

Of major clinical importance are the premalignant changes in the vulva, the intraepithelial neoplasias. A number of thorough surveys on the subject have become available recently (Crum *et al.*, 1982a,b). Scientific interest in these lesions has increased considerably during the last couple of years, concomitantly with the growing body of knowledge about the HPV–CIN relationships in uterine cervix (Meisels *et al.*, 1979; Syrjänen, 1979, 1980). In the vulva, both the cytopathic effects of HPV (koilocytosis) and viral particles have been found in 70% of cases of intraepithelial neoplasias (Crum *et al.*, 1982a). When subjected to IP-PAP staining, 50% of the polyploid and 3% of the aneuploid intraepithelial neoplasias of the vulva stained HPV-positive (Crum *et al.*, 1982b). These findings suggest that HPV may be an important etiologic factor of the intraepithelial neoplasias of the vulva, although definitive proof is still lacking. Further evidence to this important concept will undoubtedly be gained in the near future, when monoclonal antibodies against HPV6, HPV16 and 18

DNA are available for hybridization and it becomes possible to assess whether HPV genomes do exist in these vulvar lesions (Crum *et al.*, 1982a,b).

Yet another vulvular disease of possible HPV origin is Bowenoid papulosis, which has already been discussed as a penile HPV infection. As is the case with penile infection, spontaneous regression of this lesion has been reported in the vulva (Berger and Hori, 1978). The available evidence suggests that this is an HPV lesion that is distinct from the typical condyloma (Jablonska *et al.*, 1982).

Vaginal HPV infections

It is well established that HPV infection in the genital tract is frequently multicentric, i.e. the lesions involve the external genitalia as well as vaginal and cervical tissue (Schmauz *et al.*, 1978). This finding is in agreement with the reports that vaginal squamous cell carcinoma *in situ* is associated with similar lesions elsewhere in the genital tract in a high percentage (88%) of cases (Hummer *et al.*, 1970). The multicentricity of invasive squamous cell carcinomas in the genital tract has also been emphasized in the literature (Jimerson and Merrill, 1970). Although the literature dealing with the condylomas in the vagina is less extensive than that of the vulva and cervix, there seems to be little doubt that the vaginal mucosa is frequently involved in HPV infections of the genital tract. Consequently, the presence of all three types of HPV lesions (flat, inverted, and papillomatous) may be anticipated in the vagina, and there is no reason to expect that HPV would not be involved in vaginal intraepithelial neoplasia or carcinoma, if once established at other sites of the genital tract.

Cervical HPV infections

The existence of the classic venereal wart (condyloma acuminatum) within the uterine cervix has long been recognized and subjected to detailed descriptions (Woodruff and Peterson, 1958). The number of reported cases has increased steadily; only 23 well-documented papillomatous condylomas had been reported in 1952, but that number had increased to 254 by 1974 (Syrjänen, 1980). The pathology of cervical condyloma has undergone a complete re-evaluation since 1976, when cytologic and histologic evidence revealed two entities quite distinct from the papillomatous condyloma (Meisels and Fortin, 1976; Purola and Savia, 1977). These new entities were subsequently termed flat and inverted (endophytic) condylomas. Following those reports, a series of extensive surveys on the subject were published (Meisels *et al.*, 1977, 1979; Syrjänen, 1979, 1980; Syrjänen *et al.*, 1981; Ludwig *et al.*, 1981; Reid *et al.*, 1982), and at present it is amply documented that three distinct types of HPV lesions exist in the uterine cervix.

Numerous studies have reported a frequent close association between the HPV lesions and CIN (Meisels *et al.*, 1977, 1979; Syrjänen, 1979, 1980; Syrjänen *et al.*, 1981; Ludwig *et al.*, 1981; Reid *et al.*, 1982), thus lending morphological evidence substantiating the concept of HPV as a possible cause of human cervical carcinoma. Other facets of evidence will be discussed later.

To summarize the present state of knowledge, cervical HPV infection is characteristically limited to young women (the peak prevalence of the disease is at 22–24 years of age), who are sexually active and who have poor hygiene. It is frequently accompanied by cytologic and histologic signs of CIN and sometimes even by an invasive carcinoma. The venereal mode of transmission has been irrefutably established (Oriel, 1977, 1981). The clinical course of the disease and the factors modifying it, e.g. why some of the lesions disappear spontaneously while some seem to progress towards more severe forms of CIN and eventually into a squamous cell carcinoma, are less well understood. Because of their clinical importance, however, these factors will, undoubtedly, be the subject of very intense study during the years to come.

DIAGNOSTIC METHODS

Gross appearance

The gross appearance of a venereal wart is familiar to anyone treating patients with genitourinary diseases. Excellent descriptions on the gross morphology of these lesions are available (Pitkin and Kent, 1963; Woodruff and Peterson, 1958). Reference has already been made to the appearance of the giant condyloma, or B-L tumor, in the penis and vulva. The diagnosis of flat and endophytic condylomas, however, is very difficult to establish by gross appearance alone. There seems to be a consensus that HPV lesions cannot be reliably differentiated from the classic *in situ* carcinomas, or CIN of milder degree, on the basis of visual inspection alone (Meisels *et al.*, 1977, 1979; Reid *et al.*, 1982). This is because, in the majority of cases, they are invisible to the naked eye. Thus, other measures have to be used to diagnose the flat and endophytic condylomas, whatever their location in the genital tract is.

Colposcopy

HPV lesions in the vagina and uterine cervix may be seen using colposcopic techniques. A number of excellent descriptions are available (Meisels *et al.*, 1977, 1979). The colposcopic diagnosis of the classic papillomatous condyloma is readily made. The condyloma presents as a thick, white epithelial entity with finger-like projections showing irregular surface contours (Meisels *et al.*, 1979). The visualization of a regular capillary loop in each of these projections after the acetic acid has worn off is the most important diagnostic feature.

More diagnostic problems are encountered, however, when the lesion is in an early stage, with only small projections that look like asperities. In such instances, capillary loops are seldom visualized; instead, dilated vessels (punctation) are evident. At first glance the morphology mimics CIN, but the presence of surface asperities should alert the colposcopist to the possibility of an early condyloma acuminatum.

Flat and inverted condylomas are, on the other hand, practically indistinguishable from the lesions of CIN (Meisels *et al.*, 1977; Reid *et al.*, 1982). They usually appear as a white epithelium (Grade I or II, rarely III) in the transformation zone. The surface is flat, as the name implies, and mosaic and/or punctation can be found. The borders of these growths are less clearly defined than those in CIN, however. A diagnosis of HPV should be considered if they are multiple and outside the transformation zone, if the surrounding squamous epithelium shows dilated capillaries, and, of course, if condylomas are found elsewhere in the genital tract. It is clear, however, that there are HPV lesions small enough to escape detection by colposcopy alone (Purola and Savia, 1977), thus underscoring the need to include colposcopic biopsy in making the diagnosis.

Cytology

Although the term 'koilocytotic atypia' was introduced in 1956 (Koss and Durfee, 1956), it was 20 years before the cytologic pattern of the HPV lesions had been fully elucidated. The events that preceded this development have recently been reviewed (Syrjänen, 1980). Concomitant with the discovery of these lesions in biopsy specimens, it also became possible to identify them in the PAP smear with a high degree of certainty (Meisels and Fortin, 1976; Purola and Savia, 1977). The cytologic pattern of cervical HPV infection has been extensively reviewed (Ludwig et al., 1981; Syrjänen, 1980; Syrjänen et al., 1981). According to our experience, HPV lesions of the cervix, as well as those of the vagina, frequently exfoliate cells that may be classified as dyskeratotic superficial cells (either single cells or clusters). These cells have an orangeophilic cytoplasm, and they may show morphological features of dyskaryosis, especially in cases of concomitant CIN (Syrjänen et al., 1981). The typical cytologic morphology of HPV infection is the koilocyte, or balloon cell, which is usually an intermediate cell characterized by an enlarged, hyperchromatic nucleus and surrounded by a distinct cytoplasmic clear zone called the halo (Meisels and Fortin, 1976; Purola and Savia, 1977) (Fig. 1). At the margins of

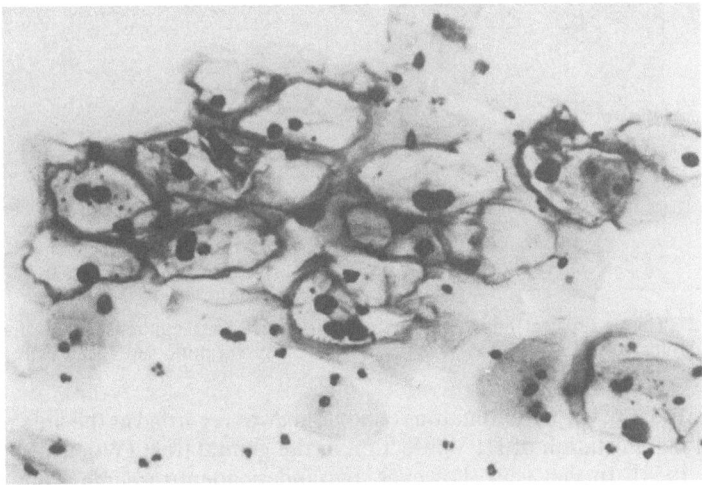

Fig. 1 A PAP smear showing a cellular pattern characteristic to an HPV infection in the cervix. A large cluster of typical koilocytes is seen with enlarged nuclei and large perinuclear halos. (Papanicolaou stain, original magnification ×250)

the halo the cytoplasm is condensed and may display an ambophilic staining pattern. Not infrequently the superficial dyskeratotic cells undergo a koilocytotic change. Both of the described cells above may appear in bi- or multinucleated forms. In addition, cells known as condylomatous intermediate cells (Purola and Savia, 1977) are encountered in a small percentage of cases (Syrjänen *et al.*, 1981). We additionally have found cells with strongly degenerated nuclei in 5% of HPV lesions in PAP smear (Syrjänen *et al.*, 1981). At present, koilocytotic cells are considered the most reliable criterion of HPV infection in the genital tract. In cases where the lesion fails to shed the characteristic cells, biopsy becomes the next alternative for establishing the diagnosis.

Histology

As was noted earlier, the histology of the classic papillomatous condyloma has been well described (Pitkin and Kent, 1963; Woodruff and Peterson, 1958). The papillomatous genital wart is characterized by papillomatosis, acanthosis, elongation and thickening of the rete pegs, parakeratosis, and cytoplasmic cavuolization (koilocytosis). In practice, this lesion is indistinguishable from the squamous cell papilloma, although the latter term is no longer applied to uterine cervical lesions (Fig. 2).

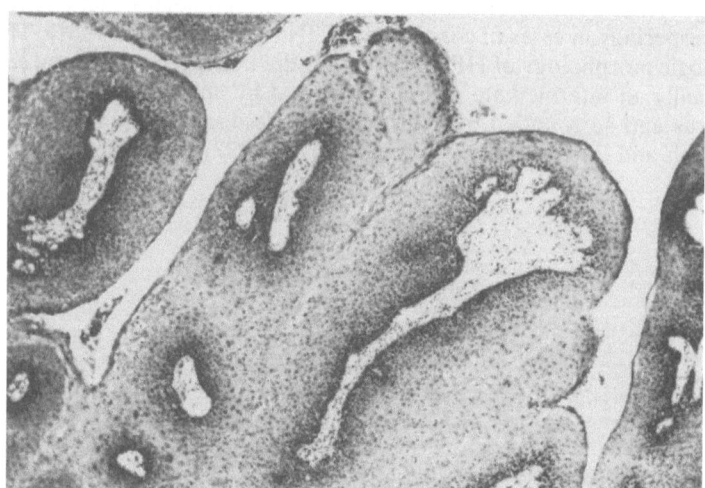

Fig. 2 This is atypical papillomatous condyloma showing epithelial projections crowded with koilocytotic cells, and covered by layers of dyskeratotic superficial cells. (H and E, original magnification ×40)

Until 1976, the papillomatous condyloma was regarded as the only morphological manifestation of HPV infection in the genital tract (Woodruff and Peterson, 1958). In that year, however, two independent research groups (Meisels and Fortin; Purola and Savia) discovered epithelial changes with cytologic features identical to condyloma acuminatum but without their papillary appearance. The two newly discovered lesions were tentatively named flat and inverted (endophytic) condylomas by these authors, and their HPV etiology has subsequently been established by electron microscopy, immunohistochemistry, and DNA hybridization experiments (Syrjänen, 1980; Ludwig *et al.*, 1981; Reid *et al.*, 1982; Gissmann *et al.*, 1982). The flat condyloma presents a flat focus of acanthotic epithelium with accentuated rete pegs, and elongated dermal papillae. There usually is a striking contrast between the deep layers of the epithelium and the more superficial ones, which are crowded with koilocytotic

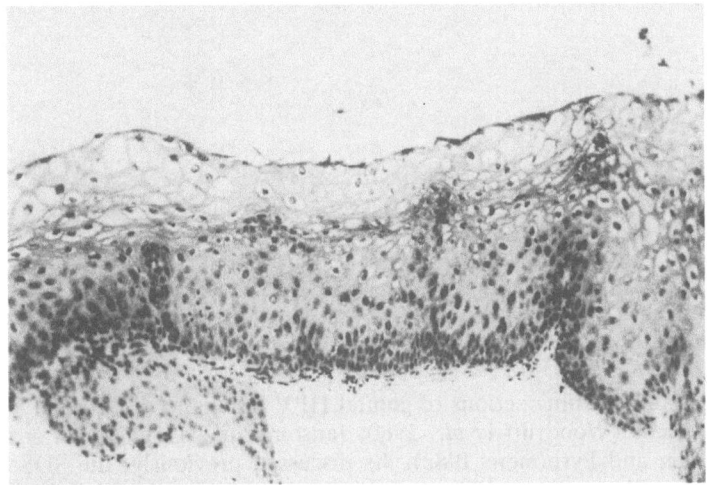

Fig 3. A quite characteristic flat type condyloma is shown, depicting all the features given in the text. Note the sharp contrast between the deeper layers and the more superficial layers of koilocytotic cells. (H and E, original magnification ×100)

cells (Fig. 3). The lesion is covered by layers of varying thickness of superficial dyskeratotic cells with nuclear pyknosis and abnormalities of varying degrees. Whenever changes consistent with CIN are encountered within or adjacent to the HPV lesion, they can be called 'atypical condylomas', 'condylomatous atypias', 'condylomas with CIN' or 'condylomatous dysplasia' (Meisels *et al.*, 1979; Ludwig *et al.*, 1981; Syrjänen, 1979, 1980; Reid *et al.*, 1982). Although the nomenclature is not in complete accord, most workers agree that HPV lesions are frequently accompanied by CIN and sometimes by an invasive squamous cell carcinoma as well.

The third condyloma type, the inverted or endophytic condyloma, is in most respects identical to the flat type, but shows additional features of pseudoinvasive penetration into the underlying stroma and/or glandular openings (Fig. 4). Thus, it shares many of the morphological features of an *in situ* carcinoma, with which it indeed seems to be frequently associated (Syrjänen, 1979).

Immunohistochemistry

Immunofluorescence techniques have been used for years to detect viral antigens and antibodies due to HPV. Only recently have IP-PAP techniques been

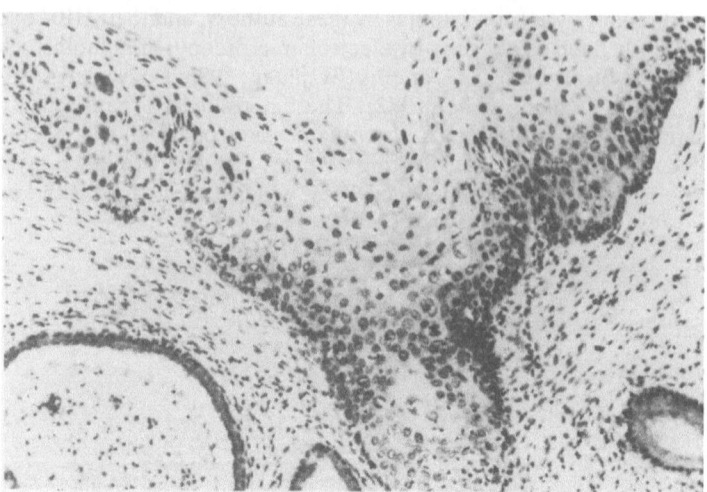

Fig. 4 An inverted (endophytic) condyloma mainly identical with the flat type, but showing as an additional feature pseudoinvasive penetration into the glandular openings of the underlying stroma. (H and E, original magnification ×100)

applied on paraffin sections of genital HPV lesions to disclose HPV antigens in the cells (Woodruff *et al.*, 1980; Jenson *et al.*, 1980; Morin *et al.*, 1981; Syrjänen and Pyrhönen, 1982). As discussed previously, the SDS-disrupted virions of PVs possess common group-specific antigens that give rise to antisera capable of cross-reacting against PV antigens of man and most animal species (Jenson *et al.*, 1980). Such an antiserum has proved a valuable tool in assessing a variety of squamous cell lesions for PV antigens. Another approach made by our group is to raise the antiserum against the highly purified viral particles from a pooled wart tissue collected from different anatomical locations of more than 20 individuals (Pyrhönen, 1978; Syrjänen and Pyrhönen, 1982). As shown before (see Table 1), such a pool contains most, if not all, of the HPV types that are known to elicit antisera against the type-specific antigens of the respective HPV types. The applicability of such a serum has been recently verified, and the staining results are identical to those obtained with sera against SDS-disrupted virions (Morin *et al.*, 1981; Syrjänen and Pyrhönen, 1982). In HPV-positive cases the epithelial cells show a dark brown precipitate that is confined exclusively to the nuclei of the koilocytes and superficial dyskeratotic cells (Fig. 5). The IP-PAP technique is currently used routinely in many laboratories to survey the squamous cell lesions of suggested HPV etiology for the presence of viral antigens. The IP-PAP method is much less time-consuming than electron microscopy.

Electron microscopy

On electron microscopy, PV particles have a characteristic appearance (Dunn and Ogilvie, 1968; Rowson and Mahy, 1967; Fig. 6) They can be visualized either in the wart tissue homogenates, or in the intact lesions prepared for

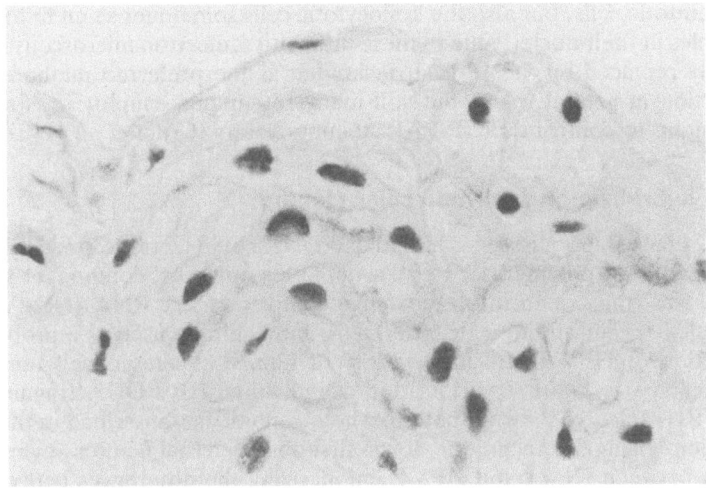

Fig. 5 A detail of a flat condyloma stained for HPV antigens with the IP-PAP technique. Most of the koilocytes show a positive reaction confined to their nuclei. (IP-PAP for HPV, no counterstain, original magnification ×400)

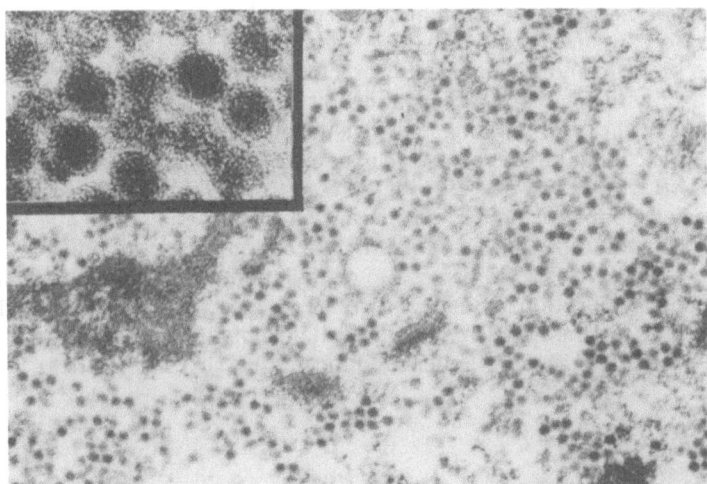

Fig 6 A detail of the nucleus of an HPV-infected cell as found in a case of papillomatous condyloma. The entire nucleus is crowded with typical HPV particles, which on higher power (inset) show a dense core and a less dense envelope. (Electron micrograph, original magnification ×25 000; the inset, ×100 000)

electron microscopy. In case of genital tract HPV infections, however, this technique of virus detection is difficult and time-consuming because of the extreme scarcity of HPV particles in genital warts. Thus, there may be lesions in which only very few cells contain the virus, which is always confined to the cell nuclei only. In most cases, viral particles are found in the superficial dyskeratotic cells, but also the koilocytotic cells sometimes seem to harbor the particles in their nuclei. Due to these difficulties, electron microscopy has been largely replaced by the IP-PAP technique as the preferred method of HPV detection in genital warts, but still many researchers employ it as a parallel technique to control ther IP-PAP staining results (Crum et al., 1982a,b).

DNA hybridization and molecular cloning

In 1974, zur Hausen observed that HPV DNA could be transcribed by *Escherichia coli* RNA polymerase. In subsequent experiments, component I of HPV DNA was transcribed into radioactive complementary RNA (cRNA), which annealed specifically to wart viral DNA and could be used as a probe for the detection of HPV DNA in a variety of human squamous cell tumors (zur Hausen, 1977, 1980). Hybridization of individual HPV DNA fragments with this cRNA clearly showed that the whole genome is transcribed in the *in vitro* reaction. Using this technique, it was first observed that no cross-hybridization exists between HPV1 and HPV4, emphasizing the differences between these two HPV types. This procedure has now been used to study a wide variety of human tumors, to detect whether any homology between the known HPV DNA probe and DNA of the tumor studied is detectable under conditions of various stringency (zur Hausen 1976, 1977, 1980; Gissmann et al., 1982). The findings of these studies are summarized in Table 1. Genital warts were recently shown to contain HPV6 DNA (Gissmann et al., 1982).

The biologic and biochemical characterization of HPVs has been seriously impeded by the lack of a tissue culture system for their *in vitro* production. To circumvent these limitations, researchers have constructed recombinant DNA molecules containing the complete genome of HPV using the certified plasmid vector pB322 in *E. coli* K-12 (de Villiers et al., 1981; Howley, 1982). Such a molecular cloning technique has permitted further analysis of the viral DNA thus obtained, using the various restriction endonucleases to refine the physical maps of these viruses, to assess the methylation sites of DNA, and finally to determine the location and sequence of the proteins coded by the virus (Howley, 1982). It is in this particular field that the major progress in the study of papillomaviruses is to be anticipated during the next few years.

EPIDEMIOLOGY

Modes of transmission

The natural history of genital warts has been elucidated in detail (Oriel, 1971, 1977, 1981) on several occasions since Barrett et al. (1954) first established that they were sexually transmissible. At present there is no doubt that the genital wart is a venereally transmitted disease. Current evidence suggests that the genital wart is a disease of sexual maturity and that the age of onset parallels that of gonorrhea. The sites at which genital warts appear are those most frequently injured during coitus, and there is a high incidence of genital warts among those with sexual partners suffering from this disease (Oriel, 1971). The incidence of genital warts steadily increased throughout the 1970s; and this rise has been linked to the increasing number of sexually active young females. The link between genital warts and those of the skin has not been clearly established, but there is some evidence of an epidemiologic association between these two entities, as well as between maternal genital warts and laryngeal papillomas in early childhood (Oriel, 1981),.

What has been stated thus far only applies to the classic venereal wart, condyloma acuminatum (Oriel, 1981); the natural history of the flat and endophytic condylomas is not known yet. Thus, the prevalence of these new lesions in women with vulvar warts has not been established, and the outcome is uncertain. Our laboratory is currently collecting epidemiologic data, including data on the sexual behavior associated with the development of genital HPV infection. We are also exploring the natural outcome of these lesions in prospective follow-up studies.

Human papillomavirus and cancer

There is an abundance of circumstantial evidence suggesting that HPV might be associated with the development of human squamous cell carcinoma. This evidence has arisen from different sources, including animal experiments, case reports of malignant conversion, HPV–CIN association studies, and epidemiological surveys. A detailed survey of all these findings, however, falls outside the scope of this chapter; the reader may refer to any of a number of recent surveys on this subject (zur Hausen, 1977, 1980; Powell, 1978; Oriel, 1977, 1981; Syrjänen, 1980).

HPV infection in the uterine cervix and vulva have been associated with CIN and, in rare cases, with invasive squamous cell carcinoma (Meisels et al., 1979; Syrjänen, 1979, 1980; Syrjänen et al., 1981; Ludwig et al., 1981; Reid et al., 1982). It is currently thought that this association is not simply accidental, but that some cause and effect relationship exists. Yet, the definitive evidence that HPV is an agent responsible for human cervical cancer is missing. The evidence is convincing, however, that human cervical cancer is a venereal disease (Kessler, 1976; King, 1980). Indeed, more than 250 papers present evidence that sexual activity may be linked to cervical cancer under certain conditions (King, 1980). Some recent data have linked carcinoma of the penis to that of the uterine cervix, suggesting that these two lesions might have a common, possibly viral, etiology (Smith et al., 1980). If cervical cancer is proved to be a venereal disease, venereally transmitted HPV will have to be seriously considered as one of the possible etiologic factors of the genital cancer in man.

At the present level of understanding, three factors should be considered when PVs are to be linked with malignant transformation of the cell (zur Hausen, 1980). These factors include: (a) malignant transformation depends on HPV type, e.g., none being ascribable to HPV1; (b) malignant transformation most probably is dependent on synergistic effects between the virus and chemical or physical carcinogens; and (c) genetic disposition (genetically regulated immune mechanisms) significantly contributes to the appearance of malignant proliferations.

TREATMENT

Surgery

Treating genital warts by surgery is associated with a high rate of recurrence, even after radical therapy. Despite this drawback, some authors advocate surgery (via excision and electrocoagulation) as the treatment of choice. Further details of the currently used cryosurgical techniques are available in a recent review (Powell, 1978).

Immunotherapy

Immunotherapy with autologous wart vaccine was introduced in the 1920s and utilized as a treatment over the next 20 years. A revival of the method took place in the 1970s, when favorable results were reported in cases of warts refractory to other treatment modalities. The present status of the technique, as well as the results obtained, have been summarized recently (Powell, 1978). The large number of recent reports on the success of autologous vaccine therapy, especially in eradicating laryngeal papillomatosis, may indicate that this mode of treatment will soon be applied to the treatment of genital warts, possibly in combination with other therapeutics.

Interferon

Interferons are potential antiviral, antiproliferative, and immunomodulating agents. Since their discovery in 1957, they have been extensively studied in the hope that they might lead to an efficient remedy against the viral diseases. Leukocyte interferon (α–IFN) therapy was recently instituted in patients with laryngeal papillomas that were refractory to usual treatment (Haglund et al., 1981); some success was achieved. There is no information at this time on the efficacy of such treatment in patients with genital warts and the role of interferons in the control of this disease remains to be proved.

Chemotherapy and podophyllin

One of the traditional methods of eradicating condylomas has been to topically apply 20% podophyllin. Unfortunately this substance has side-effects, both local and systemic. In clinical practice the incidence of side-effects appears related to the amount applied. This mode of therapy was recently subjected to extensive reappraisal to improve the efficacy and safety (von Krogh, 1981) (see Chapter 13).

Over the past decade or so a variety of cancer chemotherapeutic agents have been applied in an attempt to cure genital warts, including bleomycin, thiotepa, and 5-fluorouracil (5-FU) (Powell, 1978). The use of 5% 5-FU cream proved effective in some lesions refractory to other kinds of eradication (von Krogh, 1981). Some quite recent findings suggest that oral retinoid treatment might be beneficial in eradicating the lesions of HPV5-induced EV. When applied topically to lesions of CIN, it proved highly toxic, however.

Carbon dioxide laser

Since the mid-1970s the carbon dioxide laser has been used in some clinics to treat HPV lesions in the genital tract and larynx. Recent reports also advocate its use in eradicating intraepithelial lesions of the vagina and uterine cervix (Burke, 1982). In both applications the overall success rate has been very high (near 90%). It is our belief that the carbon dioxide laser currently offers the most satisfactory and appealing means of managing HPV lesions in the genital tract. Its advantages are its precision, its rapid and complete healing without scarring, and its safety when applied during pregnancy.

CONCLUSIONS

Human papillomavirus consists of a heterogenic group of viruses which are responsible for squamous cell papillomas (warts) in the skin and on mucous membranes of the respiratory, gastrointestinal, and genital tracts. The most common genital manifestation of HPV is the venereal wart, condyloma acuminatum, which has been recognized since antiquity. The more recently described genital manifestations of HPV infection have been defined as flat and endophytic condylomas. As has been proved in the case of condyloma acuminatum, a venereal mode of transmission has been suggested for these new condyloma types, which are frequently found in association with CIN and occasionally with invasive squamous cell carcinoma. These findings, together with reports on malignant transition of HPV lesions in the skin and genital tract as well as data from animal experiments and epidemiologic surveys, have aroused suspicion that HPV might be an etiologic agent in the development of human squamous cell carcinoma.

At the moment, HPV lesions are the subject of intense study; and morphological, immunohistochemical, biochemical, and molecular biologic methods (including DNA hybridization and molecular cloning) have been employed to further elucidate this possible relationship. Ongoing studies are also attempting to accumulate data on the natural outcome of the genital HPV infection, as well as on the factors (largely immunological), that affect its course. Currently, rapid progress is being made, and this chapter will likely need revision within a couple of years or so.

ACKNOWLEDGMENTS

This work has been supported in part by research grants from The Medical Research Council of the Academy of Finland (RG 07/014) and from the Finnish Cancer Organizations. This support is gratefully acknowledged.

References

Barrett, T. J., Silbar, J. D. and McGinley, J. P. (1954). Genital warts: a venereal disease. *J. Am. Med. Assoc.*, **154**, 333

Berger, B. W. and Hori, Y. (1978). Multicentric Bowen's disease of the genitalia: spontaneous regression of lesions. *Arch. Dermatol.*, **114**, 1698

Boxer, R. J. and Skinner, D. G. (1977). Condylomata acuminata and squamous cell carcinoma. *Urology*, **9**, 72

Burke, L. (1982). The use of the carbon dioxide laser in the therapy of cervical intraepithelial neoplasia. *Am. J. Obstet. Gynecol.*, **144**, 337

Crum, C. P., Braun, L. A., Shah, K. V. *et al.* (1982a). Vulvar intraepithelial neoplasia: Correlation of nuclear DNA content and the presence of a human papilloma virus (HPV) structural antigen. *Cancer*, **49**, 468

Crum, C. P., Fu, Y. S., Levine, R. U. *et al.* (1982b). Intraepithelial squamous lesions of the vulva: biologic and histologic criteria for the distinction of condylomas from vulvar intraepithelial neoplasia. *Am. J. Obstet. Gynecol.*, **144**, 77

Debenedictis, T. J., Marmar, J. L. and Praiss, D. E. (1977). Intraurethral condyloma acuminata: management and review of the literature. *J. Urol.*, **118**, 767

de Villiers, E.-M., Gissmann, L. and zur Hausen, H. (1981). Molecular cloning of viral DNA from human genital warts. *J. Virol.*, **40**, 932

Dunn, A. E. G. and Ogilvie, M. M. (1968). Intranuclear virus particles in human genital wart tissue: Observations on the ultrastructure of the epidermal layer. *J. Ultrastruct. Res.*, **22**, 282

Gissmann, L., de Villiers, E.-M. and zur Hausen, H. (1982). Analysis of human genital warts (condylomata acuminata) and other genital tumors for human papillomavirus type 6 DNA. *Int. J. Cancer*, **29**, 143

Gross, G., Pfiste, H., Hagedorn, M. *et al.* (1982). Correlation between human papillomavirus (HPV) type and histology of warts. *J. Invest. Dermatol.*, **78**, 160

Haglund, S., Lundquist, P.-G., Cantell, K. *et al.* (1981). Interferon therapy in juvenile laryngeal papillomatosis. *Arch. Otolaryngol.*, **107**, 327

Howley, P. (1982). The human papillomaviruses. *Arch. Pathol. Lab. Med.*, **106**, 429

Hummer, W. K., Mussey, E., Decker, D. G. *et al.* (1970). Carcinoma in situ of the vagina. *Am. J. Obstet. Gynecol.*, **108**, 1109

Jablonska, S., Orth, G. and Lutzner, M. A. (1982). Immunopathology of papillomavirus-induced tumors in different tissues. *Springer Semin. Immunopathol.*, **5**, 33

Jenson, A. B., Rosenthal, J. D., Olson, C. *et al.* (1980). Immunologic relatedness of papillomaviruses from different species. *J. Natl. Cancer Inst.*, **64**, 495

Jimerson, G. K. and Merrill, J. A. (1970). Multicentric squamous malignancy involving both cervix and vulva. *Cancer*, **26**, 150

Kessler, I. I. (1976). Human cervical cancer as a venereal disease. *Cancer Res.*, **36**, 783

Kimura, S., Hirai, A., Harada, R. *et al.* (1978). So-called multicentric Bowen's disease: Report of a case and a possible etiologic role of human papilloma virus. *Dermatologica*, **157**, 229

King, J. F. W. (1980). Sexual activity as environmental cancer hazard. *NY St Med. J.*, **96**, 1253

Koss, L. G. and Durfee, G. R. (1956). Unusual patterns of squamous epithelium of the uterine cervix: cytologic and pathologic study of koilocytotic atypia. *Ann. NY Acad. Sci.*, **63**, 1245

Kraus, T. K. and Perez-Mesa, C. (1966). Verrucous carcinoma: Clinical and pathologic study of 105 cases involving oral cavity, larynx and genitalia. *Cancer*, **19**, 26

Ludwig, M. E., Lowell, D. M. and Livolsi, V. A. (1981). Cervical condylomatous atypia and its relationship to cervical neoplasia. *Am. J. Clin. Pathol.*, **76**, 255

Meisels, A. and Fortin, R. (1976). Condylomatous lesions of the cervix and vagina. I. Cytologic patterns. *Acta Cytol.*, **20**, 505

Meisels, A., Fortin, R. and Roy, M. (1977). Condylomatous lesions of cervix. II. Cytologic, colposcopic and histopathologic study. *Acta Cytol*, **21**, 379

Meisels, A., Roy, M., Fortier, M. *et al.* (1979). Condylomatous lesions of the cervix: Morphologic and colposcopic diagnosis. *Am. J. Diagn. Gynecol. Obstet.*, **1**, 109

Morin, C., Braun, L., Casas-Cordero, M. *et al.* (1981). Confirmation of the papillomavirus etiology of condylomatous cervix lesions by the peroxidase-antiperoxidase techniques. *J. Natl. Cancer Inst.*, **66**, 831

Oriel, J. D. (1971). Natural history of genital warts. *Br. J. Vener. Dis.*, **47**, 1

Oriel, J. D. (1977). Genital warts. *Sex. Transm. Dis.*, **4**, 153

Oriel, J. D. (1981). Genital warts. *Sex. Transm. Dis.*, **8**, 326

Pitkin, R. M. and Kent, T. H. (1963). Papillary squamous lesions of the uterine cervix: A difficult problem in diagnosis. *Am. J. Obstet. Gynecol.*, **85**, 440

Powell, L. C. (1978). Condyloma acuminatum: Recent advances in development, carcinogenesis and treatment. *Clin. Obstet. Gynecol.*, **21**, 1061

Purola, E. and Savia, E. (1977). Cytology of gynecologic condyloma acuminatum. *Acta Cytol.*, **21**, 26

Pyrhönen, S. (1978). Antibody Response Against Human Papilloma Viruses. *(M.D. thesis)*. University of Helsinki. 1–41

Reid, R., Stanhope, C. R. and Herschman, B. R. *et al.* (1982). Genital warts and cervical cancer. I. Evidence of an association between subclinical papillomavirus infection and cervical malignancy. *Cancer*, **50**, 377

Rhatigan, R. M. and Saffos, R. O. (1977). Condyloma acuminatum and squamous carcinoma of the vulva. *S. Med. J.*, **70**, 592

Rowson, K. E. K. and Mahy, B. W. J. (1967). Human papova (wart) virus. *Bacteriol. Rev.*, **31**, 110

Schmauz, R., Elsässer, E., Lalwak, A. *et al.* (1978). Spitze Kondylome und Karzinome der Vulva, Vagina und des Penis. *Geburtsh. u. Frauenheilk.*, **38**, 342

Smith, P. G., Kinlen, L. J., White, G. C. *et al.* (1980). Mortality of wives of men dying with cancer of the penis. *Br. J. Cancer*, **41**, 422

Syrjänen, K. J. (1979). Morphologic survey of the condylomatous lesions in dysplastic and neoplastic epithelium of the uterine cervix. *Arch. Gynecol.*, **227**, 153

Syrjänen, K. J. (1980). Current views on the condylomatous lesions in uterine cervix and their possible relationship to cervical squamous cell carcinoma. *Obstet. Gynecol. Surv.*, **35**, 685

Syrjänen, K. J. (1983). Immunocompetent cells in uterine cervical lesions of human papillomavirus (HPV) origin. *Gynecol. Obstet. Invest.*, **16**, 327

Syrjänen, K. J., Heinonen, U.-M. and Kauraniemi, T. (1981). Cytological evidence of the association of condylomatous lesions with the dysplastic and neoplastic changes in uterine cervix. *Acta Cytol.*, **25**, 17

Syrjänen, K. J. and Pyrhönen, S. (1982). Immunoperoxidase demonstration of human papilloma virus (HPV) in dysplastic lesions of the uterine cervix. *Arch. Gynecol.*, **233**, 53

Syrjänen, K. J. and Pyrhönen, S. (1983). Demonstration of human papilloma virus (HPV) antigens in a case of urethral condyloma. *Scand. J. Urol. Nephrol.*, **17**, 267

Väyrynen, M., Romppanen, T., Koskela, E. *et al.* (1981). Verrucous squamous cell carcinoma of the female genital tract: Report of three cases and survey of the literature. *Int. J. Gynecol. Obstet.*, **19**, 351

von Krogh, G. (1981). Podophyllotoxin for condylomata acuminata eradication: Clinical and experimental comparative studies on Podophyllum lignans, colchicine and 5-fluorouracil. *Acta Dermatol. Venereol. Suppl.*, **98**, 1

Wade, T. R., Kopf, A. W. and Ackerman, A. B. (1979). Bowenoid papulosis of the genitalia. *Arch. Dermatol.*, **115**, 306

Woodruff, J. D. and Peterson, W. F. (1958). Condylomata acuminata of the cervix. *Am. J. Obstet. Gynecol.*, **75**, 1353

Woodruff, J. D., Braun, L., Cavalieri, R. *et al.* (1980). Immunologic identification of papillomavirus antigen in condyloma tissues from the female genital tract. *Obstet. Gynecol.*, **56**, 727

zur Hausen, H. (1976). Condylomata acuminata and human genital cancer. *Cancer Res.*, **36**, 530

zur Hausen, H. (1977). Human papillomaviruses and their possible role in squamous cell carcinomas. *Cur. Topics Microbiol. Immunol.*, **78**, 1

zur Hausen, H. and Gissmann, L. (1980). Papillomaviruses. In: G. Klein (ed.) *Viral Oncology*, p. 433. (New York: Raven Press)

zur Hausen, H., Meihof, W., Schreiber, W. *et al.* (1974). Attempts to detect virus specific DNA sequences in human tumors. I. Nucleic acid hybridizations with complementary RNA of human wart virus. *Int. J. Cancer*, **13**, 650

13
The biology of genitoanal warts with special reference to therapy and malignant potential

G. VON KROGH

INTRODUCTION

Condylomata acuminata occur at an increasing rate at present. As is the case with the epidemiologically associated airway papillomata, condylomata represent warts with a clearcut malignant potential. This chapter elucidates their clinical significance within the broad scope of human papilloma virus-induced mucocutaneous warts, and critically evaluates the therapeutic modalities that are currently available, including the use of various topical chemotherapeutic approaches. The inefficacy of routine applications of podophyllin at weekly intervals and the risk of serious systemic side-effects associated with this modality is also discussed. The advantages of safer alternative treatment, which is based on self-medication with 0.5% podophyllotoxin preparations continuously for 3–4 days or more, is emphasized. The use of carbon laser treatment for eradication of otherwise recalcitrant lesions and the use of autogenous vaccine preparations are also discussed.

CONDYLOMATA ACUMINATA – A DISTINCT CLINICAL ENTITY WITHIN THE BROAD SCOPE OF MUCOCUTANEOUS WARTS

Species-specific warts afflict several animals; in man, they are classified according to morphology, distribution, and epidemiology. Verrucae (skin warts) involve keratinized epithelia and are generally associated with varying degrees of macroscopically evident hyperkeratosis. Their significance is largely limited to a cosmetic problem. Verrucae vulgares (common warts) most frequently afflict the hands but may occur on any part of the skin, including the face and the genitals, where they are often filiform. Verrucae plantares frequently cause

175

ambulatory pain because they predominantly occur on weight-bearing areas of the feet. Verrucae planae are most common on the hands, limbs, and faces of children and young adults. The term mosaic warts refers to plaque-like growths usually afflicting the soles, heels, palms, and periungual areas; these are generally recalcitrant to treatment (Bunney, 1982). Condylomata acuminata represent warts of anogenital areas; histologically similar papillomata also affect the oral, laryngeal, tracheobronchial, or esophageal epithelium (von Krogh, 1983). Clearcut disparities exist with respect to peak incidence for various types of warts; nevertheless, each type may afflict individuals of any age. While skin warts are most common in school children, the peak incidence of condylomata is in the age group 19–22 years (Bunney, 1982; Oriel, 1971).

CLINICAL APPEARANCE OF ANOGENITAL WARTS

Anatomical location

Condylomata are not uniformly distributed over the genitals. Those anatomical substructures that are subjected to trauma during coitus are most frequently affected (Oriel, 1971).

Among noncircumcised males, the lesions most commonly appear in the preputial cavity, i.e. the glans penis, coronal sulcus, fraenum, and inner aspect of prepuce (Fig. 1a,b). The urinary meatus (Fig. 1c) and genital skin areas (Fig. 1d) may also be affected. Anal affliction is not uncommon and – contrary to common belief – is not restricted to males who engage in anal intercourse (von Krogh, 1982). The distribution is somewhat different among circumcised males. While warts in the urinary meatus are as common as in noncircumcised males, the shaft of the penis is more commonly engaged than the glans. Extensive wart formation is most common in uncircumcised males (Oriel, 1971a).

In females, warts appear most often at or near the posterior fourchette (Fig. 1e) and on the adjacent parts of vulva or perineum. The urinary meatus is less frequently involved than in males, while anal affliction occurs in up to one-third of cases. At least 15% of women have simultaneous growths in the vagina (Oriel, 1971a; von Krogh, 1982a).

Human papillomavirus (HPV) infection of the genitoanal areas has traditionally been thought to be limited to these anatomical sites. However, a spate of recent reports from Australia, Europe, and North America has challenged this view. In 1976 it became apparent that portiocervical warts occur more frequently than formerly suspected; they are easily overlooked by examination with the naked eye and sometimes even by colposcopy. In most such subclinical cases, they represent small white spots or plaques with minimal epithelial asperity, rather than the classically elevated lesions (Subclinical Papillomavirus Infection: SPI). An unexpectedly high prevalence has been found in recent cytological screening programs. In Quebec, for example, portiocervical warts occur in 1.5% of the female population. External female condylomata are associated with concurrent portiocervical lesions in up to 40% of cases; at least 15% reveal the latter type of lesion alone (Purola and Savia, 1977; Meisels et al., 1981).

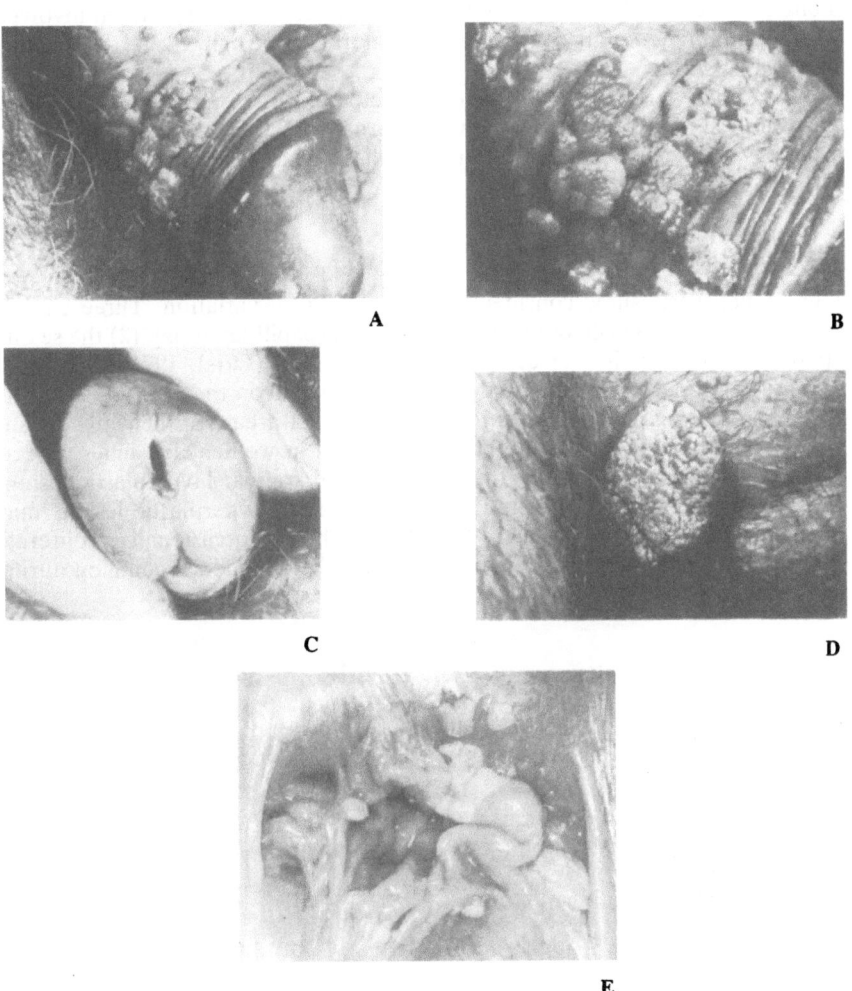

Fig. 1 **A** and **B**: typical papillomatous warts of the preputial cavity; **C**: urinary meatus wart; **D**: condyloma in the groin; **E**: condylomata of the introitus vagina

177

Although growth in or around the urinary orifice is common, dissemination to the urethra or to the bladder is extremely rare. Routine screening cannot be recommended, unless urethral dysfunction such as hematuria, recalcitrant urethritis, or voiding problems are present. In such cases, palpable masses along the urethra should be sought; the posterior urethra is seldom involved without simultaneous growth of anterior tumors (von Krogh, 1982a; de Benedictis *et al.*, 1977).

When anal warts are encountered, proctoscopy is essential to exclude the possibility of involvement beyond the external sphincter. Anal coitus or other types of anal sexual stimulation may predispose to such contamination (von Krogh, 1982a; Oriel, 1971b).

Macromorphology

Genitoanal warts show considerable morphological variation. Three clinical types can be distinguished: (1) the hyperplastic (papillomatous), (2) the sessile (papular), and (3) the verruca vulgaris-like variant (Oriel, 1971a). To some extent, the appearance of a particular type depends on the affected site. The hyperplastic type predominates in relatively moist areas. In men, this means the preputial cavity or the urinary meatus, and in women, the inner aspects of the vulva, the vestibulum, the introitus, and vagina. Hyperplastic lesions are also commonly encountered in the anal area. Hyperplastic lesions may coalesce into confluent plaques (Fig. 2), which may occasionally proliferate luxuriously into cauliflower-like tumors. This phenomenon is common during pregnancy.

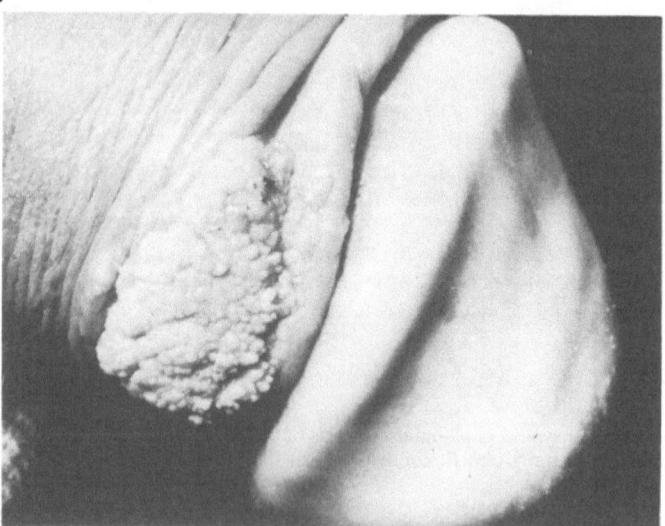

Fig. 2 Confluent plaques of condyloma in the preputial cavity

Sessile warts are not uncommon and often coexist with the hyperplastic variant; in males they usually occur on the penile shaft, and in females in the vulvoperineal areas (von Krogh). They are often multiple but tend to remain disseminated (Oriel, 1971a). In some cases hyperplastic lesions may, wherever located, gradually turn into the sessile variant in the course of time. Such warts are often pigmented or erythematous (von Krogh, 1982a).

Lesions resembling *verrucae vulgares* are the least common variant of genito-anal warts; they may be seen on areas covered by fully keratinized skin, such as the penile shaft, the outer aspects of labiae majorae, and perianal areas (Oriel, 1971; von Krogh, 1982a).

Warts that affect the portiocervix are usually flat, or grow in an endophytic manner, rather than being typically papillomatous ('atypical' condylomata corresponding to SPI) (Meisels *et al.*, 1981).

In very rare instances, condylomata of the outer genitoanal areas proliferate rapidly into a semimalignant giant variant, the Buschke–Löwenstein tumor, which simultaneously grows in an exo- and endophytic manner, penetrating underlying tissues by compression (Hudson *et al.*, 1973); subsequent malignant conversion is quite unusual, however (zur Hausen, 1977).

PATHOGENESIS

Evidence for a predominantly sexual transmission for condylomata was first documented in the US–Korean war, when the wives of American soldiers who acquired penile warts during their foreign service regularly developed vulvovaginal condylomata 4–6 weeks after their husbands' homecoming (Barret and Silbar, 1954). Subsequent studies revealed an incubation period varying from 1 to 8 months, with a mean of 3 months. Two-thirds of condylomata patients' partners contract the disease, which is most contagious during the first months of existence (Oriel, 1971a; Teokarov, 1962). In some cases, however, a nonsexual pathogenesis may be involved. This entails transmission via objects such as towels and digital auto-inoculation from one site to another in the genitoanal areas (Bunney, 1981; von Krogh, 1982a). When condylomata occasionally occur in prepubertal children (Fig. 3), the latter explanation seems rational in most cases, although the recognition of possible sexual abuse should be an essential responsibility for the involved physician (de Jong *et al.*, 1982).

ETIOLOGY

The 52–55 nm large human papilloma viruses (HPV) belong to the papova group of intranuclearly replicating DNA viruses; they have morphologically homologous capsids and supercoiled circular genomes. Polyoma viruses represent another oncogenic genus, which is responsible for a variety of animal neoplasms (Fenner *et al.*, 1974). HPV research has been hampered by a lack of *in vitro* cell culture systems or animal models for experimental viral replication; studies have been confined to extraction of capsid or genetic material directly from human warts. The fact that HPV replication frequently is absent in warts older than a year represents an additional difficulty to researchers (Barrero-Oro *et al.*, 1962; Shirodario and Matthews, 1975). Although the virus is only found intranuclearly at the stratum granulosum level,

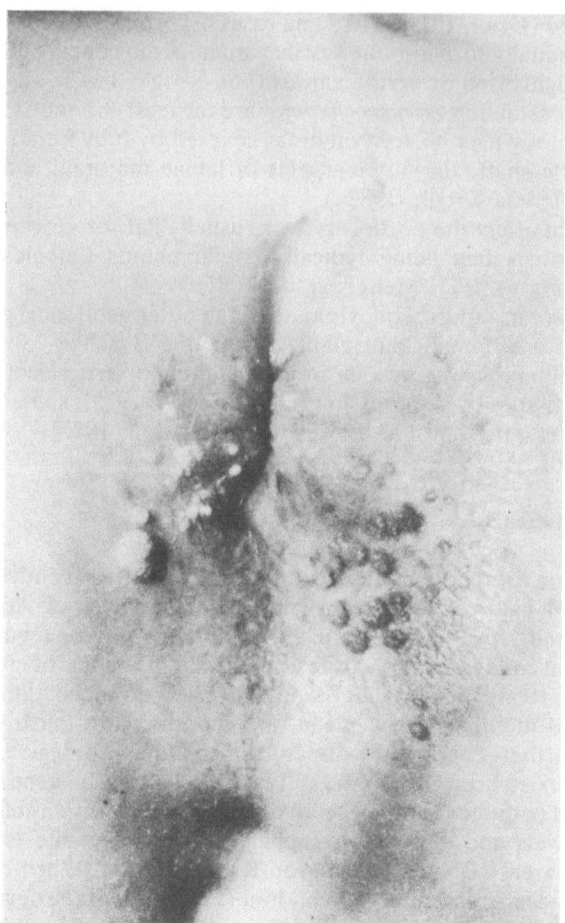

Fig. 3 Perianal warts in a 2-year-old boy

its spread into the cytoplasm has been observed at higher levels of the epidermis. In the stratum corneum it lies free within the keratin (Bunney, 1982). Due to morphologic identity for virions from clinically different wart types, it was long held that all of these tumors were caused by a single viral strain. The application of refined modern investigative tools, however, such as restriction endonuclease cleavage techniques, or nucleic acid hybridization assays for mapping of DNA nucleic acid sequences, and highly sensitive immunologic methodology for capsid characterization, has led to a considerable progress in defining a new wart biology in recent years. The new knowledge entails a HPV plurality previously unsuspected: the number of documented HPV strains is now 18 (Table 1). Their numerical designation corresponds to the chronological order of their discovery; this designation may change in the future.

Verrucae correlate to HPV types 1 to 4; HPV-1 is most frequently found in plantar lesions, HPV-2 in common skin warts located elsewhere, and HPV-3

Table 1 Preferential association of HPV type with clinical lesion

HPV type	Preferential clinical lesion
1	Verrucae plantares
2	Verrucae vulgares
3	Verrucae planae
4	Verrucae vulgares/plantares
5, 8, 9, 10, 12, 14, 15	Verrucae planae/pityriasis versicolor lesions in ED
6, 11	Condylomata; Laryngeal papillomata
6, 18	Condylomata
13	Oral focal hyperplasia
16	Bowenoid papulosis of the genitals

in plane warts. Overlap exists, however, as HPV-2 has been isolated from plantar and HPV-1 from other verrucae; furthermore, an entirely distinct type, HPV-4, has been identified in skin warts in adults. In epidermodysplasia verruciformis, an uncommon hereditary skin disorder associated with the occurrence of widely distributed warty lesions, benign warts are associated with HPV types 3, 5, 8, 9, 10, 12, 14 and 15 while a frequent existence of premalignant skin lesions in such individuals is associated with either HPV-5 or 8. HPV-5 has also been identified in wart-afflicted renal allograft recipients. HPV-7 has been found in hand warts among meat handlers (zur Hausen, 1977; Howley, 1982; Jablonska et al., 1983). The classification of the HPV types associated with condylomata acuminata has been hampered by the infrequency of virion replication in genitoanal warts, a finding that may correlate with some local factor(s) in afflicted epithelia, such as pH, temperature, or absence of significant keratinization. However, sufficient amounts of free, unintegrated HPV DNA have been traced for preliminary assessment of HPV type(s) being involved. Although the available data are quite fragmentary, recent introduction of viral DNA cloning in bacterial vectors such as Escherichia coli has opened up the possibility of producing standardized reagents in quantities sufficient for studying the HPV strains associated with condylomata in the near future – a fascinating challenge in the light of the evidence suggesting a malignant potential for these lesions.

It is plausible that multiple HPVs may potentially habitate the genitoanal areas in the same patient. Not only do morphologically distinct wart types exist in these regions, but genitoanal warts are also one of few neoplasmata in man that develop on a multiclonal basis (Friedman and Fialkow, 1976).

The genitoanal area represents an epidermal transitional zone between fully keratinized ectodermal skin and mucous membranes lined with non-keratinized epithelium of entodermal origin (Bloom and Fawatt, 1975; Langman, 1975). As Table 2 shows, the entodermally derived epithelia are commonly affected in females with genital warts and in patients with anal warts (von Krogh, 1982a). Recently, it has become evident that several HPV strains may indeed habitate these epithelia. HPV types 1 and 2, which preferentially have a tropism for hands and feet, have been isolated in a few cases of genital warts. However, the predominant number of typical condylomata acuminata seem to be caused by HPV-6 and 11 (Gissman et al., 1982). Quite recently, two additional different HPV types have been identified in warty lesions of the genitals:

Table 2 Genitoanal condylomata acuminata; anatomical distribution with respect to embryologic origin of afflicted epithelia[a]

Wart type	Afflicted germ layer(s) (%)		
	Ectodermis only[b]	Entodermis only[b]	Ecto- and entodermis simultaneously
Genital			
Males	100	0	0
Females	53	8	39
Anal			
Males	60	0	40
Females	95	0	15

[a] From von Krogh, 1982.
[b] Ectodermal origin refers to epithelium covering the perineal and the outer genital areas of both sexes, including the meatus and fossa navicularis of the urethra and the anal area accessible to inspection without proctoscopy. In the female, entodermal origin corresponds to the vestibulum, the introitus, vagina, and the portiocervical part of the uterus.

HPV-16 and 18. HPV types 6 and 11 have also been identified in laryngeal papillomatosis and type 16 from Bowenoid papulosis of the genitals (Durst *et al.*, 1983; Gissman *et al.*, 1983; Ikenberg *et al.*, 1983; Singer *et al.*, 1984). It is likely that other strains or subtypes also may exist with tropism for the genitoanal area and that more than one type may coexist in one and the same patient with condylomata. Due to the unexpected degree of genetic diversity of various HPVs that has been unmasked in recent years, it has been postulated that a propensity may exist for these viruses to accumulate mutations by mechanisms such as genetic drift or acquisition of specific information by exchange of genetic material (Danos *et al.*, 1983).

ASSOCIATED AIRWAY PAPILLOMATA

The association between certain airway papillomata and HPV infection is based upon histologic features, a strong epidemiologic link to genitoanal warts, and the recent demonstration of HPV in some of these lesions. Through the years, a number of case reports have focused on occasional occurrence of wart-like lesions intraorally (Oriel, 1978; Judson, 1981; von Krogh, 1983; Shaffer *et al.*, 1980). While previously considered quite unusual and mainly of academic interest, condylomata of ororespiratory epithelia have received increasing attention, with the consequent discovery of a higher incidence and morbidity than had been thought.

Multiple papillomas are the most common benign tumor of the larynx in childhood and among the most frequently encountered benign laryngeal growths at any age. In childhood they represent a serious clinical challenge, since they are responsible for episodes of acute respiratory obstruction that often require emergency tracheostomy and repeated surgery. About 60% of these children are delivered by mothers afflicted with clinically apparent condylomata. Since the virus may be transmitted at birth, routine screening for condylomata in pregnant women is now recommended; it aims at preventing neonatal infection through cesarian section (Quick *et al.*, 1980; *Lancet* editorial, 1980). Some of these children have concurrent intraoral condylomatous growths (Cohen *et al.*, 1980).

Recent studies have revealed the intralesional existence of HPV in more than half of the cases of juvenile laryngeal papillomatosis (Costa *et al.*, 1981; Lack *et al.*, 1980; Lancaster and Jenson, 1981).

So far HPV-6 and 11 have been identified from these warts, i.e. two of the four strains which have been found in genital lesions (Gissman *et al.*, 1983).

Some airway papillomas in adults may be pathogenetically related to sexual activity, such as fellatio, cunnilingus, and ano-oral contact; several HPVs may reveal a tropism for genitoanal as well as airway epithelia. Futhermore, HPVs with predilection for the skin may also occasionally induce papillomas in the transitional areas towards nonkeratinized airway epithelium, such as in the oral cavity. Morphologically, three distinct patterns have been described for oral papillomata: (1) focal papillomatous epithelial hyperplasia, (2) verruca vulgaris-like lesions, and (3) condylomata-like tumors. HPV-specific material has been identified in about one-half of such lesions (Jenson *et al.*, 1982). Systematic attempts to correlate occurrence of a preferential HPV species to histological type have not been performed; preliminary data indicate that focal papillomatous epithelial hyperplasia may be caused by either HPV-1, or a recently identified strain, HPV-13, while verruca vulgaris-like lesions may be induced by HPV-2 (Lutzner *et al.*, 1982; Jablonska, 1983).

INCIDENCE

There appears to be an alarming increase in the incidence of condylomata in the West, establishing this entity as a major venereal disease. The most reliable data for this concept come from England; during the period 1971 to 1978, the annual incidence of reported cases almost doubled from 29.8 to 50.3 per 10,000, representing a present morbidity rate amounting to more than 40% of that for gonorrhea (von Krogh, 1982). So far, reported cases in males have outnumbered those in females, with a M/F ratio of 2:1. The correct ratio may be closer to 1:1 in light of the existence of exclusively portiocervical growth in some women, in which cases the lesions may remain unrecognized.

HISTOPATHOLOGY

Warts represent a variable exaggeration of normal skin architecture with preservation of all cell layers, rather than a conglomeration of tumor cells. Compared to verrucae, condylomata commonly exhibit features suggestive of a relatively high cellular growth fraction (Schmauz and Owor, 1980).

In young lesions, capillary proliferation in the fibrovascular core of the dermal pedicle is a prominent feature associated with capillary loops projecting into the overlying epithelium. In flat portiocervical warts, the vessels often reach the epithelial surface, producing colposcopically visible, irregularly distributed spikes. The epidermis reveals prominent papillomatosis and acanthosis and a number of mitotic figures. In typical cases there is a basal and parabasal cell hyperplasia with broadened and elongated rete pegs (Reid *et al.*, 1982).

Within the intermediate and superficial cell layers, and usually delineated by a sharp border towards the deeper layers, viral replication results in a characteristic cellular degeneration that represents a pathognomonic hallmark for an active HPV infection and a prerequisite for the diagnosis. This cellular degeneration is manifested by the appearance of koilocytes, i.e., cells displaying variable degrees of nuclear collapse and perinuclear vacuolization. When vacuolization is modest, the term 'halo cells' is used to describe this appearance; in more advanced cases, most of the cytoplasm is displaced peripherally and the cells are classified as 'balloon cells'. The nuclei of some koilocytes, especially in areas overlying subepidermal capillary loops, may contain basophilic inclusion bodies, representing crystalline arrays of viral particles. Some nuclei are slightly enlarged, but they are usually somewhat condensed, with hyperchromatosis and angulated or stellate outlines. Koilocytes displaying pronounced degeneration may have pyknotic or karyorrhectic nuclei. Bi- or multinucleation is common (Meisels *et al.*, 1981; Pilotti *et al.*, 1981).

In *verrucae*, these changes are invariably associated with a prominent thickening of the stratum corneum. In condylomata, hyper- and parakeratosis is of a much lower magnitude and occurs less often in vaginal and portiocervical lesions, compared with other genitoanal warts. Individual cell dyskeratosis, however, is a common feature; accumulation of abnormal keratin is reflected by the presence of eosinophilic cytoplasmatic inclusion bodies. In portiocervical lesions of the flat type, the surface is only covered by a few layers of such dyskeratocytes.

Quite distinct from the typical papillomatous, exophytic ('acuminate') lesions seen elsewhere, portiocervical condylomata most commonly constitute flat tumors with an undulating, almost unmodified epithelial structure. In some cases the warts rather grow in an inverted, endophytic pattern and extend pseudoinvasively into the openings of underlying endocervical glands and of the stroma. Intermediate forms are often encountered. Ferenczy *et al.* (1981) found the frequency of flat, exophytic, and endophytic condylomata in the portiocervical region to be 70%, 27%, and 3%, respectively. Morin *et al.* (1981) found these corresponding frequencies to be 69%, 23%, and 9%, respectively. Such warts were usually misdiagnosed as cervical intraepithelial neoplasia in the past.

In typical cases, portiocervical warts characteristically shed off koilocytes, permitting an unequivocal cytologic identification. In a Papanicolaou smear, dyskeratotic cells stain orangophilic. However, a number of such lesions are associated with cytological atypia of a magnitude that necessitates a biopsy for the exclusion of cervical intraepithelial neoplasia which may coexist with benign warts. Colposcopic criteria for the differentiation between the two conditions are given in Table 3 and Figure 4 (Reid *et al.*, 1980). Although these criteria represent a useful guideline for the trained clinician, they are often inadequate for planning therapy. The atypical cells mostly emanate from the parabasal cell layer: they often have an amphophilic cytoplasm and a large, somewhat irregular, darkly stained, and sometimes karyorrhectic nucleus with

Table 3 Principal features in colposcopic differentiation between cervical intra-epithelial neoplasia (CIN) and atypical warts of the portiocervix[a]

	CIN	*Warts*
Surface contour	Flat, except in major lesions	Sometimes flat, but distinctive irregularities common
Color on acetic acid staining	Dull gray	Shiny white
Topography	Within transformation zone	Not always confined to transformation zone
Vascular atypia	Punctate or mosaic pattern in sharply localized areas of white epithelium	Usually poorly formed patterns with less defined borders

[a] From Reid *et al.*, 1980.

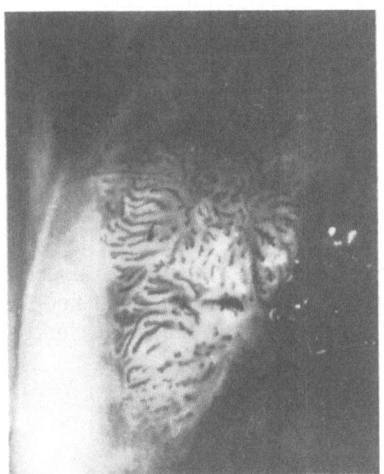 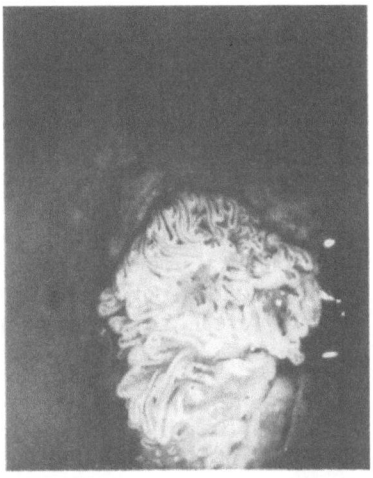

A   B

Fig. 4 Warts on the uterine portio; colposcopic appearance. **A:** Untreated; within each bud of wart hyperplasia a punctate capillary loop pattern is encountered; **B:** the capillary pattern is better visualized after the application of acetic acid. (Submitted with the courtesy of Eva Rylander, M.D., Department of Gynecology, University of Umeå, Sweden)

a smudged chromatin pattern. The presence of very pleomorphic mature squamous cells may obscure a correct diagnosis, since such cytologic findings may closely mimic the existence of dysplastic changes or carcinoma *in situ* of the endocervix.

HPV infection and intraepithelial neoplasia of genitoanal areas may coexist and may sometimes merge imperceptibly. Meisels *et al.* (1981), Crum *et al.* (1982a), have stressed that the occurrence of koilocytes in a cytologic smear does not exclude a coexisting malignancy, and enlarged hyperchromatic nuclei may occasionally be present in patients exclusively with HPV infection. When a case of intraepithelial neoplasia is suspected, evidence of abnormal mitotic processes should be sought. Although condylomata may show cells in division or with bi-multinucleation, the lesion is not associated with the existence of abnormal mitotic processes. Histologic norms for differentiation between benign warts and intraepithelial neoplasia of genitoanal epithelia are outlined

Table 4 Condylomata versus intraepithelial neoplasia of genitoanal epithelia; histological criteria for differential diagnosis[a]

	Condylomata	*Intraepithelial neoplasia*
Hyperplasia	+	+
Maturation	Discernible all layers	Atypia: often preserved in upper one-third; carcinoma *in situ*: disorderly in all layers
Koilocytes	Present from just above the parabasal layer; even distribution	Present in upper one-third; various degrees of haphazard, focal distribution
Nuclei	Pleomorphism and nuclear enlargement absent or minimal Mitosis normal	Pleomorphism and nuclear enlargement present Mitosis abnormal

[a] From Reid *et al.*, 1980; Crum *et al.*, 1982.

in Table 4. Unfortunately, histologic criteria are sometimes inadequate for evaluating cases of incipient malignant transition, since Crum *et al.* (1982a, b) have found that HPV antigen occurs in 50% of cases of condylomata and in 12.5% of clearcut atypia.

Microspectrometric determination of cellular DNA content represents a valuable measurement in such cases; HPV infection is consistently associated with diploid or polyploid DNA distribution, while intraepithelial neoplasia usually reveals an aneuploid pattern (Crum *et al.*, 1982a; Shevchuk and Richart, 1982).

MALIGNANT POTENTIAL

Sexually transmitted diseases and genital squamous cell carcinoma are associated with early sexual activity and increasing numbers of sexual partners. Speculations on a causal association between genitoanal intraepithelial neoplasia and various venereal diseases have particularly entailed herpes simplex type 2 (HSV-2), cytomegalovirus (CMV), and HPV. The frequent multicentric origin of squamous cell atypia in the genitoanal areas (Rastkar *et al.*, 1982) supports the theory of an infectious agent as a carcinogen. Interest has long been focused on HSV-2 as the carcinogen in question; its etiologic role, however, has never been confirmed.

The possible oncogenic role of HPV has been the subject of renewed interest in recent years due to impressive epidemiologic data. A final proof of a causal relationship between HPV infection and genitoanal epithelial neoplasia would require a longitudinal epidemiologic survey to show that infection is indeed followed by a significant incidence of neoplasia.

A new entity which affects individuals 15–30 years of age has been identified in genitoanal epithelia. Designated 'Bowenoid papulosis', this process involves a multifocal occurrence of erythematous or pigmented verruccoid papules with histologic changes suggestive of an incipient carcinoma *in situ* (Berger and Hori, 1978; Katz *et al.*, 1978; Wade and Kopf, 1979). Bowenoid changes have indeed been observed in close association with benign genital warts (von Krogh, 1984; Laohadtanaphorn *et al.*, 1979). HPV-16 DNA has been extracted from such histologically malignant lesions (Ikenberg *et al.*, 1983).

Although no prospective studies have been undertaken, a number of retrospective reports on malignant conversion of longstanding cases of classical genitoanal condylomata have recently appeared (Prasad and Abcarian, 1980; Syrjänen, 1980a). Both sexes may be affected. Particularly convincing are reports of vulvar carcinoma in 14-year-old girls that had suffered from vulvar warts since infancy (zur Hausen, 1977; Orth *et al.*, 1977).

Modern cytologic screening programs have traced a high and currently increasing prevalence of dysplastic or clearly malignant changes of the uterine cervix in young women. Also, some reports indicate a clearcut, up to fourfold increase in the relative frequency of warty carcinomata among all vulvar epithelial malignancies in the past decade (Rastkar *et al.*, 1982). There is mounting support for the theory that HPV represents the major infectious agent of pathogenetic significance (Reid *et al.*, 1982). Portiocervical warts often coexist and merge into areas of either atypia of various degrees or carcinoma *in situ* and frankly invasive squamous cell carcinoma of the uterine cervix (Syrjänen, 1980a,b; Syrjänen *et al.*, 1981). The most suggestive causal link between condylomata and cervical neoplasia has been reported by Reid *et al.* (1982) in a study where histologic samples from women treated by hysterectomy for malignant and premalignant changes of the uterine cervical epithelium were examined for the presence of condylomatous growths. Evidence of concurrent condylomata were found in 91% (73/80) of females with cervical intraepithelial neoplasia compared to only 12.5% (10/80) of matched controls, a highly significant difference. Furthermore, dysplastic and malignant changes develop at a significantly younger age in women with than in those without concomitant portiocervical condylomata. Moreover, among females under the age of 20 years, dysplastic changes have not been found without coexisting portiocervical warts. The highest rate of dysplastic/malignant changes of the uterine cervix occurs in such females around 30 years of age compared to around 40 years of age in condylomata-free counterparts. Malignant degeneration of portiocervical warts occurs more frequently and after a considerably shorter latency period in females 40 years or older compared to in younger women. In Uganda, malignant conversion of portiocervical condylomata was found to occur in 2.5% (6/237) of middle-aged women within a mean observation period of 6 months (Syrjänen *et al.*, 1981; Schmauz and Owor, 1978). The malignant potential may possibly be strongest for the flat or inverted atypical variant of portiocervical warts; classical papillomatous warts on this site are most commonly encountered in relatively young age groups, while the atypical lesions tend to occur in females older than 30 years (Syrjänen, 1980a,b).

In an analogous manner, a number of reports have focused on squamous cell carcinomata occurring in recurrent laryngeal and tracheal papillomata of children and adults. Atypia has been demonstrated in up to 40% of juvenile laryngeal papillomata (Cohen *et al.*, 1980). In longitudinal studies on the adult lesions, the rate of malignant transformation is above 20% (Syrjänen and Syrjänen, 1981). Malignant change seems to take place predominantly in those patients who have had their papillomata treated radiologically. When biopsy specimens from laryngeal squamous cell carcinomata in adults were rescrutinized with reference to the concurrent existence of epithelial changes fulfilling the histologic criteria of condylomata, areas with flat, exophytic or endophytic condylomatous growths were identified in 42% of samples (Syrjänen and Syrjänen, 1981). These findings support similar observations on invasive bronchial squamous cell carcinomata, in which condylomata were identified histologically in 35% of the materials (Syrjänen, 1980c). Condylomata and squamous cell carcinomata of airway epithelia coexist predominantly in males (M/F ratio 8/1) 30–80 years of age with a peak rate at 50–70 years.

The scope of HPV-associated malignancy is broadened even further by the recent identification of concurrent condylomatous lesions in 40% of cases of esophageal squamous cell carcinoma. Squamous cell papillomata of the esophagus, a poorly understood entity, bear a close histologic resemblance to condylomata. Their premalignant potential has been documented experimentally (Syrjänen, 1982).

In contrast with other well-studied DNA virus, HPV-induced tumors are in general not associated with integration of the viral genome in the host chromosome. Instead, the genetic information is present as a double-stranded, circular extrachromosomal DNA molecule even when replication of the capsid has subsided (Law et al., 1981). Quite recently, the DNA from HPV types 11, 16, and 18 has been identified in a number of cases of squamous cell malignancies of the female genital tract, in particular from neoplastic tissue from the uterine cervix (Durst et al., 1983; Ikenberg et al., 1983; Singer et al., 1984). These findings indicate that HPV may not merely act as a passenger throughout malignant transformation of warts but may have a causative role for the development of squamous cell neoplasia of the genitals. The existence of HPV-16 also in Bowenoid papulosis of the genitals is further indicative for an etiologic association between malignant change and certain HPVs that induce condylomata.

Absence of HPV DNA integration into the chromosomes of benign warts does not mean that any integration does not exist under certain circumstances; in malignant tissue subgenomic fragments may very well be integrated although they are not detectable with current methodology. In this respect, a synergistic effect may perhaps take place beteen HPV and other infectious agents such as HSV-2 (zur Hausen, 1982). This process may also be enhanced by cocarcinogens such as roentgenographic irradiation and smoking in the case of airway epithelia (Syrjänen and Syrjänen, 1981), and products related to sexual activity and/or smoking for the genitoanal areas, of which the uterine cervix evidently represents a locus minoris (Fenoglio and Ferenczy, 1982). Very likely, the process is facilitated by immunosuppressive factors in the host.

CLINICAL EVALUATION

Concurrent sexually transmitted diseases (e.g. syphilis, gonorrhea, and infections with *Chlamydia, Trichomonas*, and *Candida* organisms) should preferably be diagnosed and treated prior to condylomata therapy. Warts of long duration, or papulous and macroscopically atypical condylomata, should be biopsied to rule out the existence of atypia or malignant transformation. In females, routine procedures should include examination of the vagina and the portiocervix and a Pap smear. If there is evidence of portiocervical lesions, a colposcopy-directed biopsy should be performed; if the first examination is negative, females should be reexamined 3–6 months later due to the long incubation time. When anal warts are encountered, proctoscopy is essential for adequately determining the extent of involvement.

THERAPY

Physician treatment with crude podophyllin

Until the advent of topical podophyllin treatment condylomata therapy involved tedious and frequently unsuccessful surgical interventions. It was Culp and Kaplan (1944) who first discovered that topical application of a 25% resinic extract of *Podophyllum* species in mineral oil could induce necrosis and resolution of genitoanal warts. Although their procedure elicited varying degrees of inflammatory reactions in the tumor bases and adjacent unafflicted areas to which the mineral oil preparation easily spread, it was initially well received because of the high cure rates claimed in the early publications. The occurrences of painful local adverse reactions 2–3 days after the applications were increasingly recognized, however, and various changes were introduced to reduce the local toxic effect. Such procedures included washing off surplus medication 3–4 hours after application, protecting the surrounding epithelia with inert pastes, creams or ointments, and incorporating the drug into alternative vehicles that could better confine its activity to diseased areas. Despite these precautions, inpatient treatment was initially recommended by some investigators. In cases in which retreatment was needed, a few days' interval between applications was suggested, but it was later advocated that at least a week should elapse. A regimen based on weekly applications of 20–25% podophyllin resin in ethanol or in benzoic tincture was subsequently recommended as the treatment of choice for genitoanal warts. Objections have been raised, however, over the course of years due to the variable frequency of severe local toxic reactions, the lack of reproducibility of the efficacy originally claimed, and most seriously, the substantial risk of inducing severe systemic intoxication when applying abundant podophyllin quantities on large condylomata plaques (von Krogh, 1982a).

The podophyllin used worldwide is based mostly on resinic extracts from *Podophyllum peltatum* rhizosomes. In England, a closely related species, *P. emodi*, which is indigenous to Himalayan areas, is imported for extraction in condylomata therapy. Resins from the two plants differ markedly with respect to the chemical structure of their lignans, a class of compounds having a dibenzylbutane skeleton (Fig. 5). The cytodestructive properties of podophyllin and its activity in condylomata eradication are based on the lignans. These agents may induce lesional necrosis 3–5 days after topical administration, primarily because of their antimitotic cellular activity.

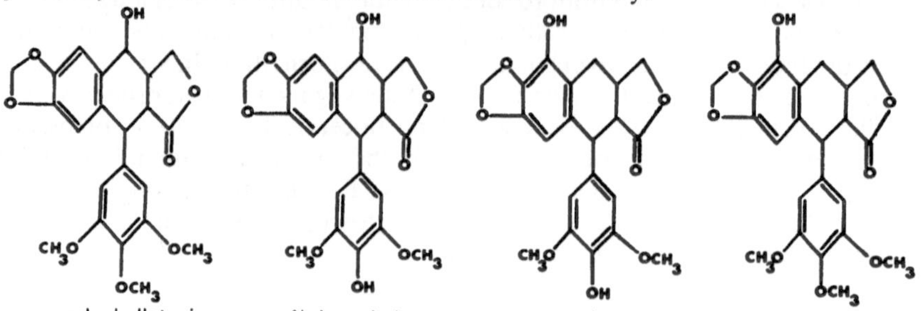

	podophyllotoxin	4'-demethyl-podophyllotoxin	α-peltatin	β-peltatin
P. peltatum	+	–	+	+
P. emodi	+	(+)	–	–

Fig. 5 *Podophyllum* lignans

The development of modern chromatographic methods for lignan purification (Treppendahl and Jacobsen, 1980; Cairnes *et al.*, 1981) has made it possible to use a more standardized lignan preparation for topical condylomata therapy. Treatment recommendations for crude podophyllin preparations must be revised in light of two important considerations: the low efficacy associated with the regimen currently recommended and the significant risk of inducing systemic side-effects due to transepidermal absorption of hazardous podophyllin ingredients.

Initial reports on podophyllin treatment of condylomata recounted a 96% cumulative cure rate of predominantly penile lesions after one or two applications. However, the reliability of these results was greatly compromised by the fact that the clinical observations were performed on soldiers and their partners and long-term follow-up data could not be accumulated. In studies with more careful long-term follow-up, recurrence rates of up to 35–50% over a 3-month period have been reported, especially in cases of numerous or relatively large tumors. A number of investigators have reported that more than one podophyllin application is regularly needed for complete cure (von Krogh, 1982a). In one study, 36% of patients required more than four applications, and condylomata were still present in 7% of cases 1 year after podophyllin treatment had been started (von Krogh, 1975). In an investigation comparing the long-term (3 months) efficacy of *P. peltatum* preparations with those based on *P. emodi* resin, only 19–24% of all patients were cured after the first application and another 13–19% when treatment was repeated on residual warts. Efficacy was similar for the two preparations despite a considerable difference in the total lignan content. The cumulative effect from two applications was somewhat better (49%) for an 8% preparation of purified podophyllotoxin, which represents the maximal possible lignan concentration in 20% podophyllin (von Krogh, 1978). The cumulative tumor destructive effect from

8% podophyllotoxin was also sustained when all lesions were treated twice at an interval of 72 hours; 54% of patients were cured of all penile lesions and 65% of at least preputial cavity warts (Table 5). As was the case when the application interval was a week, more than three-fourths of the men experienced no discomfort from the latter treatment, although involution of large or numerous warts was associated with somewhat painful epithelial erosions (von Krogh, 1981).

Table 5 Percentage cure ($\geq$ 3 months' follow-up) of penile condylomata acuminata using various procedures for topical treatment[a]

Treatment procedures	Preparation		Cure rate (%)	
			All lesions	Preputial cavity lesions
Physician application once or twice with about a 1-week interval	P. peltatum	20%	32 (15/47)	41 (16/39)
	P. emodi	20%	43 (25/58)	48 (25/52)
	Podophyllotoxin	8%	49 (35/72)	56 (36/64)
Physician application twice with 72 hours interval	Podophyllotoxin	8%	54 (22/41)	65 (24/37)
Self-application twice-thrice daily for 3 days	Podophyllotoxin	1%	51 (37/73)	66 (39/59)
	Podophyllotoxin	0.5%	46 (46/100)	70 (57/82)
Self-application twice daily for 4 days[b]	Podophyllotoxin	0.5%	70 (26/37)	80 (28/35)

[a] From von Krogh, 1981; von Krogh, 1978. These investigations were performed at the Karolinska Institute at Södersjukhuset, Department of Dermatology, Stockholm, Sweden
[b] Previously unpublished material

The tissues most sensitive to podophyllin treatment are those that have a high degree of cellular proliferation. With respect to potential systemic side-effects, the bone marrow, lymph follicles, and intestinal mucosa represent highly susceptible organs of concern. However, the functions of the nonproliferating nervous cells are also most susceptible to the influence of these drugs, which may ultimately inhibit axoplasmic flow (Filliatreau and Giamberardino, 1981; Filley et al., 1982). This fact is important for the comprehension of the toxicologic risks associated with systemic lignan side-effects; a narrow gap exists between doses sufficient to cause transient damage of organs exhibiting a high mitotic rate and those sufficient to be neurotoxic and potentially lethal. Cancer patients have received daily i.v. injections of 0.5–1.0 mg/kg for up to 2 weeks without developing clinical injury beyond transitory bone marrow and gastrointestinal disturbances. On the other hand, accidental ingestions of not much larger quantities may have caused death (Savel, 1964; Dudley, 1980; Peterson and Haines, 1923). Other agents of CNS depression such as alcohol and general anaesthetics, seem to enhance the neurotoxic effects of lignans (von Krogh, 1982a).

Acute side-effects, which may appear within a few hours after treatment, include dizziness, general weakness or lethargy, emesis, and diarrhea. These symptoms are accompanied by changes in blood pressure, pulse, and respiration. More alarming central nervous system (CNS) disturbances, sometimes commencing with a hallucinatory psychosis, may soon develop, and the following days may be critical for life. In advanced cases, stupor, depressed respiration, progressive peripheral neuropathy, urine retention, paralytic ileus, internal bleedings, and vascular crisis associated with electrolyte disturbances, may occur. Transient hepatic dysfunction and maturation disturbances of bone marrow elements or pancytopenia, may follow within a week. Nevertheless, repeated treatment with smaller doses may be well tolerated, with only temporary effects on cells in highly proliferative tissues, such as the bone marrow and intestinal mucosa. Nonlethal damage is fully reversible within days or weeks, with the exception of neuropathy, which may persist for several months (Filley *et al.*, 1982; von Krogh, 1982b, McFarland and McFarland, 1981; Leslie and Shitamoto, 1982; Cassidy *et al.*, 1982).

The systemic absorption of hazardous quantities of one or more of the cytotoxic ingredients in podophyllin preparations is well documented. A number of patients have developed serious acute systemic intoxication after applying large doses of podophyllin on extremely large condylomata. The very nature of these lesions favors a high degree of percutaneous absorption. They afflict intertriginous regions delineated by thin epidermis and subjected to occlusive factors, and their ruffled, papillomatous surface may represent a substantial absorbing area. Furthermore, systemic distribution is facilitated by their highly vascularized base. Therefore, when calculating safety margins for topical lignan treatment, the possibility for a 100% absorption must be considered (von Krogh, 1982b).

The available data on toxicity margins for lignan administration indicate that topical treatment should not exceed 0.5 mg/kg per application. This amount corresponds to a maximum volume of 20% podophyllin of 0.9–1.2 ml for preparations based on *P. peltatum* and 0.4–0.5 ml for *P. emodi*-based remedies (von Krogh, 1982b). Nevertheless, during the 35-year period that podophyllin has been used worldwide, many patients have doubtlessly received one or more treatments with considerably larger volumes without developing clinical manifest injuries even to the most sensitive organs, indicating that a complete systemic absorption of lignans seldom occurs.

Self-treatment with 0.5% podophyllotoxin for 3–4 days, or more

As animal experiments demonstrate, divided doses of a given lignan quantity is toxicologically much safer than administration of the same amount as a single dose (Sullivan *et al.*, 1951; Philip *et al.*, 1948; Greenspan and Leiter, 1949). In an attempt to reduce the risk of systemic toxicity and the number of time-consuming and expensive physician consultations associated with current use of crude podophyllin preparations, our research group has initiated an evaluation of a regimen based on repeated self-applications with low-dose, topical podophyllotoxin preparations. The selection of podophyllotoxin*, the only lignan occurring in podophyllin of any origin, is based on evidence that this compound tends to elicit a superior cutaneous cytodestructive response on animal skin compared to the other lignans (von Krogh, 1982; von Krogh and Maibach, 1982).

* Available from: Pharma-Medica A-S, Herlev, Denmark.

Males afflicted with penile warts were provided with 5 ml of 0.5% or 1.0% podophyllotoxin in ethanol to be applied with a cotton-wool swab; 0.05% methylrosaniline dye was added as a color indicator so that treated areas could be visualized. The overall cure rate (48%) was similar to results achieved in physician-treatment regimens, in which two applications of 8% podophyllotoxin were separated by 72 hours (see Table 5), and was significantly higher than the 22% cure rate based on clinical treatment of penile warts with various single-dose 20% podophyllin preparations. The outcome was the same whether 0.5% or 1.0% podophyllin was used or whether the men applied the medication two or three times daily. All preputial cavity warts were eradicated in 66–70% of the cases; the method had a comparably lower efficacy when warts grew in the urinary meatus (32%) or on penile skin (13%) (von Krogh, 1981). The cure rate was inversely proportional to tumor duration or lesional bulk; condylomata that coalesced into plaques were particularly recalcitrant to treatment (Table 6). When an ethanolic preparation of 0.5% podophyllotoxin was applied twice daily for 4 days, the efficacy increased further; 70% of those in a preliminary study (von Krogh, unpublished data) were cured of all penile warts (See Table 5).

Table 6 Factors influencing the outcome of previously untreated penile condylomata acuminata treated with ethanolic podophyllotoxin preparations repeatedly applied within a 3-day period

Factor	Prognosis	
	Favorable	Unfavorable
Distribution	Preputial cavity	Urinary meatus
	'Transitional area' of prepuce	Skin
Number	≤5	>5
Growth pattern	Disseminated	Plaques
	Relatively small lesions	Relatively large lesions
Duration	≤6 months	>6 months

From: von Krogh, 1981.

Repeated topical treatments with podophyllin are generally well tolerated. When this agent is repeatedly administered during the phase of drug-induced involution, however, therapeutic benefits will inevitably be accompanied by an associated discomfort due to the presence of necrotizing tumor cells and a destructive influence on the adjacent epithelium to some degree. Minor complaints, including localized erythema, superficial ulceration, and/or some tenderness were observed for a few days in 45–72% of patients in our series. These conditions responded quickly to mild adjunctive topical anti-inflammatory therapy (von Krogh, 1982a, 1981, 1978). A small percentage (6–8%) of patients exhibiting a relatively large tumor bulk complained of either some pain in the treated area for a few days, or a severe, temporary burning from the ethanolic vehicle in association with reapplications of the medication during the third or fourth day of therapy. The latter complication may be overcome by incorporating the drug into an alternative vehicle, such as a cream or an ointment. This alternative has been pursued because of the encouraging therapeutic results from recent studies on penile warts. Moreover, the non-liquid preparation may be useful to patients with vulvar and anal warts, for whom self-treatment with a liquid is not feasible. From preliminary studies on vulvar and anal lesions, using physician application of 0.5% podophyllotoxin-ethanol once daily for 3 consecutive days, cure rates have not been comparable to those obtained by self-medication for penile warts twice daily for the same period of time. The inferior outcome may be due to the lower number of applications or to a dilution of the drug's effect *in situ* because of the higher degree of moisture in vulvar and anal areas. The use of a cream vehicle may hinder any diluting and, thereby, render drug penetration into the lesions more effective.

Daily self-treatment with a low-dose podophyllotoxin preparation until genitoanal warts disappear represents a practical approach, but the optimal treatment duration for various morphological condylomata types and lesions afflicting the numerous genital–anatomical substructures has not yet been established. It is likely that treatment in excess of 3–4 days may be required for many of the problem warts, such as those in the urinary meatus, papulous lesions, and relatively large lesions, especially those coalescing into plaques.

The safety and potential systemic effects of this type of self-treatment were evaluated by using high-performance liquid chromatography (HPLC) to search for traces of drug quantities in serum. We also monitored some relevant clinical toxicological parameters, such as levels of aminotransferase enzymes; leukocyte, erythrocyte, and thrombocyte counts; pulse, blood pressure; respiration; and general condition and comfort, including frequency of bowel emptying (von Krogh, 1982). The drug was undetectable using individual doses in the magnitude of 0.05 ml. The use of 0.1 ml doses, a volume which is quite sufficient to treat even numerous tumors, gave rise to a serum peak level of up to 5 ng/ml within a couple of hours and subsequent levels of up to 3 ng/ml for 4 hours. When extraordinarily large condylomata with plaques were literally drenched with 0.5% podophyllotoxin-ethanol, peak levels of up to 17 ng/ml were measured within a few hours and were followed by traceable nanogram quantities for 12 hours or more (Table 7). These results confirm that podophyllotoxin may enter the blood rapidly after topical administration to genitoanal areas but that the compound does not tend to accumulate in the serum. Studies on closely related compounds indicate that excretion is mainly through the hepatobiliary system (Emenegger *et al.*, 1961), which appears to be well protected against toxic effects from lignans (Kiso *et al.*, 1982). In no case did any signs occur indicating hazardous toxic effects from 3 days' twice-daily administration of individual podophyllotoxin doses in the magnitude of up to 7.5 mg (see Table 7), a quantity which in terms of mg/kg is equivalent to about 0.1 per application or 0.2 per day. This dose is still far below the critical level of 0.5 mg/kg body weight of individual lignan doses, which is considered dangerous. In the majority of cases, volumes of up to about 0.2 ml are sufficient to treat all lesions in individual patients. Such doses are far below dangerous levels; they are 18–36 times smaller than the podophyllotoxin quantities found to elicit transient functional depression of highly proliferative tissues after i.v. injection of a single dose into humans.

The significance of the detected serum quantities of podophyllotoxin in the self-treatment regimen is better appreciated when it is correlated to existing

Table 7 Correlation between topical dose of 0.5% podophyllotoxin-ethanol applied twice daily for 3 days on genitoanal condylomata plaque, and magnitude and duration of subsequent drug levels in serum[a]

Dose		Serum podophyllotoxin concentration (ng/ml) at time after application			
Preparation (μl)	Podophyllotoxin (mg)	1–2 h	4 h	8 h	12 h
≤50	0.25	0	ND[b]	ND	ND
100	0.50	0–5.0	0–3.0	0–0.5	0
150	0.75	1.0–5.0	0.5–3.5	0	0–1.0
300	1.50	8.0	ND	ND	0
600	3.00	7.5	4.0	2.0	ND
800	4.00	9.0–17.0	10.0	ND	2.0
1100	5.50	7.5–9.0	7.0	3.5	0.5
1500	7.50	5.0–9.0	5.0–7.0	3.0–4.5	3.5

[a] From von Krogh, 1982b
[b] ND = not determined

reports on the *in vitro* effect of lignans on cell cultures. When amnion cells in stationary growth phase are submitted to the potent antimitotic lignan deoxypodophyllotoxin, up to 11,000 ng/ml may be tolerated for up to 4 days without causing evident cyctotoxicity, in spite of the fact that as minute quantities as 1 ng/ml may significantly suppress cellular thymidine incorporation transitorily (Markanen *et al.*, 1981, 1982). Cells in log phase of cellular proliferation are considerably more sensitive. Metaphasic arrest of fibroblasts in log phase may be accomplished by podophyllotoxin in quantities of 3 ng/ml when exposure time is up to 6 hours (von Krogh, 1982b; Emenegger *et al.*, 1961). Proliferating bone marrow cells seem somewhat less vulnerable; incubation with 2 ng of the drug/ml for 1 week suppresses growth by only 5%, while an increase in concentration to about 20 ng/ml leads to total inhibition of cultures (Smissmann *et al.*, 1976). On the other hand, mature marrow elements are considerably more sensitive than blast forms and early precursors, which are well preserved during acute intoxication. Hematologic resolution seems to follow invariably in patients surviving systemic intoxication (Leslie and Shitamoto, 1982). Potential CNS disturbances from minute podophyllotoxin quantities represents a major concern, but there were no signs of pathological CNS function in any of the patients in our series who demonstrated continuous drug levels up to 3.5 ng/ml for 12 hours (von Krogh, 1982b).

These data indicate that self-treatment with 0.5% podophyllotoxin twice daily for 3–4 days, or more, is highly satisfactory in terms of efficacy and safety. Nevertheless, only volumes sufficient to cover all lesions should be used; excessive medication should be avoided. As noted earlier, this treatment modality must be refined prior to general use by a broad range of patients with condylomata of the outer genitoanal area. In any event, the high susceptibility of proliferating cells to even minute quantities of podophyllotoxin represents a clear contraindication against using this drug in pregnant women because of its potential for damaging the fetus and placenta (Chamberlain *et al.*, 1972; Karol *et al.*, 1980).

Other chemotherapeutic modalities

As the shortcomings of traditional podophyllin treatment have gained recognition, other chemotherapeutic modalities for topical condylomata treatment have been sought. Successful treatment with topical colchicine has been reported, but most studies have dealt with small series, and practical details with respect to appropriate regimens have been sparse (Bourg and Dustin, 1945, Sullivan and King, 1947; Wiedeman-Erfurt, 1959; Gigax and Robison, 1971). Although colchicine has *in vitro* pharmacokinetic properties that are similar to those of lignans, investigations on large patient groups demonstrate that its therapeutic activity against condylomata is lower and that unacceptable local adverse effects occur considerably more often. Accordingly, colchicine is not recommended in the routine treatment of genitoanal warts (von Krogh and Ruden, 1980).

Newer chemotherapeutic agents, such as thiotepa and bleomycin, have only limited usefulness in condylomata management. Thiotepa therapy has been used experimentally for the management of extensive intraurethral lesions, which are otherwise particularly hard to manage, even with repeated surgery (Halverstadt and Perry, 1969). Topical application of bleomycin has been tried with poor results (von Krogh, 1984); when injected intralesionally, up to 70% cure rates have been achieved but only after numerous repeated administrations over periods of several months (Figueroa and Gennaro, 1980).

A number of workers have reported on the use of 5-fluorouracil (5-FU) in condylomata treatment. The results have been somewhat controversial; cure rates in the range of 33–70% have been reported after daily applications for up to 8 weeks. However, cure is usually obtained at the cost of painful epithelial ulcerations. For this reason, primary use of 5-FU in condylomata therapy is not justified, with the exception of lesions of the urinary meatus, which may disappear in up to 90% of cases when 5-FU ointment is applied after each voiding for 2–3 weeks. On this site, the medication can be confined to a limited area, and subsequent ulcerations merely cause dysuria (von Krogh, 1982a, 1976).

Various caustic agents have also been used in condylomata therapy over the years. Their efficacy has been poorly documented. The most commonly used compounds are bi- and trichloracetic acid, both of which rapidly penetrate and cauterize the skin. Maximum benefit from such treatment occurs when application is performed at weekly intervals. However, numerous treatments are required, and the procedure is in no way superior to podophyllin with the exception of its lack of systemic toxicity (Swerdlow and Salvati, 1971; Willcox, 1977). Caustic lesional destruction is particularly valuable during pregnancy.

Surgical intervention

While simple surgical excision and electrocautery are convenient methods for eradication of a few solitary and discrete lesions, these techniques are unfeasible for routine treatment of relatively large or numerous condylomata, when several repeated sessions are usually necessary. Surgical intervention, however, represents an important alternative during pregnancy, in patients with otherwise inaccessible warts of the anal canal, the vagina and the portiocervix, and in cases refractory to topical chemotherapy (Graver et al., 1967; Lewis, 1973).

Cryosurgery represents a useful modality for primary treatment of intravaginal condylomata (Townsend et al., 1971; Simmons et al., 1981) and in the management of recalcitrant lesions, especially those of the urinary meatus (von Krogh, 1983) and anal area. Several visits generally are required for total clearance.

Modern CO_2 laser surgery, the surgeon's 'light scalpel', represents a considerable technical advance. Tissue cauterization and evaporation is accomplished while cutting; the heat from the laser beam tends to seal off small severed blood vessels, thereby minimizing the amount of bleeding from these richly vascularized tumors. The high accuracy of the procedure allows normal tissues to be spared and healing to occur with minimal scar formation. Cure rates of up to 63–86% have been reported for genitoanal warts after only one session, although larger tumors require staged operations (Baggish, 1980; Hahn, 1981; Calkins et al., 1982; Rosenberg et al., 1982). Laser instruments are expensive, however, and their use requires special clinical experience and skill; the method, therefore, is presently limited to larger medical centers. Although this technique may not represent a therapeutic tool for routine office use, it has proven valuable for primary eradication of portiocervical and intraurethral growths, as well as for giant condylomata occurring during pregnancy and for relatively quick surgical treatment of otherwise recalcitrant tumors. CO_2 laser evaporation of laryngeal papillomata has also proven to be superior to simple surgical removal, which is associated with a frustratingly high degree of recurrences and postoperative complications such as laryngeal edema and disturbances of vocal quality. When combined postoperatively with podophyllin painting of the tumor bed in order to prevent papilloma reimplantation, up to about 40% long-term remission has followed (Dedo and Jackler, 1982).

Immunotherapy

The role of humoral responses against HPV particles in the etiology of wart diseases has been somewhat controversial. From animal studies it is known that the antiviral defense against DNA viruses is mediated mainly by antibodies to capsid antigens (Fig. 6). While IgM is the first antibody type to appear, IgG dominates the later stages of inoculation. Small quantities of viral particles only elicit a transitory IgM response without producing an immunologic memory capability, while larger doses give rise to specific IgG antibodies and an established antiviral humoral immunologic memory associated with various degrees of protection against reinfection. However, once inside intact cells, such as is the case with HPV-induced tumors, the viral particles seem well protected against the action of specific immunoglobulins (von Krogh, 1979).

The prevalence of HPV antibodies in human sera varies from 21% to 66% in various investigations. In healthy controls, only IgG has been found; it can be traced years after a known wart infection. It is also present in a number of cases with a negative wart history. The prevalence of HPV-IgG is significantly higher during the first year or so of wart duration, when the intracellular yield of particles tends to be highest. The presence of HPV-IgG antibodies represents

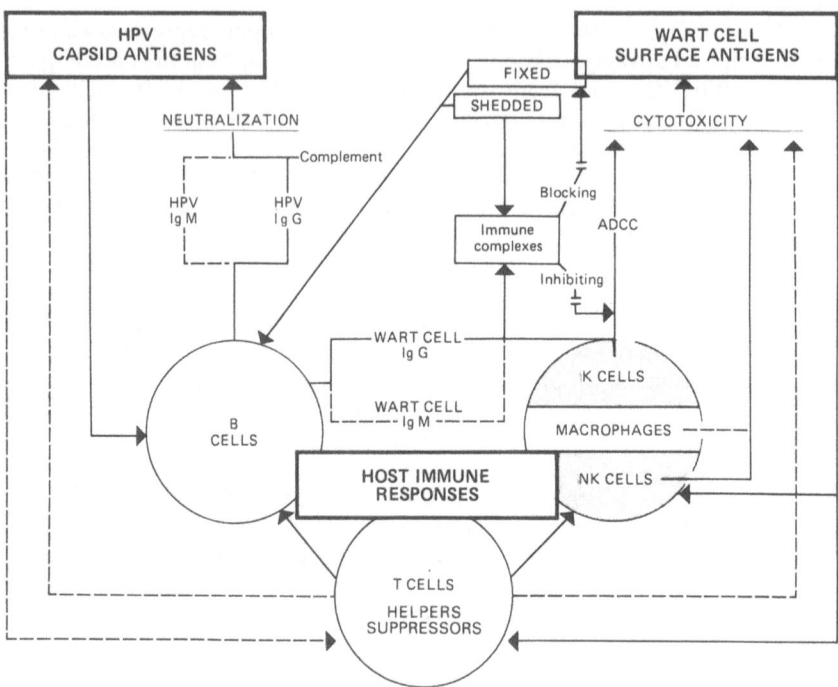

Fig. 6 The figure represents a simplified illustration of major immunological events being potentially elicited during the course of warts. Intracellular HPV particles are protected from the action of host immune defense; occurrence of HPV capsid antibodies in association with wart cure seem to reflect a liberation of viral particles secondary to wart cell destruction. Nevertheless, HPV antibodies, predominantly of the IgG class, may contribute to limit the tumor bulk during wart establishment in various epithelia through complement-dependent neutralization of the virus. When spontaneous wart rejection occurs, humoral and cell-mediated immune responses directed against tumor surface antigens are believed to represent the major effector mechanisms inducing a cytotoxic response. In this respect, NK cells and macrophages are the predominant components of cell-mediated resistance; macrophages may contribute non-specifically, while clones of NK cells are coded for specific cognizance of tumor neoantigens and other surface markers. K cells effectuate antibody-dependent cell-mediated cytoxocity (ADCC) through cognizance of tumor cell-specific IgG on the wart cells, to which K cells attach due to their possession of Fc receptors; the reaction may be inhibited by the occurrence of circulating immune complexes due to shedding of wart cell antigens, or blocked by immune complexes of coating the tumor. The figure does not account for the immune modulating influence of e.g. interferons and lymphokines. (© Geo. von Krogh)

a prognostically favorable sign but is in no way required for successful therapy or spontaneous resolution. Of 173 patients examined regularly during a 6-month period of active therapy, 75–94% of IgG-positive cases were cured within 2 months and all were cured within 3 months. Only 16–46% with IgM solely and 37–64% without any HPV antibodies were cured within the 2-month period (Pyrhönen and Johansson, 1975; Pyrhönen and Penttinen, 1972). It is believed that the favorable prognostic association with presence of HPV-IgG reflects secondary events during wart cure, when tumor cell destruction leads to the cellular release of viral material. The persistence of HPV-IgG in the serum is not associated with full protection from further wart attacks (Cubie, 1972), although it may contribute to a restriction of tumor bulk when reinfection occurs (von Krogh, 1979).

Two types of new antigens (neoantigens) appear on the cell surface of virus-induced tumors: oncofetal antigens (OFA) and tumor-specific transplantation antigens (TSTA). OFA represent nonspecific, tumor-associated embryonic determinants common to the organ of origin of the tumor, having 'disappeared' from adult cells (von Krogh, 1979). Crossreactive antigens of this type appear in such varying epidermal tumors as warts, keratoacanthomata, and squamous cell carcinomata (Pass *et al.*, 1971). TSTA has not been identified for wart tumors but may possibly be crossreactive for various HPV-induced tumor types.

Both humoral and cell-mediated immune responses are evoked against these antigens (see Fig. 6). Their reciprocal importance is at present the subject of investigation, and the long-standing theory that humoral responses merely played a minor role and that cell-mediated responses were mediated predominantly by T cells has recently been reevaluated. The latter concept was supported by such findings as the presence of impaired T cell function in individuals with a high incidence of recalcitrant tumors, a phenomenon which has been clearly demonstrated in wart patients.

The incidence of persistent warts is greater among subjects with cell-mediated immune defects, as well as during immunosuppressive treatment. The delayed cutaneous hypersensitivity reaction against tuberculin is weaker in children with warts than in healthy controls of the same age. Patients with warts of a long duration have generally reduced *in vitro* cell-mediated immunologic responses against mitogenic substances as compared with controls (von Krogh, 1979). Nevertheless, the majority of wart patients seem to represent fully immunocompetent individuals; this has been demonstrated on condylomata patients using evaluation of epicutaneous challenge responses for dinitrochlorobenzene (DNCB) subsequent to sensitization with the compound (von Krogh, 1982a, 1981).

The concept that T cells are the prevailing defenders against neoplastic cells has been challenged by some intriguing experimental findings, such as the fact that there is no major increase in tumor incidence in nude athymic mice or in neonatally thymectomized mice and an absence of specific cytotoxic T cells in many patients with malignant tumors (Herbeman, 1980).

The discovery and incipient characterization of natural killer (NK) cells, which are a separate and unique developmental lineage within the lympho-reticular system, represent a marked shift from their prior classification as 'null cells' to the present appreciation of their positive features. These new theories have opened new avenues for the understanding of immune surveillance and tumor resistance. Although potential assistance from cytotoxic T cells has not been dismissed, it is now believed that NK cells and macrophages represent the most significant components of cell-mediated tumor resistance. While macrophages are nonspecific in their action, clones of NK cells may specifically seek tumor targets by recognizing neoantigens and other surface markers. NK cells seem to most effectively deal with a small number of tumor cells; individuals with well established tumors may for obscure reasons have significantly decreased NK-cell activity, compared to normal controls (Herbeman, 1980).

It seems quite clear at present that humoral responses against tumor cells may contribute significantly to resistance against warts and other tumors. Such responses are largely mediated by another type of killer cells, the K cells, which seem developmentally related to NK cells. K cells represent the predominant effector cell for antibody-dependent, cell-mediated cytotoxicity (ADCC); they may exert a cytotoxic effect on IgG-coated target cells (see Fig. 6) due to their possession of membrane Fc receptors with avidity for the activated Fc region of IgG. ADCC may to some extent also be mediated by small subpopulations of NK cells and macrophages exhibiting surface Fc receptors. Target-cell selectivity of ADCC resides in the specificity of the coating antibody and not in the effector lymphocyte; due to extreme economy in use of IgG, the reaction may contribute significantly to immunological tumor rejection. The phenomenon is easily blocked by immune complexes (von Krogh, 1979; Herbeman, 1980; Berman and Frankfort, 1982).

The functions of NK cells, K cells, and macrophages are greatly enhanced by the lymphokine *interferon*, which plays a central role as an immunomodulatory link in the host defense against tumors. Interferon comprises a group of secretory proteins that can potentially be produced by a high number of cells; lymphocytes, leukocytes, macrophages and fibroblasts are particularly productive in response to various stimuli such as exposure to virally infected cells and tumor-transformed cells. Interferon may thereby induce a direct suppression on virus replication, as well as cell proliferation, in addition to an augmentation of the host's cytotoxic immune responses (Herbeman, 1980). The multiplicity of immunological factors of potential significance for the influence on the growth and rejection of warts is summarized visually in Figure 6.

The two major types of interferon are Type I (alpha and beta), which are induced by viruses, and Type II (gamma), which is induced by antigens or mitogens. At present, alpha-Type I interferon of leukocyte origin has been the main source for clinical trials. It has been used successfully as an ointment (4000 u/g) against recalcitrant genitoanal warts. Although 90% cure rates have been claimed, treatment is tedious and expensive as five to six daily applications are required for up to 8 weeks (Ikic *et al.*, 1975). Alpha-interferon has also been given im (2 million U daily) against laryngo-tracheobronchial papillomatosis with beneficial clinical effect in a large number of cases, although complete cure has seldom occurred. Again, the treatment is not very practical, since daily or alternate day injections were required for several months; furthermore, all patients experienced drug-related side effects during treatment (Goepfert *et al.*, 1982).

Other types of immunomodulatory treatments, such as administration of *cimetidine*, which may inactivate T-suppressor cells to some extent, have a negligible effect on condylomata (Rampen and Everdingen, 1982). Somewhat more encouraging results have been achieved with methods that attempt to attract potentially cytotoxic effector cells to the site of tumor growth. Injection of BCG into condylomatous lesions is technically difficult and associated with intense local pain; alternative injection into para-lesional genitoanal areas is better tolerated but does not assure cure (Malison and Salkin, 1981). The possibility exists of using tuberculin jelly for topical application in future trials. This procedure has led to cure of recalcitrant common warts in 57% of cases. The method is not attractive for routine use because applications several times a week for many months seem necessary (Lahti and Hannuksela, 1982).

Patience and numerous consultations are also required when topical DNCB applications are attempted in DNCB-sensitized individuals. The fact that the magnitude of challenge doses required for cure will induce an incipient dermatitic response in the sensitive genitoanal areas indicates that the regimen is quite unsuitable for condylomata therapy (von Krogh, unpublished data).

Potential use of vaccine therapy with wart tissue components represents an old concept which was first tested by Biberstein in 1925. High cure rates were achieved for wart patients after injection with crude wart extracts. A dispute in the literature ensued when these results could not be reproduced by others, and the technique was long forgotten. During the past decade, however, the method has been reevaluated in condylomata patients who received subcutaneous injections of autogenous tumor homogenates repeatedly for about 6 weeks. Although initial reports indicated cure rates of more than 80% (Abcarian *et al.*, 1976; Abcarian and Sharon, 1977; Eftaiha *et al.*, 1982) a dispute has again arisen with respect to the scientific background for current use of such techniques. It has recently been documented that autogenous wart vaccine does not seem to induce a higher frequency of wart rejection than use of 'placebo' vaccine prepared from patients' own normal skin (Malison *et al.*, 1982). This is not to say that the immune system does not play a role in the resolution of wart disease; it rather focuses on what specific cellular factors are capable of enhancing the efficacy of the immune system. Injections of homogenates from normal epidermis may stimulate a focal attraction of nonspecific cytotoxic cells through induction of interferon production (Herbeman, 1980). Research in this area seems to reach a crescendo phase, providing hope that more scientifically monitored vaccine programs may eventually be developed for a range of various HPV papillomata.

References

Abcarian, H., Smith, D. and Sharon, N. (1976). The immunotherapy of anal condylomata acuminatum. *Dis. Colon Rect.*, **19,** 237

Abcarian, H. and Sharon, N. (1977). The effectiveness of immunotherapy in the treatment of anal condylomata acuminatum. *J. Surg. Res.*, **22,** 231

Baggish, M. S. (1980). Carbon dioxide laser treatment for condylomata acuminata venereal infection. *Obstet. Gynecol.*, **55,** 711

Barrero-Oro, J. G., Kendall, O. S. and Melnick, J. L. (1962). Quantitation of papova virus particles in human warts. *J. Natl. Cancer Inst.*, **29,** 583

Barret, T. J. and Silbar, J. D. (1954). Genital warts – a venereal disease. *J. Am. Med. Assoc.*, **154**, 333

Berger, B. W. and Hori, Y. (1978). Multicentric Bowen's disease of the genitalia. *Arch. Dermatol.*, **114**, 1698

Berman, B. and Frankfort, H. M. (1982). The human interferon system. *Int. J. Dermatol.*, **21**, 12

Biberstein, H. (1925). Versuche über Immunotherapie der Warzen und Kondylome. *Klin. Wochenschr.*, **4**, 638

Bloom, W. and Fawatt, D. W. (eds.). (1974). *A Textbook of Histology*, 10th edn., Chap. 3, pp. 27, 31 (Philadelphia, London, Toronto: W. B. Saunders)

Bourg, R. and Dustin, P. (1945). Le traitement des papillomes vulvaires par l'application locale de colchicine. *Presse Med.*, **53**, 578

Bunney, M. H. (ed.). (1982). *Viral Warts. Their Biology and Treatment*, p. 1. (New York, Toronto: Oxford University Press)

Cairnes, D. A., Kingston, G. I. and Rao, M. M. (1981). High performance liquid chromatography of podophyllotoxins and related lignans. *J. Nat. Prod.*, **44**, 34

Calkins, J. W., Masterson, B. J., Magrina, J. F. *et al.* (1982). Management of condylomata acuminata with the carbon dioxide laser. *Obstet. Gynecol.*, **59**, 105

Cassidy, D. B., Drewry, J. and Fanning, J. P. (1982). Podophyllum toxicity: A report of a fatal case and a review of the literature. *J. Toxicol. Clin. Toxicol.*, **19**, 35

Chamberlain, M. J., Reynolds, A. L. and Yeoman, W. B. (1972). Toxic effect of podophyllum application in pregnancy. *Br. Med. J.*, **3**, 391

Cohen, S. R., Seltzer, S., Geller, A. K. *et al.* (1980). Papilloma of the larynx and tracheobronchial tree in children. A retrospective study. *Ann. Otolaryngol.*, **89**, 497

Costa, J., Howley, P. M., Bowling, M. C. *et al.* (1981). Presence of human papilloma viral antigens in juvenile multiple laryngeal papilloma. *Am. J. Clin. Pathol.*, **75**, 194

Crum, C. P., Braun, L. A., Shah, K. V. *et al.* (1982a). Vulvar intraepithelial neoplasia: Correlation of nuclear DNA content and the presence of a human papillomavirus (HPV) structural antigen. *Cancer*, **49**, 468

Crum, C. P., Fu, Y. S., Levine, R. U. *et al.* (1982b). Intraepithelial squamous lesions of the vulva: Virologic and histologic criteria for the distinction of condylomas from vulvar intraepithelial neoplasia. *Am. J. Obstet. Gynecol.*, **144**, 77

Cubie, H. A. (1972). Serological studies in a student population prone to infection with human papillomavirus. *J. Hyg. Camb.*, **70**, 677

Culp, O. S. and Kaplan, I. W. (1944). Condylomata acuminata: 200 cases treated with phodophyllin. *Ann. Surg.*, **120**, 251

Danos, O., Engel, L. W., Chen, E. Y. *et al.* (1983). Comparative analysis of the human type 1a and bovine type 1 papillomavirus genomes. *J. Virol.*, **46**, 557

de Benedictis, T. J., Marmar, J. S. and Praiss, D. E. (1977). Intraurethral condyloma acuminata: management and review of the literature. *J. Urol.*, **118**, 767

Dedo, H. H. and Jackler, R. K. (1982). Laryngeal papilloma: results of treatment with the CO_2 laser and podophyllum. *Ann. Otol. Rhinol. Laryngol.*, **91**, 425

de Jong, A. R., Weiss, J. C. and Brent, R. L. (1982). Condyloma acuminatum in children. *Am. J. Dis. Child.*, **136**, 704

Durst, M., Gissman, L., Ikenberg, H. *et al.* (1983). A papillomavirus DNA from a cervical carcinoma and its prevalence in cancer biopsy samples from different geographic regions. *Proc. Natl. Acad. Sci.*, **80**, 3812

Dudley (1980). (Quoted by Slater, G. E., Rumak, B. H. and Peterson, R. G., 1978). Podophyllin poisoning. Systemic toxicity following cutaneous application. *Obstet. Gynecol.*, **52**, 94

Editorial. Multiple papillomas of the larynx in children. *Lancet*, **1**, 367

Eftaiha, M. S., Amshel, A. L. and Shonberg, I. L. *et al.* (1982). Giant and recurrent condyloma acuminatum. *Dis. Colon Rect.*, **25**, 136

Fenner, F., McAuslan, B. R., Mims, G. A. *et al.* (1974). *The Biology of Animal Viruses*, 2nd edn. (London: Academic Press)

Fenoglio, C. M. and Ferenczy, A. (1982). Etiologic factors in cervical neoplasia. *Seminars in Oncology*, **9**, 349

Ferenczy, A., Braun, L. and Shah, K. V. (1981). Human papillomavirus (HPV) in condylomatous lesions of cervix. A comparative ultrastructural and immunohistochemical study. *Am. J. Surg. Pathol.*, **5**, 661

Figueroa, S. and Gennaro, A. (1980). Intralesional bleomycin injection in treatment of condyloma acuminatum. *Dis. Colon Rect.*, **23**, 550

Filley, C. M., Graff-Radford, N. R., Lacy, J. R. *et al.* (1982). Neurologic manifestations of podophyllin toxicity. *Neurology*, **32**, 308

Filliatreau, G. and Giamberardino, L. di. (1981). In vivo reassembly of axonal microtubules: A fast unidirectional process. *Biol. Cell*, **41**, 63

Friedman, J. M. and Pialkow, P. J. (1976). Cell marker studies of human tumorigenesis. *Transplant Rev.*, **28**, 17

Gigax, J. H. and Robison, J. R. (1971). The successful treatment of intraurethral condyloma acuminata with colchicine. *J. Urol.*, **105**, 809

Gissman, L., Villiers, E-M. de and Hausen, H. zur (1982a). Analysis of human genital warts (condylomata acuminata) and other genital tumors for human papillomavirus type 6 DNA. *Int. J. Cancer.*, **29**, 143

Gissman, L., Diehl, V., Schultz-Coulon *et al.* (1982b). Molecular cloning and characterization of human papillomavirus DNA derived from a laryngeal papilloma. *J. Virol.*, **44**, 393

Gissman, L., Wolnik, L., Ikenberg, H. *et al.* (1983). Human papillomavirus types 6 and 11 DNA sequences in genital and laryngeal papillomas and in some cervical cancers. *Proc. Natl. Acad. Sci.*, **80**, 560

Goepfert, H., Gutterman, J. U., Dichtel, W. J. *et al.* (1982). Leucocyte interferon in patients with juvenile laryngeal papillomatosis. *Ann. Otol. Laryngol.*, **91**, 431

Graber, E. A., Barber, H. R. K. and O'Rourke, J. J. (1967). Simple surgical treatment for condyloma acuminatum of the vulva. *Am. J. Obstet. Gynecol.*, **29**, 247

Greenspan, E. M. and Leiter, J. (1949). Toxicity and hematological changes produced by alpha-peltatin, beta-peltatin and podophyllotoxin. *Proc. Am. Ass. Cancer Res.*, **9**, 629

Hahn, G. A. (1981). Carbon dioxide laser surgery in treatment of condyloma. *Am. J. Obstet, Gynecol.*, **141**, 1000

Halverstadt, R. B. and Parry, W. L. (1969). Thiotepa in the management of intrauaurethral condylomata acuminata. *J. Urol.*, **101**, 729

Herberman, R. B. (ed.) (1980). *Natural Cell-mediated Immunity Against Tumors* (New York, London, Toronto, Sydney, San Francisco: Academic Press)

Howley, P. M. (1982). The human papillomaviruses. *Arch. Pathol. Lab. Med.*, **106**, 429

Hudson, H. C., Holcomb, F. L. and Gates, W. (1973). Giant condylomata acuminata of the penis: a case report and review. *J. Urol.*, **110**, 301

Ikenberg, H., Gissman, L., Gross, G. *et al.* (1983). Human papillomavirus type-16A related DNA in genital Bowen's disease and in Bowenoid papulosis. *Int. J. Cancer*, **32**, 563

Ikic, D., Orescanin, M., Krusic J. *et al.* (1975). Preliminary study of the effect of human leucocytic interferon on condylomata acuminata in women. In: Proceedings of the Symposium on Clinical Use of Interferons. Yugoslavia Academy of Science and Arts, p. 223.

Jablonska, S. (1983). Morphology and immunology of warts and tumors induced by human papillomaviruses. Lecture at the Swedish Society of Dermatology, Falun, Sweden

Jablonska, S., Orth, G., Obalek, S. *et al.* (1983). Oncogenic potential of human papillomaviruses epidermodysplasia verruciformis; a counterpart of Shope papilloma–carcinoma complex. *Arch. Geschwulstforsch.*, **53**, 207

Jensen, A. B., Lancaster, W. D., Hartmann, D. P. *et al.* (1982). Frequency and distribution of papillomavirus structural antigens in verrucae, multiple papillomas, and condylomata of the oral cavity. *Am. J. Pathol.*, **107**, 212

Judson, F. N. (1981). Condyloma acuminatum of the oral cavity: a case report. *Sex. Transm. Dis.*, **8**, 213

Karol, M. D., Conner, C. S. and Murphrey, K. J. (1980). Polophyllum: suspected teratogenicity from topical application. *Clin. Toxicol.*, **16**, 283

Katz, H. I., Pasalaky, Z. and McGinley, D. (19778). Pigmented penile papules with carcinoma *in situ* changes. *Br. J. Dermatol.*, **99**, 155

Kiso, Y., Konno, C., Hikino, H. *et al.* (1982). Liver-protective actions of desoxypodophyllotoxin and its analogs. *J. Pharm. Dyn.*, **5**, 638

Lack, E. E., Janson, A. B., Smith, H. G. *et al.* (1980). Immunoperoxidase localization of human papillomavirus in laryngeal papillomas. *Intervirol.*, **14**, 148

Lahti, A. and Hannuksela, M. (1982). Topical immunotherapy with tuberculin jelly for common warts. *Arch. Dermatol. Res.*, **273**, 153

Lancaster, W. D. and Jenson, A. B. (1981). Evidence for papillomavirus genus-specific antigens and DNA in laryngeal papilloma. *Intervirology*, **15**, 204

Langman, J. (ed.). (1975). *Medical Embryology*, 3rd edn., Chap. 11-13. (Baltimore: Williams & Wilkins)

Laohadtanaphorn, S., Hunter, J. C. and Ansell, L. D. (1979). Multicentric, pigmented carcinoma *in situ* of the vulva in association with vulval conduloma acuminata. *Aust. NZ. J. Obstet. Gynecol.*, **19**, 249

Law, M-F., Lowry, D. R., Dvoretzky, I. *et al.* (1981). Mouse cells transformed by bovine papillomavirus contain only extrachromosomal viral DNA sequences. *Proc. Natl. Acad. Sci.*, **78**, 2727

Leslie, K. O. and Shitamoto, B. (1982). The bone marrow in systemic podophyllin toxicity. *Am. J. Clin. Pathol.*, **77**, 478

Lewis, M. I. (1973). Treatment of extensive condyloma acuminata of the anal canal. *Int. Surg.*, **58**, 412

Lutzner, M., Kuffer, R., Blanchett-Bardon, C. *et al.* (1982). Different papillomaviruses as the causes of oral warts. *Arch. Dermatol.*, **118**, 393

Malison, M. D. and Salkin, D. (1981). Attempted BCG immunotherapy for condylomata acuminata. *Br. J. Vener. Dis.*, **57**, 148

Malison, M. D., Morris, R. and Jones, L. W. (1982). Autogenous vaccine therapy for condylomata acuminatum. A double-blind controlled study. *Br. J. Vener. Dis.*, **58**, 62

Markkanen, T., Mäkinen, M. L., Nikoskelainen, J. *et al.* (1981). Antiherpetic agent from Juniper tree (juniperus communis), its purification, identification, and testing in primary human amnion cell cultures. *Drugs. Exp. Clin. Res.*, **7**, 691

Markkanen, T., Mäkinen, M. L., Miettinen, J. *et al.* (1982). Antiviral effects of deoxypodophyllotoxin on HSV-infected amnion cell cultures. *Drugs Exp. Clin. Res.*, **8**, 27

Meisels, A., Roy, M., Fortier, M. *et al.* (1981). Human papillomavirus infection of the cervix: the atypical condylomata. *Acta Cytol.*, **25**, 7

Morin, C., Braun, L., Casas-Cordero, M. *et al.* (1981). Confirmation of the papillomavirus etiology of condylomatous cervix lesions by the peroxidase–antiperoxidase technique. *J. Natl. Cancer Inst.*, **66**, 831

McFarland, M. F. and McFarland, J. (1981). Accidental ingestion of Podophyllum. *Clin. Toxicol.*, **18**, 973

Oriel, J. D. (1971a). Natural history of genital warts. *Br. J. Vener. Dis.*, **47**, 1

Oriel, J. D. (1971b). Anal warts and anal coitus. *Br. J. Vener. Dis.*, **47**, 1

Oriel, J. D. (1978). Genital warts. *Sex. Transm. Dis.*, **5**, 153

Orth, G., Breitburd, F., Favre, M. *et al.* (1977). Papillomaviruses: possible role in human cancer. In: J. Watson (ed.), *Origins of Human Cancer*, p. 1043 (New York: Cold Spring Harbor)

Pass, F., Janis, R. and Marcus, D. M. (1971). Antigens of human wart tissue. *J. Invest. Dermatol.*, **56**, 305

Peterson, F. and Haines, G. (1923). Quoted by Slater, G. E., Rumak, B. H. and Peterson, R. G. (1978). Podophyllin poisoning. Systemic toxicity following cutaneous application. *Obstet. Gynecol.*, **42**, 94

Philips, F. S., Chenoweth, M. B. and Hunt, C. C. (1948). Studies on the toxicology of podophyllotoxin and related substances. *Fed. Proc.*, **7**, 249

Pilotti, S., Rilke, F. and Palo, G. de (1981). Condylomata of the uterine cervix and koilocytosis of cervical intraepithelial neoplasia. *J. Clin. Pathol.*, **34**, 532

Prasad, M. L. and Abcarian, H. (1980). Malignant potential of perianal condyloma acuminatum. *Dis. Colon Rectum.*, **23**, 191

Purola, E. and Savia, E. (1977). Cytology of gynecologic condyloma acuminatum. *Acta Cytol.*, **21**, 26

Pyrhönen, S. and Johansson, E. (1975). Regression of warts. An immunological study. *Lancet*, **1**, 592

Pyrhönen, S. and Penttinen, K. (1972). Wart-virus antibodies and the prognosis of wart disease. *Lancet*, **2**, 1330

Quick, C. A., Watts, S. L., Krzyzek, R. A. *et al.* (1980). Relationship between condylomata and laryngeal papillomata; clinical and molecular virological evidence. *Ann. Otolaryngol*, **89**, 467

Rampen, F. H. J. and Everdingen, J. J. E. van (1982). Inefficacy of cimetidine in condylomata acuminata. *Br. J. Vener. Dis.*, **58**, 275

Rastkar, G., Okagaki, T., Twiggs, L. B. *et al.* (1982). Early invasive and *in situ* warty carcinoma of the vulva: clinical, histologic, and electron microscopic study with particular reference to viral association. *Am. J. Obstet. Gynecol.*, **143**, 814

Reid, R., Laverty, C. R., Coppleson, M. *et al.* (1980). Noncondylomatous cervical wart virus infection. *Obstet. Gynecol.*, **55**, 476

Reid, R., Stanhope. P. and Herschman, B. R. *et al.* (1982). Genital warts and cervical cancer. I. Evidence of an association between subclinical papillomavirus infection and cervical malignancy. *Cancer.*, **50**, 377

Rosenberg, S. K., Jacobs, H. and Fuller, T. (1982). Some guidelines in the treatment of urethral condylomata with carbon dioxide laser. *J. Urol.*, **127**, 906

Savel, H. (1964). Clinical experience with intravenous podophyllotoxin. *Proc. Am. Assoc. Cancer Res.*, **5**, 56

Schmauz, R. and Owor, R. (1980). Condylomatous tumors of vulva, vagina and penis. *J. Clin. Pathol.*, **33**, 1039

Shaffer, E. L., Reimann, B. E. and Oysland, W. B. (1980). Oral condyloma acuminatum. A case report with light microscopic and ultrastructural features. *J. Oral Pathol.*, **9**, 163

Shevchuk, M. M. and Richart, R. M. (1982). DNA content of condyloma acuminatum. *Cancer*, **49**, 489

Shirodario, P. V. and Matthews, P. S. (1975). An immunofluorescent study of warts. *Clin. Exp. Immunol.*, **21**, 329

Simmons, P. D., Langlet, F. and Thin, R. N. T. (1981). Cryotherapy versus electrocautery in the treatment of genital warts. *Br. J. Vener. Dis.*, **57**, 273

Singer, A., Walker, P. and McCance, D. J. (1984). Genital wart virus infections: nuisance or potentially lethal? *Br. Med. J.*, **288**, 735

Smissman, E. E., Murray, R. J. and McChesney, J. D. (1976). Podophyllotoxin analogs. I. Synthesis and biological evaluation of certain trans-2-aryl-trans-6-hydroxymethyl-3-cyclohexene-carboxylic acid lactones as antimitotic agents. *J. Med. Chem.*, **19**, 148

Sullivan, M. and King. L. (1947). Effects of resin of podophyllum on normal skin, condylomata acuminata and verrucae vulgares. *Arch. Dermatol. Syphil.*, **56**, 30

Sullivan, M., Follis, R. H. and Hilgartner, T. (1951). Toxicology of podophyllin. *Proc. Soc. Exp. Biol. Med.*, **77**, 269

Swerdlow, D. B. and Salvati, E. P. (1971). Condyloma acuminatum. *Dis. Colon Rect.*, **14**, 226

Syrjänen, K. J. (1980a). Current views on the condylomatous lesions in the uterine cervix and their possible relationship to cervical squamous cell carcinoma. *Obstet. Gynecol. Survey*, **35**, 685

Syrjänen, K. J. (1980b). Condylomatous epithelial changes in uterine cervix and their relationship to cervical carcinogenosis. *Int. J. Obstet. Gynecol.*, **17**, 415

Syrjänen, K. J. (1980c). Epithelial lesions suggestive for a condylomatous origin found closely associated with invasive bronchial squamous cell carcinomas. *Respiration*, **40**, 150

Syrjänen, K. J. and Syrjänen, S. M. (1981). Histological evidence for the presence of condylomatous epithelial lesions in association with laryngeal squamous cell carcinoma. *ORL*, **43**, 181

Syrjänen, K. J., Heinonen, U-M. and Kauraniemi, T. (1981). Cytologic evidence of the association of condylomatous lesions with dysplastic and neoplastic changes in the uterine cervix. *Acta Cytol.*, **25**, 17

Syrjänen, K. J. (1982). Histological changes identical to those of condylomatous lesions found in esophageal squamous cell carcinomas. *Arch. Geschw.*, **52**, 283

Teokharov, B. A. (1962). (Abstract). *Vestn Vener.*, **36**, 56

Townsend, D. E., Ostergard, D. R. and Lickrish, G. M. (1971). Cryosurgery for benign disease of the cervix. *J. Obstet. Gynecol.*, **78**, 667

Treppendahl, S. and Jacobsen, P. (1980). Isolation of α- and β- peltatin and podophyllotoxin by liquid chromatography and analysis by high-performance liquid chromatography. *J. Chromat.*, **189**, 276

von Emenegger, H., Stähelin, H., Rutschmann, J. *et al.* (1961). Zur Chemie und Pharmakologie der Podophyllumglucoside und ihrer Derivate. *Arzneim Forsch.*, **11**, 327

von Krogh, G. (1975). Lokalisation, spridningssättoch behandling av Condylomata acuminata. *Läkartidningen* (Stockholm), **72**, 2167

von Krogh, G. (1976). 5-fluorouracil cream in the successful treatment of therapeutically refractory condylomata acuminata of the urinary meatus. *Acta Dermatol. Venereol.*, **56**, 297 von Krogh, G. (1978). Topical treatment of penile condylomata acuminata with podophyllin, podophyllotoxin and colchicine. *Acta Dermatol. Venereol.*, **58**, 163

von Krogh, G. (1979). Warts; Immunologic factors of prognostic significance. *Int. J. Dermatol.*, **18**, 195

von Krogh, G. (1981). Penile condylomata acuminata: an experimental model for evaluation of topical self-treatment with 0.5–1% ethanolic preparations of podophyllotoxin for three days. *Sex. Transm. Dis.*, **8**, 179

von Krogh, G. (1982a). Podophyllotoxin for condylomata acuminata eradication. Clinical and experimental comparative studies on Podophyllum lignans, colchicine and 5-fluorouracil. *Acta Dermatol. Venereol. Suppl.*, **98**, 1

von Krogh, G. (1982b). Podophyllotoxin in serum: absorption subsequent to three-day repeated applications of a 0.5% ethanolic preparation on condylomata acuminata. *Sex. Transm. Dis.*, **9**, 26

von Krogh, G. (1983). Condylomata acuminata 1983: an updated review. *Seminars Dermatol.*, **2**, 109

von Krogh, G. Unpublished materials

von Krogh, G. and Maibach, H. I. (1982). Cutaneous cytodestructive potency of lignans. I. A comparative evaluation of influence on epidermal and dermal DNA synthesis and on dermal microcirculation in the hairless mouse. *Arch. Dermatol. Res.*, **274**, 9

von Krogh, G. and Rudén, A-K. (1980). Topical treatment of penile condylomata acuminata with colchicine at 48-72 hours intervals. *Acta Dermatol. Venereol.*, **60**, 87

Wade, T. R. and Kopf, A. W. (1979). Bowenoid papulosis of the genitalia. *Arch. Dermatol.*, **115**, 306

Wiedeman-Erfurt, G. (1959). Erfahrungen mit der externen Colchicin-behandlung in der Dermatologie. *Arch. Klin. Exp. Dermatol.*, **206**, 686

Willcox, R. R. (1977). How suitable are available pharmaceuticals for the treatment of sexually transmitted diseases? (2) Conditions presenting as sores or tumors. *Br. J. Vener. Dis.*, **53**, 340

zur Hausen, H. (1977). Human papillomaviruses and their possible role in squamous cell carcinomas. *Curr. Top. Microbiol. Immunol.*, **78**, 1

zur Hausen, H. (1982). Human genital cancer; synergism between two virus infections or synergism between a virus infection and initiating events? *Lancet*, **2**, 1370

14
Animal models for the study of human genital infection

E. KITA

THE NEED FOR ANIMAL MODELS IN THE STUDY OF STDs

Although the incidence of sexually transmitted diseases (STDs) has increased in many countries, our knowledge about the immunobiology of the etiologic agents is inadequate to develop effective vaccines and minimize the incidence of these infections. Because most of the etiologic agents of STDs are pathogenic only for humans, experimental infectivity studies are limited. Why these organisms infect only humans and not other vertebrates is not known, but it is possible to speculate on the microbial factors that are involved.

To clarify the roles of these factors in genital infections, we must develop practical animal models that can reproduce the same natural infections that occur in humans. Although there are reports of infections by STD pathogens in animal models, the sites of these infections are different from those of natural infections. Few animal models are adequate for a laboratory study of genital infections, but many are available for determining the immunologic features of etiologic agents in these infections. Space limitations dictate that only the most common be discussed here.

CURRENT EXPERIMENTAL ANIMAL MODELS IN CURRENT USE

Gonorrhea

Chimpanzee model

A male chimpanzee developed gonococcal urethritis after inoculation with a pure culture of colony type T1 and T2 *N. gonorrhoeae* (Lucas *et al.*, 1971). This was the first report on the virulence of *N. gonorrhoeae* in chimpanzees after the investigation of morphological types of gonococcal colonies in artificial media (Kellog *et al.*, 1963) and in human volunteers (Kellog *et al.*, 1968). In this study the urethral exudate collected from five male patients with gonococcal urethritis was pooled and suspended in trypticase–soy broth. The exudate–broth suspension was then injected via a catheter into the urethra and the catheter was clamped and left in place for 30 minutes. Postinoculation cultures were taken on days 4, 7, 10, 14, 18, 20, 25, and 30. Using this manipulation, the infection produced was clinically and bacteriologically similar to that occurring in human males with gonococcal urethritis. This model subsequently was used to determine the effect of immunization with homologous and heterologous isolates of *N. gonorrhoeae* (Arko *et al.*, 1974). Systemic immunization with a formalinized gonococcal antigen protected against a localized urethral infection with a homologous strain, but this immunity was strain-specific. The infection was venereally transferred to a female cage-mate, as was demonstrated by cervical culture and development of gonococcal antibodies.

Subcutaneous chamber model

Subcutaneous chambers implanted in various animals (rabbits, guinea-pigs, hamsters, mice, and rats) were infected with various colonial types of *N. gonorrhoeae* (Arko, 1972). Hollow polyethylene practice golf balls with holes in their walls were sterilized and surgically implanted in the subcutaneous tissue on the back of each animal. The chambers became encapsulated within the subcutaneous tissues after about 30 days; during this time they filled with transudate, which could be easily removed with a hypodermic needle and syringe. An appropriate volume of liquid culture medium, containing approximately 10^8 colony-forming units of *N. gonorrhoeae* per ml, was injected through a 25-gauge needle into the encapsulated spheres. Fluid was removed at 2- or 3-day intervals and spread over a GC plate. Inoculated plates were incubated for 18–24 hours, and the chambers were determined as being infected when gonococci could be identified in the cultures. Each chamber was sampled several times and it was regarded as being noninfected when no gonococcal growth was obtained on three successive occasions.

This technique was first applied to rabbits and a modification was used to infect guinea-pigs, hamsters, rats, and mice. Gonococci appeared to grow in chambers implanted in rabbits, despite the fact that rabbit serum has potent bacteriolytic activity for *N. gonorrhoeae* (Keefer and Spink, 1938). In the guinea-pig model, two important factors capable of affecting the susceptibility of the chamber became apparent. Both the genotype of the gonococcus and that of the guinea-pigs must be considered when this model is used, because the ability to infect guinea-pigs is strictly strain-related (Novotny *et al.*, 1978). In addition, certain lines of guinea-pigs are very sensitive to gonococcal infection in the chambers and respond to gonococcal antigens by developing complement-fixing bactericidal antibodies which appear to mediate strain-related immunity (Arko *et al.*, 1976; Brown *et al.*, 1972).

Although there is a fundamental difference between the infection site in human gonorrhea and in the subcutaneous chamber, the chamber model is useful for investigating the immunologic properties of gonococcal infections. It should be used for *in vivo* studies of the antigonococcal effects of antibiotics and other chemotherapeutic and prophylactic substances.

Chicken embryo model

The chicken embryo has been used extensively in research on many microbial pathogens, including *N. gonorrhoeae*. The chorioallantoic membranes (CAM) of 10-day embryos were used and infected with *N. gonorrhoeae* in the earlier works (Bang, 1974; Hill and Pitts, 1939). However, none of these early studies were performed in an attempt to develop the chicken embryo as an animal model for gonococcal infection.

A more extensive investigation of gonococcal infection was done by several investigators (Buchanan and Gotschlich, 1973; Bumgarner and Finkelstein, 1973) to clarify the difference in virulence between colony types T_1, T_2 and T_3, T_4. Colony types T_1 and T_2 were found to have high virulence for embryos, whereas T_3 and T_4 colony types were relatively avirulent. This was due to the differences in clearing the gonococci from the blood stream. In this model the infection with virulent colony types was primarily bacteremic.

It has been found that the 11-day chicken embryo has phagocytic capability (Karthigasu and Jenkin, 1963; Kent, 1961), although circulating leukocytes are not yet present in significant numbers (Romanoff, 1960). The age of the chicken embryos thus has a profound effect on their susceptibility to gonococci. While it is not known whether the chicken embryo model has a direct relationship with the immune state in man, it is being used to evaluate the potency of purified gonococcal vaccines (Table 1).

Table 1 Mouse protection tests using gonococcal LPS vaccines

LPS vaccine	Dose	Challenge with 10 LD_{50}		
		75004	G9	G6
75004	50 μg	22/25[a,d]	14/20[c]	16/20[d]
G9	50 μg		12/20[d]	17/20[d]
G6	50 μg		16/20[d]	14/20[c]
G6	10 μg			11/20[b]
Control		4/25	4/20	4/20

[a] Survivors/injected
[b] Significantly better ($p<0.05$) than the control in the same column
[c] Significantly better ($p<0.01$) than the control in the same column
[d] Significantly better ($p<0.001$) than the control in the same column
(From *Neisseria gonorrhoeae and Gonococcal Infections*, Report of a WHO Scientific Group, 1978, Technical Report Series No. 616, World Health Organization, Geneva, with permission of WHO Publication Office)

Mouse model

In the earlier works using mouse models, an intracerebral inoculation was used to evaluate the immunogenic activity of antigens purified from *N. gonorrhoeae* (Diena *et al.*, 1975). In this model, gonococcal lipopolysaccharide (LPS) afforded significant protection against homologous and heterologous challenges with *N. gonorrhoeae* (Table 2). However, the infection process in this model is very different from that of the natural infection in a human.

Table 2. Protection afforded by vaccination of hens with purified gonococcal LPS against challenges of embryos by *N. gonorrhoeae* and *N. meningitidis*

Vaccine	Challenge strain	CFU/dose[a]	Normal embryos	Immune embryos
LPS (GC 6-T4)	GC 6-T1	100	7/10[b]	–
		600	4/10	–
		3000	2/10	8/10
		20 000	–	7/10
LPS (GC 9-T4)	GC 9-T1	31	1/10	–
		500	1/10	10/10
		3000	–	9/10
		20 000	–	7/10
LPS (GC 6-T4)	*N. meningitidis*	2	4/8	–
		13	0/8	0/8
		72	0/8	0/8
		500	–	0/8

[a] Colony-forming units of *N. gonorrhoeae* or *N. meningitidis* per challenge dose
[b] Survivors/injected
(From *Neisseria gonorrhoeae and Gonococcal Infections*, Report of a WHO Scientific Group, 1978, Technical Report series No. 616, World Health Organization, Geneva, with permission of WHO Publication Office)

Recently, female mice (CF1) have been shown to be sensitive to a urogenital infection with gonococci during the preovulatory period of their estrous cycles (Braude *et al.*, 1978). The cell patterns in the genital tracts of normal mice at various stages of their cycles were determined by genital impression smears

Table 3 Cell pattern in genital impression smears of normal animals at various stages of the estrous cycle

Group	Animal no.	Vagina	Cervix	Right horn	Left horn
Late	1181	C+E+	C+E+	E	E
proestrus	1212	C+E++	C+E++	E	E
Early	1184	C++E±	C++	E	E
estrus	1214	C++E+	C++E	E	E
Early	1196	C+++	C++	C+	C+
metestrus	1197	C+++	C+++	E	E
Diestrus	1208	CEL++	EL++	EL	EL
	1210	EL++	EL++	EL	EL

E, nucleated epithelial cell; C, cornified epithelial cell; L, neutrophilic leukocyte.
(From Braude, A. I., Corbeil, L. B., Levine, S., Ito, J., and McCutchan, J. A. (1978). Possible influence of cyclic menstrual changes on resistance to the gonococcus. In Brooks, G. F. *et al.* (eds) *Immunobiology of Neisseria gonorrhoeae*, American Society for Microbiology, Washington, DC, p. 328, with permission of the authors and publisher)

(Table 3). The sensitivity of mice to genital infection with *N. gonorrhoeae* varies between strains. CF1 mice are fairly sensitive to gonococcus but the infection persists for only a few days.

Among other mouse strains, ddY mice are the most susceptible to a genital infection of *N. gonorrhoeae* (Kita *et al.*, 1981). The infection was observed for at least 4 weeks when mice were challenged during late proestrus or early estrus (Table 4). The minimum inoculum dose was 10^4 colony-forming units

Table 4 Relationship between estrous cycle and infectivity of *Neisseria gonorrhoeae* in strain ddY mice.

Stage of inoculation[a]		Cell population (vaginal smear)[b]			No. with positive cultures for gonococcus/no. cultured at week[c]			
		E	C	P	1	2	3	4
I	(late proestrus)	+	−	−	5/5	5/5	5/5	4/5
II	(early estrus)	±	+	−	5/5	5/5	5/5	5/5
III	(early metestrus)	−	+	+	5/5	4/5	3/5	3/5
IV	(diestrus)	+	−	+	4/5	3/5	2/5	2/5

[a] Groups of 20 mice at each estrous stage were inoculated intravaginally with 10^6 strain PH2 gonococci
[b] E, nucleated epithelial cells; C, cornified epithelial cells; P, polymorphonuclear leukocytes; (+), presence of cells; (−), absence of cells
[c] Every week for 4 weeks after challenge five of 20 mice were killed and uterine cultures performed. Data are number of mice with positive cultures of uterine specimens/number of mice studied
(From Kita, E., Matsuura, H., and Kashiba, S. (1981). A mouse model for the study of gonococcal genital infection. *J. Infect. Dis.*, **143**, 67, with permission of the authors and publisher)

for ddY mice. Infection was confirmed by culturing the vaginal discharge which appeared 2 days after inoculation. For a quantitative analysis of the multiplication of gonococcus in the uterine bodies, their homogenate is cultured and the degree of gonococcal multiplication is determined by viable counts. The infection is evidenced by the development of gonococcal antibodies as measured by passive hemagglutination (Fig. 1) and by histologic examination to demonstrate endometritis.

The mouse model of gonococcal genital infection can reproduce an infectious process similar to that in humans. Two important differences have become apparent: the first relates to the lower response of leukocytes in the genital tract of mice, compared with that of humans; the second relates to the normal vaginal flora. Both the low response of leukocytes and the normal low prevalence of detectable flora enhance the sensitivity of mice to a genital infection of *N. gonorrhoeae* (Streeter and Corbeil, 1981). Although these genetically controlled factors are not observed in the genital tract of humans, the mouse model is useful in the study of the immunobiology of *N. gonorrhoeae* infection in humans.

Syphilis

Attempts to grow virulent *Treponema pallidum* in pure culture have not yet been successful, and research efforts are now being directed towards defining the metabolic capabilities and deficiencies of this organism. Despite the failure to produce a pure culture in a synthetic medium, our knowledge about the immune response that develops during infection has increased. Experimental infections may be produced in a variety of laboratory animals. In this regard the rabbit has been a convenient model for the study of experimental syphilis.

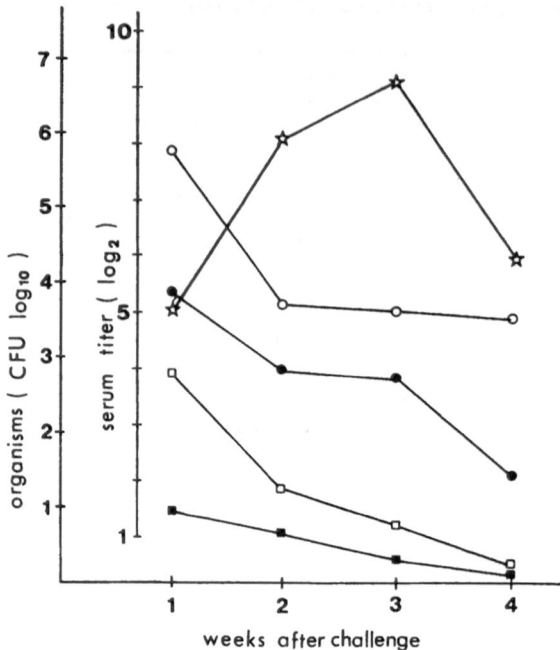

Fig. 1 Viable counts of *Neisseria gonorrhoeae* in the uteri of strain ddY mice challenged with strain PH2 at different stages in the estrous cycle. Mice challenged at stage I (o———o); mice challenged at stage II (•———•); mice challenged at stage III (□———□); and mice challenged at stage IV (■———■). Titer of antibodies to crude outer membrane complex in sera of mice challenged at stage I (✴———✴). (From Kita, E., Matsuura, H., and Kashiba, S. (1981). A mouse model for the study of gonococcal genital infection. *J. Infect. Dis.*, **143**, 67, with permission of the authors and publisher)

In early studies, human syphilitic material was inoculated into the eyes of rabbits in which local lesions developed. Chimpanzees also have been used as animal models, developing not only primary but also secondary lesions after inoculation with human syphilitic material. Guinea pigs have also been found to be sensitive to *T. pallidum*; spirochaetes reached the focal lymphnodes within 5 minutes of cutaneous inoculation of the scrotum.

Experimental syphilitic disease in rabbits, monkeys, and chimpanzees simulates the early course of the natural disease in humans. However none of the studies using these animals have employed direct inoculation of *T. pallidum* into the genital tract. Rabbits are infected by inoculation of organisms into the eye, skin, testis, or scrotum; viable organisms persist for life. Although the rabbit cannot serve as a model in which the initial pathologic changes that develop in the mucous membranes of the genital tract can be produced, it remains an economical animal model for the study of the immunologic aspects of *T. pallidum* infections (Miller, 1965, 1967, 1973; Miller *et al.*, 1963; Metzger and Smogor, 1969).

Herpes infection

To establish a test system for antiviral drugs to HSV type 2 in humans, an experimental model for genital herpes has been developed using mice. In this model (Overall *et al.*, 1975), an intravaginal inoculation with HSV type 2 (approximately 10^6 plaque-forming units) was given by means of a small plastic catheter attached to a syringe. This resulted in an initial local vaginitis with erythema, hair loss, and ulceration in the perineal area with mucopurulent discharge. Subsequently, hind limb paralysis, encephalitis and death were observed. Pregnant mice were found to be more susceptible to viral infections (Farber and Glasgow, 1968) and to HSV type 2 (Overall *et al.*, 1975). Since progesterone levels rise early in pregnancy and remain at a high level late in pregnancy (Murr *et al.*, 1974), and since maternal cell-mediated immunity is decreased during pregnancy (Andresen and Monroe, 1962; Smith *et al.*, 1972; Purtilo *et al.*, 1972), it has been suggested that progesterone might be responsible either directly or indirectly (Mori *et al.*, 1977). In this mouse model (Baker and Plotkin, 1978) progesterone treatment affects the resistance of mice to HSV type 2. Although man is the natural host for HSV type 2, a relatively wide range of animals, including guinea pigs, hamsters, rats, and rabbits, is also susceptible. In all instances the effect of the infection depends upon the route of the challenge. Intravaginal inoculation of HSV type 2 in mice is the most adequate way to produce herpes genital infection in laboratory animals.

Experimental urinary tract infection

Most of the animal models for genital tract infections have been developed for studies of STDs. But a suitable animal model for urinary tract infection in man is also required because of the clinical importance of this infection. It is easier to produce experimental urinary tract infection in male than in female animals, because male hormonal changes are not sufficient to affect the host's susceptibility.

Animals used include mice, rats, rabbits, and dogs. Organisms were instilled in the bladder. This procedure produced not only local infection, including pyelonephritis, but also bacteremia (Fierer *et al.*, 1971). This animal model using retrograde inoculation is available for studies of human urogenital infection with bacteria as well as viral etiologic agents.

FACTORS INFLUENCING THE SUSCEPTIBILITY OF EXPERIMENTAL ANIMALS

In the study of the immunologic aspects of infectious diseases, the use of inbred strains of mice has been the rule. These strains were developed and are maintained by breeding through brother–sister mating in each generation. After an uninterrupted chain of more than 20 such generations, genetic variability among the mice is usually reduced to a minimum, and the progeny can be considered to be genetically homogenous. These inbred strains allow the effective application of sophisticated genetic tests in immunology. However, these strains are not adequate to establish animal models for infectious diseases because man is not naturally inbred. The best animal models for laboratory research should be outbred animals. Although the susceptibility of inbred animals is higher than that of outbred ones, immune responses may be extremely selective in the inbred strain. Pathological changes also differ greatly. As a result, the availability of experimental data obtained from the inbred animals is limited. However, selection of the animal strain is very important in obtaining a model capable of producing an infection similar to the disease in man. For example, ddY mice are the most sensitive to gonococcus; among conventionally raised mice, CF1 mice are the next most sensitive. Also important in achieving successful results in experimental animal models is the bacterial strain. Human genital tract isolates should be stored just as they were isolated from clinical specimens. Most of the pathogenic organisms can be preserved with gelatin discs (Yamai *et al.*, 1979), a technique that preserves virulence and biologic characteristics, including plasmids, for several years at least.

In the genital tract of female animals, the reproductive hormones may have an influence in resisting invading organisms. Generally, estrogen is the factor found to enhance the growth of organisms (Salt, 1982), whereas progesterone had the opposite effect (Morse and Fitzgerald, 1974). Increases in vaginal bacterial counts were observed during the preovulatory stage when estrogen levels were the highest. Decreases in vaginal bacterial counts were related to the presence of leukocytes in the vagina after estrus (Larsen *et al.*, 1977). In guinea pigs, treatment with estradiol markedly enhanced chlamydial genital infections, producing infections of greater intensity and longer duration (Rank *et al.*, 1982). This effect was also evident in candidiasis of genital tract (Catterall, 1971; Oriel *et al.*, 1972), and in genital herpes (Baker and Plotkin, 1978). Low *in vivo* hormone concentrations in animals suggest that the effect of hormones on the animals' susceptibility to genital pathogens is mediated rather than direct. It is well known that estrogen can effect vaginal cytology, mucus secretion, vascularity, and intracellular concentrations of cyclic adenosine monophosphate – factors which may enhance the uptake of pathogens into mucosal cells.

Other potent factors that can influence the susceptibility of animals to genital infections are lysozyme and iron. Although such substances have demonstrated some biological effect on bacteria *in vitro*, their exact role *in vivo* has not yet been determined.

References

Andresen, R. H. and Monroe, C. W. (1962). Experimental study of the behavior of adult human skin homografts during pregnancy. A preliminary report. *Am. J. Obstet. Gynecol.*, **84**, 1096

Arko, R. J. (1972). *Neisseria gonorrhoeae*: experimental infection of laboratory animals. *Science*, **177**, 1200

Arko, R. J., Kraus, S. T., Brown, W. J. *et al.* (1974). *Neisseria gonorrhoeae*: effect of systemic immunization on resistance of chimpanzees to urethral infection. *J. Infect. Dis.*, **130**, 160

Arko, R. J., Wong, K. H., Bullard, J. C. *et al.* (1976). Immunological and serological diversity of Neisseria gonorrhoeae: immunotyping of gonococci by cross-protection in guinea pig subcutaneous chambers. *Infect. Immun.*, **14**, 1293

Baker, D. A. and Plotkin, S. A. (1978). Enhancement of vaginal infection in mice by Herpes Simplex Virus Type II with progesterone (40156). *Proc. Soc. Exp. Biol. Med.*, **158**, 131

Bang, F. (1941). Experimental gonococcus infection of the chicken embryo. *J. Exp. Med.*, **74**, 387

Braude, A. I., Corbeil, L. B., Levine, S. *et al.* (1978). Possible influence of cyclic menstrual changes on resistance to the gonococcus. In Brooks, G. F., Gotschlich, E. C. and Holmes, K. K. *et al.* (eds) *Immunobiology of Neisseria gonorrhoea*, p. 328 (Washington, DC: Am. Soc. Microbiol.)

Brown, W. J., Lucas, C. T. and Kuhn, U. S. G. (1972). Gonorrhea in the chimpanzee. Infection with laboratory-passed gonococci and by natural transmission. *Br. J. Vener. Dis.*, **48**, 177

Buchanan, T. M. and Gotschlich, E. C. (1973). Studies on gonococcus infection. III. Correlation of gonococcal colony morphology with infectivity for the chick embryo. *J. Exp. Med.*, **137**, 196

Bumgarner, L. R. and Finkelstein, R. A. (1973). Pathogenesis and immunology of experimental gonococcal infection: virulence of colony types of *Neisseria gonorrhoeae* for chicken embryos. *Infect. Immun.*, **8**, 919

Catterall, R. D. (1971). Influence of gestogenic contraceptive pills on vaginal candidasis. *Br. J. Vener. Dis.*, **47**, 45

Diena, B. B., Ryan, A., Ashton, F. E. *et al.* (1975). A mouse intracerebral infection with Neisseria gonorrhoeae. *Br. J. Vener. Dis.*, **51**, 22

Farber, P. A. and Glasgow, L. A. (1968). Factors modifying host resistance to virus infection. II. Enhanced susceptibility of mice to encephalomyocarditis virus infection during pregnancy. *Am. J. Pathol.*, **53**, 463

Fierer, J., Talner, L. and Brande, A. I. (1971). Bacteremia in the pathogenesis of retrograde *E. coli* pyelonephritis in the rat. *Am. J. Pathol.*, **64**, 443

Hill, J. H. and Pitts, A. C. (1939). The growth of *Neisseria gonorrhoeae* on the chorioallantoic membrane of the chick embryo. *J. Urol.*, **41**, 81

Karthigasu, K. and Jenkin, C. R. (1963). The functional development of the reticuloendothelial system of the chick embryo. *Immunology*, **6**, 255

Keefer, C. S. and Spink, W. W. (1938). Studies of gonococcal infection. IV. The effect of mucin on the bacteriolytic powder of whole blood and immune serum. *J. Clin. Invest.*, **17**, 23

Kellogg, D. S., Jr., Cohen, I. R., Norins, L. C. *et al.* (1968). *Neisseria gonorrhoeae*. II. Colonial variation and pathogenicity during 35 months in vitro. *J. Bacteriol.*, **96**, 596

Kellogg, D. S., Jr., Peacock, W. L., Jr., Deacon, W. E. *et al.* (1963). *Neisseria gonorrhoeae*. I. Virulence genetically linked to colonial variation. *J. Bacteriol.*, **85**, 1274

Kent, R. (1961). The development of the phagocytic activity of the reticulo-endothelial system in the chick. *J. Embryol. Exp. Morphol.*, **9**, 128

Kita, E., Matsuura, H. and Kashiba, S. (1981). A mouse model for the study of gonococcal genital infection. *J. Infect. Dis.*, **143**, 67

Larsen, B., Markovetz, A. J. and Galask, R. P. (1977). Relationship of vaginal cytology to alterations of the vaginal microflora of rats during the estrous cycle. *Appl. Environ. Microbiol.*, **33**, 556

Lucas, C. T., Chandler, F., Jr., Martin, J. E., Jr. *et al.* (1971). Transfer of gonococcal urethritis from man to chimpanzee. An animal model for gonorrhea. *J. Am. Med. Assoc.*, **216**, 1612

Metzger, M. and Smogor, W. (1969). Artificial immunization of rabbits against syphilis. I. Effect of increasing doses of treponemes given by the intramuscular routes. *Br. J. Vener. Dis.*, **45**, 308

Miller, J. N. (1965). Immunity in experimental syphilis. *J. Bacteriol.*, **90**, 297

Miller, J. N. (1967). Immunity in experimental syphilis. V. The immunogenicity of Treponema pallidum attenuated by γ-irradiation. *J. Immunol.*, **99**, 1012

Miller, J. N. (1973). Immunity in experimental syphilis. VI. Successful vaccination of rabbits with Treponema pallidum, Nichols strain, attenuated by γ-irradiation. *J. Immunol.*, **110**, 1206

Miller, J. N., Whang, S. J. and Fazzan, F. P. (1963). Studies on immunity in experimental syphilis. I. Immunogenic response of rabbits immunized with Reiter protein antigen and challenged with virulent Treponema pallidum. *Br. J. Vener. Dis.*, **39**, 195

Mori, T., Kobayashi, H. and Nishimoto, H. *et al.* (1977). Inhibitory effect of progesterone and 20 alpha-hydroxypreg-4-en-3-one on the phytohemagglutinin-induced transformation of human lymphocytes. *Am. J. Obstet. Gynecol.*, **127**, 151

Morse, S. A. and Fitzgerald, T. J. (1974). Effect of progesterone on Neisseria gonorrhoeae. *Infect. Immun.*, **10**, 1370

Murr, S. M., Stabenfeldt, G. H. and Bradford, G. E. *et al.* (1974). Plasma progesterone during pregnancy in the mouse. *Endocrinology*, **94**, 1209

Ng, A. B. P., Reagan, J. W. and Yen, S. S. C. (1970). Herpes genitalis: clinical and cytopathologic experience with 256 patients. *Obstet. Gynecol.*, **36**, 645

Novotny, P., Broughton, E. S. and Cownley, K. *et al.* (1978). Strain related infectivity of Neisseria gonorrhoeae for the guinea-pig subcutaneous chamber and the variability of the immune resistance in different breeds of guinea-pig. *Br. J. Vener. Dis.*, **54**, 88

Oriel, J. D., Partridge, B. M. and Denny, M. J. *et al.* (1972). Genital yeast infections. *Br. Med. J.*, **4**, 761

Overall, J. C., Jr., Kern, E. R. and Schlitzer, L. *et al.* (1975). Genital Herpesvirus hominis infection in mice. I. Development of an experimental model. *Infect. Immun.*, **11**, 476

Purtilo, D. T., Hallgren, H. M. and Yunis, E. J. (1972). Depressed maternal lymphocyte response to phytohaemagglutinin in human pregnancy. *Lancet*, **1**, 769

Rank, R. G., White, H. J. and Houch, A. J., Jr. *et al.* (1982). Effect of estradiol on chlamydial genital infection of female guinea pigs. *Infect. Immun.*, **38**, 699

Romanoff, A. L. (1960). *The Avian Embryo: Structural and Functional Development.* (New York: Macmillan)

Salt, I. E. (1982). The differential susceptibility of gonococcal opacity variants to sex hormones. *Can. J. Microbiol.*, **28**, 301

Smith, J. K., Caspary, E. A. and Field, E. J. (1972). Immune responses in pregnancy. *Lancet*, **1**, 96

Streeter, P. R. and Corbeil, L. B. (1981). Gonococcal infection in endotoxin-resistant and endotoxin-susceptible mice. *Infect. Immun.*, **32**, 105

Yamai, S., Obara, Y., Nikkawa, T. *et al.* (1979). Preservation of Neisseria gonorrhoeae by the gelatin-disc method. *Br. J. Vener. Dis.*, **55**, 90

15
Animal models of genital *Chlamydia* and *Mycoplasma* infections

C. E. SWENSON

INTRODUCTION

Bacteria within the families Chlamydiaceae and Mycoplasmataceae are biologically distinct. The former are obligate intracellular parasites with cell walls and complex life cycles; the latter live almost exclusively outside of the cell, lack cell walls, and have simple life cycles. However, in many respects the problems presented by these organisms to microbiologists and clinicians working in the field of sexually transmitted diseases (STDs) are similar.

Organisms from both families are found throughout the world in a wide range of vertebrate (and invertebrate) animals, yet the species and strains isolated from the human genital tract appear to be highly specific for that host. Organisms from both families may cause severe, acute infections, but these infections are more often chronic and clinically inapparent. Organisms from both families can be cultured *in vitro*, yet the specialized procedures necessary for this are not widely available to clinicians and their true prevalence in many populations remains to be determined. Little is known about the clinical spectrum and sequelae of these infections and even less is known about the pathogenic mechanisms involved in the production of clinical infections. It is likely that genetic or hormonal factors, other microorganisms, and/or the host's immune response all interact during infections with both families of microorganisms. Finally, both the chlamydiae and the mycoplasmas are relatively recent additions to the list of sexually transmitted pathogens in man.

That these organisms are clearly associated with conditions such as urethritis, salpingitis, infant pneumonitis and postpartum fever is enough to justify a strong effort to develop animal models to assist in their study. In addition, the possibility that these organisms may also be involved in the etiology of ectopic pregnancy, spontaneous abortion, intrauterine growth retardation, idiopathic infertility, perinatal morbidity and other serious but little understood conditions makes the search for animal models urgent.

Two major problems affect the search for animal models of genital *Chlamydia* and *Mycoplasma* infections. The first is the relative–host species specificity of these infections. Unlike some organisms which reach the reproductive tract by a hematogenous route and cause disease and abortion in both man and animals (e.g. *Listeria monocytogenes*, *Toxoplasma gondii*, *Coxiella burnetti*), *Chlamydia* and *Mycoplasma* are thought to infect the mucous membranes of the lower genital tract, at least initially, and in most cases reach the upper tract by an ascending route. STDs of this nature generally have a very narrow host range. Consequently, investigators must rely on natural animal models (when a naturally occurring infection in an animal mimics the human disease but is caused by a different species or strain of organism), and experimental animal models (when an infection occurs when the animal is inoculated with the specific agent of the human disease). This chapter describes those organisms for which the natural site of infection is the eye or respiratory tract of an animal but which also establish an infection in the genital tract when experimentally introduced there, as a natural animal infection. In the case of experimental animal models, unnatural routes of inoculation or manipulation of the animal (immunosuppressive or hormonal treatment) may be necessary to establish the infection.

The second major problem in developing appropriate animal models involves reproductive biology. Different animal species generally arise through reproductive isolation; such isolation is often achieved through the development of different types of reproductive organs or specific changes in reproductive physiology. It is therefore not surprising that sperm, eggs, endometrial cycles, placentas, etc. are more likely to differ among species than are lungs, livers, and spleens. In most cases the best models for human reproductive diseases are the primates which are more similar to humans in terms of anatomy, menstrual cycles, placentation, gestation length, etc., than are other animals. Unfortunately, primates are among the most expensive and least available animals and are generally reserved for use only in those cases where considerable evidence has already been accumulated that a particular organism produces a specific disease.

ANIMAL MODELS OF CHLAMYDIAL GENITAL INFECTION

Two species of *Chlamydia* are currently recognized: *C. psittaci* and *C. trachomatis*. With the exception of some rodent strains, man is the only known natural host for *C. trachomatis*. Human *C. trachomatis* strains can be divided into two biotypes: the lymphogranuloma venereum (LGV) strains (not discussed extensively here) and the trachoma-inclusion conjunctivitis (TRIC), or non-LGV, strains.

The non-LGV strains of *C. trachomatis* are now recognized as etiologic agents in nongonococcal urethritis (NGU), postgonococcal urethritis (PGU), acute salpingitis (AS), and cervicitis. They are strongly implicated in at least some cases of endometritis, perihepatitis and infertility due to tubal occlusion in the female, as well as epididymitis and proctitis in the male, and pneumonia in the infant. The association, if any, between *C. trachomatis* and Reiter's syndrome, enteric infections, prostatitis, cystitis, cervical dysplasia, maternal complications of pregnancy, spontaneous abortion, perinatal morbidity, or idiopathic infertility is less clear (Schachter, 1978; Taylor-Robinson and Thomas, 1980).

Natural infections

C. psittaci is a recognized abortifacient in sheep and cattle. Natural and induced chlamydial orchitis, epididymitis, and seminal vesiculitis have been demonstrated in bulls and rams (Storz *et al.*, 1976). These infections, like most caused by *C. psittaci*, are generally systemic and usually involve hematogenous dissemination of the organism. *C. trachomatis* infections of man, excluding those caused by the LGV group and possibly those in infants, appear to be restricted to epithelial cells and mucosal membrane surfaces. Hematogenous spread is unknown. Therefore, although genital chlamydial infections of domestic ruminants are intriguing, their relevance to human diseases has not been demonstrated. There are, however, two naturally occurring *C. psittaci* infections and one relatively uncommon rodent *C. trachomatis* strain that may provide insight into *C. trachomatis* genital infections in man.

Guinea pigs and the agent of guinea pig inclusion conjunctivitis

A naturally occurring eye infection in young guinea pigs is caused by a *C. psittaci* organism. Guinea pig inclusion conjunctivitis (GPIC) agent causes a mild, short-lived conjunctivitis that spontaneously resolves without damage to the cornea or conjunctiva. Studies on this organism have shown that although it belongs to a different species, its infectious process in the guinea pig is similar to human non-LGV *C. trachomatis* oculogenital infection in several respects:

(1) it causes follicular conjunctivitis and, with repeated infections, can produce a more severe disease associated with conjunctival scarring and neovascularization (pannus) of the cornea;
(2) it infects the male and female genital tract and apparently remains localized to the superficial epithelia; and
(3) venereal and eye-to-eye transmission occurs, as well as transmission to newborn guinea pigs on their passage through the birth canal (Barron, 1982).

Intravaginal inoculation of guinea pigs produces a mild, self-limited infection of the squamous and transitional epithelia of the exocervix. An acute inflammatory response, consisting chiefly of polymorphonuclear (PMN) leukocytes, occurs within 5 days, followed by a mononuclear infiltration of the subepithelial tissue at about 10 days postinoculation. The exocervix returns to a normal histologic state within 20 days.

Intraurethral inoculation of male guinea pigs results in a transient, overt disease characterized by inclusions in superficial urethral epithelial cells, a PMN response, the development of serum antibodies, and resistance to reinfection. Intraurethral inoculation may also produce an inapparent infection in which organisms cannot be recovered from urethral scrapings, serum antibodies and resistance do not develop, but which can be transmitted to the eyes of susceptible animals (Ozanne and Pearce, 1980).

Direct inoculation of the GPIC agent into the oviducts of adult guinea pigs induces an acute salpingitis. The organism infects only the lumenal epithelial cells of the oviduct. There is a marked inflammatory response, and the lumen becomes filled with purulent material and necrotic debris. The serum antibody response peaks and the inflammatory reaction subsides in 2–3 weeks. *Chlamydia* are rarely recovered from genital tract tissues beyond this period. The tubes in the majority of infected animals are permanently damaged, however, and hydrosalpinx is a regular finding in animals examined 1–2 months postinoculation (Schachter *et al.*, 1982).

Immunosuppression and hormonal treatment affects the course of GPIC infection in guinea pigs. While intravaginal inoculation of females usually results in only a limited cervical infection, treatment with cyclophosphamide or estradiol produces an ascending infection with endometrial, oviductal, and peritoneal involvement (Barron, 1982). It is thought that estradiol allows ascending infection by suppressing the local immune response (Rank *et al.*, 1982). Even though estradiol-treated animals have infections that are more widespread, last longer, and produce more inclusions in vaginal smears, the serum IgG response follows the same course and reaches the same peak titers as in untreated animals whose infection is limited to the cervix. Although immunosuppressed males (and some estradiol-treated females) develop infections of the bladder epithelium, infections of the prostate, seminal vesicles, or epididymis have not been clearly detected either in normal or immunosuppressed guinea pigs.

Electron microscopy of infected guinea pig tissues has shown that the GPIC agent enters and multiplies in epithelial cells of the conjunctiva, squamous and transitional zones of the exocervix, urethra, oviduct, and urinary bladder (Soloff *et al.*, 1982). Inclusions have also been observed by light microscopy in the epithelial cells of the uterine lumen and in peritoneal mesothelial cells. At present there is no evidence for invasion of the GPIC agent into submucosal tissues.

Genital GPIC infections induce the production of specific serum and secretory antibody, as well as delayed hypersensitivity responses. It is not clear what role humoral, local, or cellular immunity plays in the resolution of, or resistance to, infection. Serum antibody alone is not protective. The passive transfer of antibody *in utero* does not protect the newborn against infection, and killed parenteral vaccines induce serum antibody but do not protect. Most work points to a role for local, secretory antibody, although experiments summarized by Murray (1977) suggest that immunity is not entirely a local phenomenon. Thus, infection at one site (eye, urethra, vagina) results in resistance to reinfection (with moderate challenge doses) at the same site for 4–8 weeks after the primary infection. Whereas a primary infection of the eye also produces strong immunity to vaginal or urethral challenge, a primary infection of the genital tract produces only partial immunity to eye challenge. In all cases, however, immunity wanes after 3–4 months.

Mice and the agent of mouse pneumonitis

The agent of mouse pneumonitis (MoPn) was originally isolated from the lungs of mice. It is a *C. trachomatis* strain that differs significantly from human strains antigenically and in DNA-reassociation studies. MoPn infection is not found frequently in mice, but is the only known natural *C. trachomatis* infection other than those that occur in man.

Intravaginal inoculation of MoPn into adult mice produces a short-lived cervical infection (Barron *et al.*, 1981). Histologically, the inflammatory response is limited to the exocervix and inclusions are found in superficial epithelial cells.

Direct inoculation of the MoPn agent into the ovarian bursa results in an acute salpingitis (Swenson *et al.*, 1983a). The histologic picture and course of the infection is similar to that seen after oviductal inoculation of guinea pigs with the GPIC agent: i.e., an acute inflammatory response that subsides in 2–3 weeks and subsequent formation of hydrosalpinx 1–2 months postinoculation. Thus, in two rodent species, a primary oviductal infection with a single bacterial agent (*Chlamydia*) results in tubal occlusion and hydrosalpinx formation. During the acute phase of tubal infection in mice, chlamydial inclusions are present in both ciliated and nonciliated columnar epithelial cells of the oviduc-

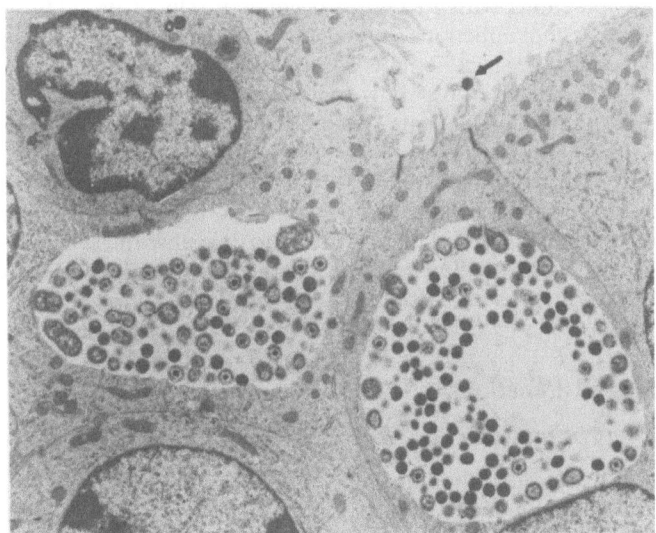

Fig. 1 *Chlamydia trachomatis* (the agent of mouse pneumonitis) inclusions in nonciliated epithelial cells of the mouse oviduct. One elementary body is free in the lumen (arrow) (D. M. Phillips, C. E. Swenson, and J. Schachter, unpublished)

tal lumen (Fig. 1) In most mice there is also evidence of endometrial infection; however, *Chlamydia* are not found in the submucosal tissues and hematogenous dissemination does not occur. Therefore, in the mouse as well as the guinea pig, *Chlamydia* are pathogens of the superficial epithelium of the genital tract; this also appears to be the case in non-LGV *C. trachomatis* infections in man.

Perhaps of greater importance, infected mice are infertile during the acute stage of the infection, as well as long after the inflammatory reaction and the disappearance of viable organisms (Swenson and Schachter, 1984). This infertility is probably due to occlusion of the oviduct by inflammatory exudate or scarring, although other mechanisms (interference with implantation?) are possible. Early antibiotic treatment of infected mice can prevent the development of salpingitis and subsequent infertility (Swenson *et al.*, 1984). Thus, the mouse model should provide an opportunity to study treatment modalities for chlamydial tubal infections that would preserve reproductive function as well as eradicate the organism.

Cats and the agent of feline keratoconjunctivitis

A naturally occurring keratoconjunctivitis in cats is caused by the feline keratoconjunctivitis (FKC) agent, a member of the species *C. psittaci*. Experimental inoculation of the eyes of cats with FKC produces an infection with clinical features similar to human trachoma. Blindness occurs after repeated inoculations of FKC in conjunction with other bacteria (normal throat flora), providing further evidence that concurrent or sequential infection with other organisms is a factor in the pathogenesis of chlamydial disease.

Genital infections with FKC also occur naturally. Kittens born to queens with natural genital infections show severe conjunctivitis early in life. Necropsy of kittens that die occasionally shows histologic evidence of pneumonia, whereas kittens that survive show some resistance to reinfection. Vaccination with egg attenuated organisms reduces the incidence and severity of disease (Shewen, 1980).

Only a few experimental studies with the FKC agent in the genital tract have been performed. Intraurethral inoculation of males results in a moderate urethritis with chlamydial shedding for up to 2 weeks. Intravaginal inoculation produces a moderate vaginitis with discharge and recovery of the organism for 2 weeks (Darougar *et al.*, 1977).

Experimental infections

Nonhuman primates

Studies on experimental genital *Chlamydia* infection in nonhuman primates have been the subject of several reviews (Barron, 1982; Møller and Mårdh, 1982; Johnson and Taylor-Robinson, 1982; Taylor-Robinson *et al.*, 1982; Gale *et al.*, 1977).

Many primate species are susceptible to experimental ocular infection with human strains of *C. trachomatis*. In most cases a self-limiting follicular conjunctivitis occurs. Repeated infections, however, can lead to more severe disease. Fewer animals have been used to study genital *Chlamydia* infections, but, at least in the case of NGU and possibly AS, this work has succeeded in fulfilling Koch's postulates.

Intraurethral inoculation of human non-LGV *C. trachomatis* strains into male nonhuman primates usually results in a persistent infection. This is demonstrated by the fact that organisms may be recovered from urethral swabs for up to 3 months postinoculation and by the serologic response. The clinical response to the infection, however, varies. Some chimpanzees and baboons, and one rhesus monkey, have shown frank urethral discharges, while other chimpanzees and baboons, as well as pig-tailed macaques, have not. Since the clinical responses in man may also vary, perhaps these results are not surprising. Urethral follicles, shown histologically to be subepithelial, granulomatous lesions consisting of plasma cells and macrophages, have been seen in the pig-tailed macaques. A submucosal lymphocytic infiltration was found in the urethra of one chimpanzee examined 3 months after inoculation (Gale *et al.*, 1977; Johnson and Taylor-Robinson, 1982).

Transperineal injection of non-LGV strains into the prostates of male grivet monkeys did not produce an inflammatory response, but inoculation directly into the spermatic cord resulted in enlargement of the testes and epididymis, inflammation of the spermatic cord, and urethral discharge (Møller and Mårdh, 1982).

Female baboons, marmosets, and grivet monkeys have been used to study the effect of cervical inoculation of *C. trachomatis*. In most cases, infection can be established. In marmosets the infection persisted for several weeks and there was a PMN response (Johnson, 1982). In grivets, repeated inoculations resulted in cervical erosions and slight dysplasia. Vaginal inoculation did not result in infection (Møller and Mårdh, 1982).

Infection of the upper female genital tract has been studied in grivets (Møller *et al.*, 1980a) and pig-tailed macaques (Patton *et al.*, 1982). Inoculation directly into the fallopian tubes (via the fimbrial os) or the uterus resulted in salpingitis. In grivet monkeys an inflammatory exudate is present within the lumen 7–14 days after inoculation. The inflammation decreases by 3 weeks, but adhesions between the mucosal folds are found and tubal occlusion may occur. If the isthmus of the oviduct is ligated prior to intrauterine inoculation, salpingitis does not occur, suggesting that *C. trachomatis* must spread canalicularly through the reproductive tract to reach the oviducts rather than via the lymphatics or some other route. In macaques, mucosal and submucosal lymphocytic infiltration is found after intratubal inoculations, but exudate is not seen within the lumen. Tubal occlusion did not occur, but Patton *et al.* (1982) found an abnormal deciliation of the endosalpinx in these monkeys 1 month after inoculation.

Immunity to genital tract infections in primates has been studied in male baboons (Gale *et al.*, 1977) and female marmosets (Johnson, 1982). After organisms can no longer be recovered from a primary urethral or cervical infection, rechallenge with the same or a different serotype results in an infection of shorter duration. It is not clear whether an anamnestic serologic response occurs, but an inflammatory reaction does occur and may persist longer than the presence of viable organisms. A strong serologic response was found in the female macaques and grivets with primary upper genital tract infections, but there are no data on the effect of reinfection on the upper tract. It is possible that in the oviducts, as in the eye, hypersensitivity reactions to reinfection play a role in the pathologic process.

Mice and other experimental models

It has not been possible to establish an infection in the lower genital tract of normal mice with human non-LGV strains of *C. trachomatis* (Taylor-Robinson *et al.*, 1982), although there is evidence that limited replication and an inflammatory response occur when organisms are inoculated into the upper genital tract (Swenson and Schachter, unpublished observations). 'Fast' (LGV) strains are also not very infectious for the lower genital tract of mice, unless the mice have been pretreated with progesterone (Taylor-Robinson *et al.*, 1982). Progesterone may suppress the cellular changes that occur in the short (4–5-day) estrus cycle and, thereby, promote infection; alternatively, the drug may produce local immunosuppressive effects. Congenitally athymic nude mice treated with progesterone and inoculated with the same LGV strain show a greater number of inclusions in vaginal smears than progesterone-treated furred mice, but the infection spontaneously resolves in both groups at about the same time (Taylor-Robinson *et al.*, 1982).

Organ culture models have also been used to study chlamydial infection. Human *C. trachomatis* strains will infect and multiply in human fallopian tube as well as in mouse trophoblast cells in culture (Hutchinson *et al.*, 1979; Banks *et al.*, 1982). The infection has little effect on the ciliary activity, histologic or ultrastructural integrity of fallopian tube tissue, suggesting that much of the pathology in *Chlamydia*-induced salpingitis may be due to the host's response rather than the direct cytotoxic or lytic effects of the bacterium itself.

ANIMAL MODELS OF *MYCOPLASMA* GENITAL INFECTION

At least seven different *Mycoplasma* species have been isolated from the human genital tract. Of those, only two are found commonly: *M. hominis* and *U. urealyticum*. A new species, *M. genitalium* (Tully *et al.*, 1983) has recently been recovered from the human urethra, but its prevalence and pathologic significance is unknown. *M. hominis* and *U. urealyticum* have been implicated in a wide variety of genital tract diseases and reproductive disorders, including NGU, urethroprostatitis, epididymitis, vaginitis, cervicitis, salpingitis, postpartum fever, chorioamnionitis, spontaneous abortion, low birth weight, and idiopathic infertility. It is generally accepted that *U. urealyticum* is an etiologic agent in NGU, but the proportion of cases due to this organism is unknown. Similarly, *M. hominis* is a recognized cause of mild postpartum fever and a probable cause of AS, but its prevalence in these conditions is unknown (Taylor-Robinson *et al.*, 1981). Proving an etiologic relationship between *Mycoplasma* infection and any disease has always been difficult because of the subtle pathogenicity of most of these organisms. In the case of the human genital mycoplasmas this task is further complicated by the lack of clear diagnostic criteria for certain disorders (e.g. idiopathic infertility) and the fact that both *M. hominis* and *U. urealyticum* can be recovered from a large number of apparently healthy adults.

Natural infections

There are currently over 70 named *Mycoplasma* species found in hosts through-out the animal and plant kingdoms. Although the names of *Mycoplasma* organisms often reflect the host or anatomic site of their original isolation, the species differ in antigenic, biochemical, and other properties in addition to their ecologic niches. Therefore, the fact that a *Mycoplasma* is responsible for a particular disease in an animal does not necessarily indicate any similar pathology in man. Nonetheless, knowledge of natural genital *Mycoplasma* diseases can provide some insight into the mechanisms of *Mycoplasma* pathogen-esis and suggest specific areas for further research in humans.

Rodents and murine mycoplasmas

M. pulmonis, the etiologic agent of murine respiratory mycoplasmosis, has been studied extensively in infection of the respiratory tract. Much of the work with this organism in rodent disease has been reviewed by Cassell and colleagues (Cassell *et al.*, 1979, 1981; Cassell, 1982). *M. pulmonis* can infect and colonize the genital tract of mice and rats. In some animal colonies up to 40% of female rats are naturally infected. Gross pathology (usually unilateral perioophoritis or salpingitis) in the upper tract, but not in the vagina or cervix, may occur in 30% of naturally infected females. Microscopically, a neutrophilic exudate is evident in the oviductal lumen and there is hyperplasia of the epithelium and lymphoid infiltration of the submucosa. *M. pulmonis* can be seen (by electron microscopy and immunofluorescence) to adhere to both squamous and nonsquamous epithelial cells of the entire tract. Organisms are not found in the submucosa.

Intravaginal, intranasal, and intravenous inoculation of pathogen-free female rats results in colonization of the upper tract in most cases and micro-scopic lesions (primarily in the oviduct) in up to 80%. Disease and viable mycoplasmas persist for up to 8 months or more postinoculation, despite the development of a cellular immune response that, when passively transferred to uninfected rats, is protective.

Although *M. pulmonis* can be recovered from the lungs, blood, and occasion-ally brain tissue of some mice, natural genital infections seem to be rare. Nonetheless, organisms localize in the genital tract, causing salpingitis and perioophoritis, after intraperitoneal inoculation. There is an acute inflamma-tory response within the oviducts and ovarian bursa that, histologically, resem-bles the acute inflammation seen after intraovarian bursa inoculation of the mouse pneumonitis biovar of *C. trachomatis*. However, viable *M. pulmonis* organisms may persist longer than *Chlamydia*, and tubal occlusion with hydro-salpinx formation has not been clearly described in mice with genital *M. pulmonis* infection. In both infections the ovary appears to be largely spared, although the function of this organ has not been assessed after infection with either organism.

Infertility and fetal wastage have been associated with naturally occurring *M. pulmonis* infections after intravenous and intraperitoneal inoculation of female rats and mice (Cassell, 1982; Taylor-Robinson *et al.*, 1975). However, these results must be interpreted with caution. *M. pulmonis* given intravenously is arthritogenic (the organism is also able to infect the brain, lung, and spleen of rodents), so it is difficult to separate the direct effect of the *Mycoplasma* and the problem of poor maternal health on the fertility and outcome of pregnancy in these studies.

M. pulmonis infection of the male genital tract has not been studied extensively, although natural urethral colonization is known to occur in rats, and intraperitoneal inoculation of mice results in acute orchitis and epididymitis.

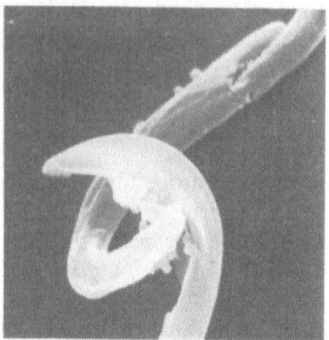 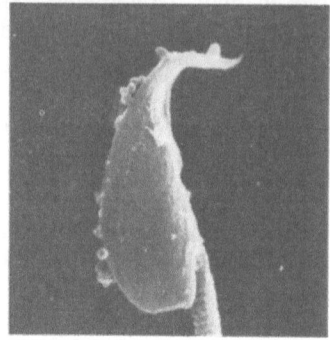

Fig. 2 Adherence of *Mycoplasma pulmonis* to rat (a) and mouse (b) spermatozoa. (C. E. Swenson, unpublished)

In vitro, *M. pulmonis* will adhere to rat and mouse spermatozoa (Fig. 2) and causes a decrease in the motility of rat sperm (Cassell *et al.*, 1981). Preincubation of mouse sperm with *M. pulmonis* reduces the fertilization rate of mouse eggs *in vitro* (Fraser and Taylor-Robinson, 1977) and *in vivo* (Swenson, 1982), although the mechanism of this effect is not clear at this time.

Cattle and bovine mycoplasmas

M. bovis is a recognized bovine pathogen capable of causing mastitis and polyarthritis under natural and experimental conditions. When *M. bovis* is inoculated into the seminal vesicles of bulls, a persistent infection with an acute and chronic inflammatory reaction results (LaFaunce and McEntee, 1982). When this agent is inoculated into the uterus of normal heifers, or mixed with semen prior to artificial insemination, varying degrees of endometritis and salpingitis are found. Intraperitoneal inoculation of pregnant cows produces placentitis, and intra-amniotic inoculation causes abortion and fetal infection (Gourlay and Howard, 1979). These results demonstrate that a known bovine *Mycoplasma* pathogen can produce disease and persist in the reproductive tract when experimentally introduced there. *M. bovis*, however, is not commonly found in the genital tract and has not been clearly associated with naturally occurring reproductive disorders.

M. bovigenitalium is a common inhabitant of the bovine urogenital tract. It is frequently found in the semen of bulls and, like other genital mycoplasmas, appears to be able to adhere to spermatozoa. Its presence has been associated with poor semen quality in some studies. In the majority of cases the presence of mycoplasmas in the semen probably represents contamination from the prepuce on ejaculation. However, in several instances *M. bovigenitalium* has been isolated from the upper tract of bulls with seminal vesiculitis, and poor semen quality is seen in bulls with subclinical vesicular *Mycoplasma* infection (Hall and McEntee, 1981; Panagala *et al.*, 1982). Experimental inoculation into the seminal vesicles produces vesiculitis and, in some cases, epididymitis (Panagala *et al.*, 1982). Experimental vulvar or uterine inoculation of normal heifers does not induce clinical disease or visible lesions. If the vulvar or uterine epithelium is scraped prior to inoculation, however, inflammatory lesions are produced.

Ureaplasmas are frequently found in the semen and vaginas of cattle. The strains recovered are distinct from human strains and have recently been designated as a separate species, *U. diversum* (Howard and Gourlay, 1982). Bovine genital ureaplasmosis has been reviewed by Doig (1980).

Ureaplasmas appear to be involved in the etiology of granular vulvitis, and the acute stage of the disease has been associated with infertility in some studies. Experimental vulvar inoculation of virgin heifers produces vulvitis, and organisms persist for up to 7 months. Uterine or cervical inoculation results in a transient (1-week) infection and inflammation of the uterus and oviducts and persistent infection of the vulva. The presence of ureaplasmas in the vulva could be a source of recontamination of the uterus at each breeding, producing sufficient alteration of the uterine environment to interfere with the development of the fertilized egg. Ureaplasmas have been recovered in pure culture from embryo transplant flushings containing fertilized but degenerate ova. A high incidence of early fetal loss has been noted in some herds with *Ureaplasma*-associated granular vulvitis, and experimental intra-amniotic inoculation of ureaplasmas results in placentitis and abortion.

Other natural infections

Cats and several nonhuman primate species have naturally occurring genital *Ureaplasma* infections. The relationship of these organisms to human and bovine ureaplasmas is not clear. In one study with feline ureaplasmas, intravaginal inoculation of queens resulted in endometrial infection, spontaneous abortion, and neonatal death (Tan and Miles, 1974). Several nonhuman primate groups harbor naturally occurring *M. hominis*. Thus far, there has been no clear association between genital mycoplasmas in nonhuman primates and disease (Somerson and Cole, 1979).

Experimental infections

Nonhuman primates

It has been possible to establish persistent urethral or vaginal infections with *U. urealyticum* in several nonhuman primate species. These include pig-tailed (Gale *et al.*, 1977) and crab-eating macaques (Bowie *et al.*, 1978; Swenson, 1980), rhesus monkeys, baboons, chimpanzees (Swenson, 1980; Taylor-Robinson *et al.*, 1978) and marmosets (Furr *et al.*, 1978). Clinically apparent urethritis has only been observed in chimpanzees inoculated with unpassaged human ureaplasmas (Taylor-Robinson *et al.*, 1981).

Grivet monkeys have been used to study the pathogenic potential of the human genital mycoplasmas in the upper genital tract. Direct inoculation of *U. urealyticum* into the tubes does not result in disease, but *M. hominis* and *M. fermentans* are able to cause an acute 'exosalpingitis' and parametritis when given by this route (Møller *et al.*, 1980a,b). At the peak of inflammatory response the tubes are swollen and the parametria are edematous. There is an intense lymphocytic and PMN infiltration of the mucosa, although the lumen is free of exudate. Viable mycoplasmas are recovered for up to 17 days from the upper tract and persist longer (up to $3\frac{1}{2}$ months) in the vagina. The reproductive organs are macroscopically normal 4–5 weeks after inoculation.

Inoculation of *M. hominis* into the cervical epithelium also produces inflammatory lesions of the tubes and parametria, but inoculation into the uterine cavity does not. If the tubes are ligated and *M. hominis* is introduced into the uterus followed by endometrial curettage, salpingitis and parametritis occur. It may be that infection of the upper tract must be preceded by mechanical injury of the epithelial barrier and that spread occurs via the blood and lymphatics (Møller *et al.*, 1980a).

Rodents and other experimental models

Intravaginal inoculation of rats and mice with *M. hominis* or *U. urealyticum* has not resulted in infection or colonization (Millar and Graber, 1974; Swenson, 1980). Intraperitoneal inoculation of pregnant rats with *M. hominis*, however, may cause a transient mycoplasmemia, with invasion of the placenta and fetus (Millar and Graber, 1974). Intraperitoneal inoculation of some mouse strains with *M. hominis* during pregnancy results in an increased number of fetal resorptions (Gabridge and Cohen, 1976). Some strains of *U. urealyticum* and *M. hominis* will multiply and persist in subcutaneous tissue cavities in mice. Both induce an inflammatory response with a giant cell reaction in and around the cavities (Krause *et al.*, 1977). Human ureaplasmas multiply in the mammary glands of several strains of mice and produce a vacuolative hyperplasia and involution (Howard *et al.*, 1975). Fallopian tube organ cultures of bovine and human origin can be infected with *U. urealyticum* and *M. hominis* and may show a decrease in ciliary activity (Swenson *et al.*, 1983b). These models, while not of genital tract infection *per se*, may be of value in differentiating pathogenic and nonpathogenic strains of the human genital mycoplasmas (if they exist) and in studying certain aspects of the host's immune response.

CONCLUSIONS

Chlamydia trachomatis is clearly pathogenic in man, yet the full clinical spectrum; the long-term sequelae; and the role of immune factors in the pathogenesis, resolution, and resistance to chlamydial infections are still largely unknown. The finding that *Chlamydia* can infect the bladder epithelium in guinea pigs and trophoblastic cells in the mouse does not indicate a similar pathology in man, but should at least stimulate further research. The fact that a primary infection of the oviducts results in the development of hydrosalpinx in guinea pigs and mice, and adhesions with possible tubal occlusion in grivet monkeys, emphasizes the possibility of severe long-term sequelae in humans with chlamydial salpingitis. The complexity of the immune response in animal chlamydial infections makes it clear that much more work must be done in model systems before vaccination of humans as a means of preventing infection or reducing its effects in the genital tract is even contemplated.

Aside from *M. pneumoniae*-induced pneumonia in man, the role of mycoplasmas in human disease is controversial. Reliable means of determining the virulence of different genital mycoplasma strains will have to be developed before the pathogenic potential of these organisms in man is fully understood. The use of subcutaneous chambers or mammary gland inoculation in mice may prove useful in this respect. A relationship beween the genital mycoplasmas and various reproductive disorders has been suggested and denied in a number of epidemiologic studies in man (and cattle). In all likelihood, the resolution of this controversy will depend at least in part on determining the mechanisms by which these organisms could produce such effects. Studies of the effect of mycoplasmas on sperm function *in vitro* and *in vivo* and subclinical endometrial or oviductal infection in rodents may provide some insight in these areas. The finding that epithelial damage promotes *Mycoplasma* infection in cows and grivet monkeys, and that intravenous or intraperitoneal inoculation of rodents with mycoplasmas results in reproductive tract infection and fetal wastage, suggests that more work should be done to determine the invasiveness and subsequent tissue tropisms of genital mycoplasmas in humans.

C. trachomatis and the genital mycoplasmas are some of the most common sexually transmitted agents in man. The development and interpretation of animal models of these infections present many problems, but their eventual utility and value in understanding these pathogens is unquestioned.

ACKNOWLEDGMENTS

I thank Dr Julius Schachter for thoughtful discussions and advice on this manuscript. This work was supported by United States Public Health Service grants EY-01205 and HD-12271 from the National Institutes of Health and the Venereal Disease Research Fund of the American Social Health Association.

References

Banks, J., Glass, R., Spindle, A. I. *et al.* (1982). *Chlamydia trachomatis* infection of mouse trophoblasts. *Infect. Immun.*, **38**, 368

Barron, A. L. (1982). Contributions of animal models to the study of human chlamydial infections. In Mårdh, P.-A., Holmes, K. K., Oriel, J. D. *et al.* (eds) *Chlamydial Infections* (Fernstrom Foundation Series), p. 357. (Amsterdam: Elsevier)

Barron, A. L., White, H. J., Rank, R. G. *et al.* (1981). A new animal model for the study of Chlamydia trachomatis genital infections: Infection of mice with the agent of mouse pnemonitis. *J. Infect. Dis.*, **143**, 63

Bowie, W. R., Digiacomo, R. F., Holmes, K. K. *et al.* (1978). Genital inoculation of male

Macaca fascicularis with *Neisseria gonorrhoeae* and *Ureaplasma urealyticum*. *Br. J. Vener. Dis.*, **54**, 235

Cassell, G. H. (1982). The pathogenic potential of mycoplasmas: *Mycoplasma pulmonis* as a model. *Rev. Infect. Dis.*, **4**, S18

Cassell, G. H., Lindsey, J. R., Baker, H. J. *et al.* (1979). Mycoplasmal and rickettsial diseases. In Baker, J. H., Lindsey, J. R. and Weisbroth, S. H. (eds) *The Laboratory Rat*, vol. 1, p. 243. (New York: Academic Press)

Cassell, G. H., Wilborn, W. H., Silvers, S. H. *et al.* (1981). Adherence and colonization of Mycoplasma pulmonis to genital epithelium and spermatozoa in rats. *Israel J. Med. Sci.*, **17**, 593

Darougar, S., Monnickendam, M. A., El-Sheikh, J. *et al.* (1977). Animal models for the study of chlamydial infections of the eye and genital tract. In Hobson, D. and Holmes, K. K. (eds) *Nongonococcal Urethritis and Related Infections*, p. 186. (Washington: American Society for Microbiology)

Doig, P. A. (1980). Bovine genital mycoplasmosis. *Can. Vet. J.*, **22**, 339

Fraser, L. R. and Taylor-Robinson, D. (1977). The effect of *Mycoplasma pulmonis* on fertilization and preimplantation development in vitro of mouse eggs. *Fertil. Steril.*, **28**, 488

Furr, P. M., Hetherington, C. M. and Taylor-Robinson, D. (1978). Studies of the specificity of ureaplasmas for marmosets. *J. Med. Microbiol.*, **11**, 537

Gabridge, M. G. and Cohen, L. J. (1976). Development of an animal model for mycoplasma-related reproductive failure. *Lab. Anim. Sci.*, **26**, 206

Gale, J. L., Digiacomo, R. F., Kiviat, M. D. *et al.* (1977). Experimental nonhuman primate urethral infection with *Chlamydia trachomatis* and *Ureaplasma* (T-mycoplasma). In Hobson, D. and Holmes, K. K. (eds) *Nongonococcal Urethritis and Related Infections*, p. 205. (Washington: American Society for Microbiology)

Gourlay, R. N. and Howard, C. J. (1979). Bovine mycoplasmas. In Tully, J. G. and Whitcomb, R. F. (eds) *The Mycoplasmas*, vol. II, *Human and Animal Mycoplasmas*, p. 50. (New York: Academic Press)

Hall, C. E. and McEntee, K. (1981). Reduced post-thawing survival of sperm in bulls with mycoplasmal vesiculitis. *Cornell Vet.*, **71**, 111

Howard, C. J. and Gourlay, R. N. (1982). Proposal for a second species within the genus *Ureaplasma*, *Ureaplasma diversum* sp. nov. *Int. J. Syst. Bacteriol.*, **32**, 446

Howard, C. J., Anderson, J. C. and Gourlay, R. N. *et al.* (1975). Production of mastitis in mice with human and bovine ureaplasmas (T-mycoplasmas). *J. Med. Microbiol.*, **8**, 523

Hutchinson, G. R., Taylor-Robinson, D. and Dourmashkin, R. R. (1979). Growth and effect of chlamydiae in human and bovine oviduct organ cultures. *Br. J. Vener. Dis.*, **55**, 194

Johnson, A. P. (1982). Genital infection of marmosets with *Chlamydia trachomatis*. In Mårdh, P.-A., Holmes, K. K., Oriel, J. D. *et al.* (eds) *Chlamydial Infections* (Fernstrom Foundation Series), p. 395. (Amsterdam: Elsevier)

Johnson, A. P. and Taylor-Robinson, D. (1982). Chlamydial genital tract infections: Experimental infection of the primate genital tract with *Chlamydia trachomatis*. *Am. J. Pathol.*, **106**, 132

Krause, S. J., Jacobs, N. F., Chandler, F. W. *et al.* (1977). Experimental animal infections with *Mycoplasma hominis* and *Ureaplasma urealyticum*. *Infect. Immun.*, **16**, 302

LaFaunce, N. A. and McEntee, K. (1982). Experimental *Mycoplasma bovis* seminal vesiculitis in the bull. *Cornell Vet.*, **72**, 150

Millar, M. and Graber, C. D. (1974). Experimental *Mycoplasma hominis*. I. Infection in the pregnant rat. *Gynecol. Invest.*, **5**, 73

Møller, B. R., and Mårdh, P.-A. (1982). The grivet monkey as animal model for the study of chlamydial infection of the urogenital tract. In Mårdh, P.-A., Holmes, K. K., Oriel, J. D. *et al.* (eds) *Chlamydial Infections* (Fernstrom Foundation Series), p. 367. (Amsterdam: Elsevier)

Møller, B. R., Freundt, E. A., Black, F. T. *et al.* (1980a). Experimental infection of the upper genital tract of female grivet monkeys with *Mycoplasma fermentans*. *J. Med. Microbiol.*, **13**, 145

Møller, B. R., Freundt, E. A. and Mårdh, P.-A. (1980b). Experimental pelvic inflammatory disease provoked by *Chlamydia trachomatis* and *Mycoplasma hominis* in grivet monkeys. *Am. J. Obstet. Gynecol.*, **138**, 990

Murray, E. S. (1977). Review of clinical, epidemiological and immunological studies of guinea pig inclusion conjunctivitis infection in guinea pigs. In Hobson, D. and Holmes, K. K. (eds) *Nongonococcal Urethritis and Related Infections*, p. 199. (Washington: American Society for Microbiology)

Ozanne, G. and Pearce, J. H. (1980). Inapparent chlamydial infection in the urogenital tract of guinea pigs. *J. Gen. Microbiol.*, **119**, 351

Panagala, V. S., Hall, C. E., Caveney, N. T. *et al.* (1982). *Mycoplasma bovigenitalium* in the upper genital tract of bulls: spontaneous and induced infections. *Cornell Vet.*, **72**, 292

Patton, D. L., Brunham, R. C., Halbert, S. A. *et al.* (1982). *Chlamydia trachomatis* salpingitis in the pig-tailed macaque. In Mårdh, P.-A., Holmes, K. K., Oriel, J. D. *et al.* (eds) *Chlamydial Infections* (Fernstrom Foundation Series), p. 399. (Amsterdam: Elsevier)

Rank, R. G., White, H. J., Hough, Jr., A. J. *et al.* (1982). Effect of estradiol on chlamydial genital infection of female guinea pigs. *Infect. Immun.*, **38**, 699

Schachter, J. (1978). Chlamydial infections. *N. Engl. J. Med.*, **298**, 428

Schachter, J., Banks, J., Sung, M. *et al.* (1982). Hydrosalpinx as a consequence of salpingitis in the guinea pig. In Mårdh, P.-A., Holmes, K. K., Oriel, J. D. *et al.* (eds) *Chlamydial Infections* (Fernstrom Foundation Series), p. 371. (Amsterdam: Elsevier)

Shewen, P. E. (1980). *Chlamydia* infection in animals: a review. *Can. Vet. J.*, **21**, 2

Soloff, B. L., Rank, R. G. and Barron, A. L. (1982). Ultrastructural studies of chlamydial infection in guinea pig urogenital tract. *J. Comp. Pathol.*, **92**, 547

Somerson, N. L. and Cole, B. C. (1979). The mycoplasma flora of human and nonhuman primates. In Tully, J. G. and Whitcomb, R. F. (eds) *The Mycoplasmas*, vol II, *Human and Animal Mycoplasmas*, p. 191. (New York: Academic Press)

Storz, J., Carroll, E. J., Stephensen, E. H. *et al.* (1976). Urogenital infection and seminal excretion after inoculation of bulls and rams with chlamydiae. *Am. J. Vet. Res.*, **37**, 517

Swenson, C. E. (1980). Studies on the association of *Ureaplasma urealyticum* and infertility in humans and laboratory animals. *Thesis, Cornell University, New York*

Swenson, C. E. (1982). Effect of *Mycoplasma pulmonis* on *in vivo* fertilization in the mouse. *J. Reprod. Fertil.*, **65**, 257

Swenson, C. E. and Schachter, J. (1984). Infertility as a consequence of chlamydial infection of the upper genital tract in female mice. *Sex. Transm. Dis.*, **11**, 67

Swenson, C. E., Banks, J. and Schachter, J. (1983a). Organ culture studies with *Mycoplasma hominis*. *Sex. Transm. Dis.*, **11**, S355

Swenson, C. E., Donegan, E. and Schachter, J. (1983b). *Chlamydia trachomatis*-induced salpingitis in the mouse. *J. Infect. Dis.*, **148**, 1101

Swenson, C. E., Sung, M. and Schachter, J. (1984). The Effect of Tetracycline Treatment on Chlamydial Salpingitis and Subsequent Fertility in the Mouse. In preparation

Tan, R. J. S. and Miles, J. A. R. (1974). Possible role of feline T-strain mycoplasmas in cat abortion. *Aust. Vet. J.*, **50**, 142

Taylor-Robinson, D., Purcell, R. H., London, W. T. *et al.* (1978). Urethral infection of chimpanzees by *Ureaplasma urealyticum*. *J. Med. Microbiol.*, **11**, 197

Taylor-Robinson, D., Rassner, C. and Furr, P. M. *et al.* (1975). Fetal wastage as a consequence of *Mycoplasma pulmonis* infection in mice. *J. Reprod. Fertil.*, **42**, 483

Taylor-Robinson, D. and Thomas, B. J. (1980). The role of *Chlamydia trachomatis* in genital tract and associated diseases. *J. Clin. Pathol.*, **33**, 205

Taylor-Robinson, D., Tuffrey, M. and Falder, P. (1982). Some aspects of animal models for *Chlamydia trachomatis* genital infections. In Mårdh, P.-A., Holmes, K. K., Oriel, J. D. *et al.* (eds) *Chlamydial Infections* (Fernstrom Foundation Series), p. 375. (Amsterdam: Elsevier)

Taylor-Robinson, D., Tully, J. G., Furr, P. M. *et al.* (1981). Urogenital mycoplasma infections of man: A review with observations on a recently discovered mycoplasma. *Israel J. Med. Sci.*, **17**, 524

Tully, J. G., Taylor-Robinson, D., Rose, D. L. *et al.* (1983). *Mycoplasma genitalium*, a new species from the human urogenital tract. *Int. J. Syst. Bacteriol.*, **33**, 387

16
Maternofetal transmission of infection

A. H. BASALAMAH and F. E. SEREBOUR

INTRODUCTION

Our present understanding of perinatal infections has mostly accrued from analyzing the perinatal outcome of pregnancy after epidemics and pandemics involving various microbes. The 1964–1965 rubella epidemic, and the thousands of congenital defects that developed as a result of it, provided some insights about pregnancy and intrauterine infections. The otherwise healthy placental barrier, which provides the germ-free and immunologically incompetent fetus with protection and warmth for survival, is compromised by perinatal pathogens. This may happen as a result of primary maternal infection or by the reactivation of a latent infection during pregnancy. The perinatal outcome varies widely, ranging from no fetal involvement to spontaneous abortions, still births, developmental defects, and chronic postnatal infections.

The cost to society for the rehabilitation of congenitally infected newborns is immense. For example, congenital toxoplasmosis among infants costs 221.9 million dollars per year (Wilson and Remington, 1980). Although the implementation of preventive measures has led to a steady decline in the incidence of congenital rubella in the United States, the annual cost remains at an estimated 50 million dollars (Schoenbaum et al., 1976).

As many as 2% of fetuses are infected in utero, and up to 10% of newborns are infected during delivery or in the immediate postpartum period. Although the importance of intrauterine infection in perinatal mortality and morbidity is declining in developed countries, this is not the case in underdeveloped countries where unexplained abortions, congenital defects, intrauterine growth retardation, and elevated levels of umbilical IgM are commonly observed in obstetric practice.

The pregnant woman who suspects that she has been exposed to teratogenic microbial agents experiences tremendous anxiety. In developing countries, where this possibility is more likely, parents must often face without governmental aid the social and economic hardships that a handicapped child brings. Measures that decrease the risk of intrauterine infection provide not only economic and social gains to society, but also a better quality of life for newborns.

DEFINITION

Maternofetal transmission may be simply defined as the mechanical transport of a microbial agent from the mother to the fetus via the placenta. The transmission of infectious disease, however, can also occur during passage of the baby through an infected cervix or birth canal or via fetal contact with maternal secretions in the immediate postpartum period. It is important to remember that maternal infection can occur without fetal involvement, and fetal involvement may not occur even if the placenta is infected. Such factors as gestational age, virulence of the microbial agent, maternal susceptibility, fetal susceptibility, and placental maturation collectively determine the perinatal outcome of these infections.

MICROBIAL AGENTS

Of the multitude of microbes capable of infecting the human adult, comparatively few may be transmitted to the fetus or the newborn and cause infection. Table 1 presents the microbial agents that may be involved in intrauterine infection. While intrauterine pathogenicity of rubella (Gregg, 1941), cytomegalovirus, *Toxoplasma gondii* and *Treponema pallidum* are well proven, the maternofetal transmission of microbes such as hepatitis A, influenza, and measles and so on, and their pathogenicity on the fetus, remains to be clarified.

Table 1 Perinatal pathogens

Viruses	*Protozoa*	*Bacteria*
Rubella virus	*Toxoplasma gondii*	*Listeria monocytogenes*
Cytomegalovirus	*Plasmodia* ssp	*Treponema pallidum*
Herpes simplex virus	*Trypanosoma* ssp	*Mycobacterium tuberculosis*
Varicella-zoster	*Filaria* ssp	*Mycobacterium leprae*
Variola		
Epstein–Barr virus		
Poliovirus		
Hepatitis B		
Hepatitis A		
Non A-non B hepatitis		
Measles virus		
Enteroviruses		
Rabies virus		
Mumps virus		

TORCH agents

The acronym 'TORCH' which stands for TOxoplasmosis, Rubella, Cytomegalo-virus, Herpes simplex virus and others, including syphilis, listeriosis, aseptic meningitis, and enteroviral infections was adopted by A. J. Nahmias in 1971 to emphasize the fact that, despite the differences in genera, structure, and biochemical constitution, these microbes exhibit a similar pathology.

TORCH characteristics:

1. The infection tends usually to be harmless or subclinical in normal adults.
2. Despite the presence of specific IgG anamnestic antibody, reactivation of latent infection can occur (Stagno et al., 1977; Schopfer et al., 1978). In such cases, however, placental infection tends to be less intense and fetal involvement less severe.
3. These organisms cause clinically indistinguishable diseases, which can only be confirmed serologically by using specific sensitivity tests.
4. Congenital infections with these agents leads to early synthesis of IgM by the fetus, which then leads to elevated cord IgM in all symptomatic neonates.
5. The pathogens show specific organ trophism with predilection for the eye, CNS, heart, and reticuloendothelial system.

THE EPIDEMIOLOGY OF MICROBIAL AGENTS INVOLVED IN MATERNOFETAL INFECTION

Although the prevalence of microbial antibodies in various adult populations is high, intrauterine infections do occur, as maternal immunity does not totally guarantee protection against future intrauterine transmissions. Such factors as age, socioeconomic class, and parity also play a role in determining the prevalence of intrauterine infections in the community.

The incidence of congenital toxoplasmosis is rare in the United Kingdom, where about 5 cases per 100,000 live births are reported. Higher incidences have been reported elsewhere, including 130 per 100,000 in New York, 300 per 100,000 in Paris, 650 per 100,000 in Netherlands, 700 per 100,000 in Vienna, and 600 per 100,000 in Jeddah, Saudi Arabia (Basalamah and Serebour, 1981). Interestingly, our prevalence of 30% in antenatal screening using the latex agglutination test is comparable to a similar population in New York, yet the incidence of congenital toxoplasmosis is higher in our community. While the consumption of raw meat is the main etiologic factor in most western countries, it is the propagation of the *T. gondii* oocyst in cat feces that is responsible for most cases of congenital toxoplasmosis in Saudi Arabia.

Cytomegalovirus (CMV) is the most common cause of intrauterine infections in man, despite the high prevalence of antibody in adults. Maternal immunity to CMV ranges from 100% in Ivory Coast (Africa) to 98% in Saudi Arabia, 83% in Japan, 52% in Denmark, around 60% in upper socioeconomic class and 85% in low socioeconomic class in Alabama (USA), to a low 25% in Manchester, UK (Stagno et al., 1982). Despite the high prevalence of its antibody, CMV is responsible for approximately 1% of the infections in all neonates, Seroepidemiologic studies show that the incidence of infection is indirectly proportional to the socioeconomic class of the mother. The young unmarried woman generally has a higher risk of infection (MacDonald and Tobin, 1978). Recurrent CMV infection in pregnancy due to reactivation of latent infection rather than reinfection with different strains is very common in highly immune populations (Stagno et al., 1977). From 3% to 28% of pregnant women may show reactivation of latent infection (Hanshaw and Dudgeon, 1978).

The immunity provided by rubella 'wild' virus or vaccines seems to be long-lasting. Reactivation of a latent infection has occurred, but only in rare cases (Eilard and Stannegard, 1974; Forsgren et al., 1979). Seroepidemiologic surveys range from ideal immunity in Chile (Dowdle et al., 1970), 98% in USSR (Kantorovic et al., 1979), 85% in most European countries (Horstmann, 1971; Rawls et al., 1967), 73% in Nigeria (Odelola, 1978), to 57% in Japan and 50% in Trinidad and Panama (Cockburn, 1969).

Despite the fact that a vaccination program against rubella has not been established in Saudi Arabia, the 'wild' virus is prevalent there. Our survey of antenatal samples showed a 93% prevalence of hemagglutination inhibition antibodies. The seronegative mothers are at higher risk of primary infection in our gregarious society during pregnancy.

The seriousness of congenital infections caused by agents such as herpes simplex viruses, measles, and enteroviruses and their perinatal outcome cannot be overemphasized.

MATERNAL SUSCEPTIBILITY DURING PREGNANCY

The mechanism by which it is possible for the genetically incompatible fetus to defy the laws of tissue transplantation and to be tolerated by the mother is intriguing. Pregnancy is associated with physiologic immunosuppression of both humoral and cellular immunity. This immunosuppression, however, is not manifested by a reduction in T- and B-lymphocyte numbers (Birkeland et al., 1977; Cornfield et al., 1979) nor in their proliferative response to mitogens (Gehrz et al. 1981). Olding and Oldstone (1974, 1976) have described the suppression of maternal mixed lymphocyte cultures (MLC) during pregnancy. A soluble suppressor factor produced by the fetal suppressor cells may be responsible for this maternal hyporeactivity response (Toivanen et al., 1980).

Other hormones associated with pregnancy, such as progesterone and human chorionic gonadotrophin (HCG), have an immunosuppressive role in the in vitro inhibition of lymphocyte proliferation (Kaye and Jones, 1971) and might also exert some immunosuppression in vivo. α-fetoprotein is thought to induce the production of suppressor lymphocytes in the fetus. This may contribute to the fetal tolerance of the mother (Murgita, 1976). Virus-specific cytotoxic responses seem to be depressed in maternal lymphocytes during pregnancy (Thong et al., 1973; Rola-Pleszczynski et al., 1977). The role of these factors in the suppression of maternal immunity during pregnancy and the subsequent susceptibility to infection remains to be fully elucidated.

As a result of this physiologic immunosuppression during pregnancy, micro-bial agents such as varicella, influenza, polio, smallpox (when it existed), and herpesviruses tend to be more severe in pregnancy than in the nonpregnant state. Other factors, such as maternal age, socioeconomic class, nutrition, and parity, also play a role in perinatal infections and reproductive outcome.

FETAL IMMUNITY AND SUSCEPTIBILITY TO INFECTION

The development of the fetal immune system begins at the time of conception (Stiehm, 1975). By 3–4 weeks' gestation the multipotential stem cell in the yolk sac has migrated to the fetal liver and bone marrow. The identity of T cells in the cortex of thymus can be established as early as 6–8 weeks' gestation, and IgM- and IgG-producing B lymphocytes can be identified in the peripheral blood by 12 weeks' gestation.

The main source of fetal immunity is derived by the transfer of maternal IgG through the placenta. The mechanism of transfer is conferred by the intrinsic nature of the Fc, rather than the Fab portion, of the immunoglobulin (Ovary, 1974). This is an active process in which Fc receptors on the trophoblast play a role in the recognition. The bound IgG is transported across the plasma membranes into phagosomes, where vesicles protect them against lysosomal degradation. Fetal IgG concentration remains at a low 10% of the mean adult concentration (MAC) up to 20 weeks' gestation. Around the 27th week, IgG levels rise rapidly so as to parallel adult levels by birth. The other immunoglobulins, i.e., IgA, IgM, IgE and IgD, are not known to cross the placenta.

The elevation of IgM in the cord blood is a sign of intrauterine infection. Maternal IgG provides the major line of defense against fetal infections during pregnancy and the neonatal period. Lack of maternal antibody to certain microbes, such as varicella and group-B streptococci, can lead to devastating infections in the fetus and the newborn. Fetal susceptibility is therefore in-directly proportional to maternal immunity.

DIAGNOSIS OF MATERNAL INFECTIONS

Maternal infections cannot be diagnosed on clinical grounds alone, and sero-logic assays may not be adequate. The subclinical processes of many infections and the clinically indistinguishable presentation of others mean that the obstetri-cian is dependent on the laboratory for diagnosis. For example, clinical observa-tion of TORCH signs and symptoms fails to identify as high as 95% of cases of primary cytomegalovirus infections and 90% of *Toxoplasma gondii* infections.

A variety of serologic assays are now available for TORCH infections in pregnancy, but since positive diagnosis may lead to anxiety and therapeutic abortion, it is advisable that reagents should be standardized and trained personnel involved with testing and interpretation of the tests. New enzyme-linked immunosorbent assay (ELISA) methods for the detection of IgM is quickly replacing the hemagglutination, latex agglutination, indirect fluorescence, and complement-fixation tests. These latter tests require two samples taken 14 days apart. A fourfold rise in the IgG titer of the two samples tested at the same time indicates recent infection. ELISA and radioimmunoassay (RIA) methods have made it possible to confirm specific IgM elevation in the mother on the basis of a single sample. The following sections summarize our recommendations of some of the tests for diagnosis of TORCH infections.

Toxoplasmosis

Various screening methodologies are available for toxoplasmosis, including the dye test (Sabin–Feldman test), complement fixation tests, indirect hemagglutination tests, and indirect fluorescence test. We have adopted the recommendation of Desmonts and Couvreur (1974), by which all pregnant women are screened for *Toxoplasma* antibody at first antenatal visit (usually during the first trimester) using the latex agglutination test (Toxotest*). All seronegative mothers are retested around the 20th to 22nd week and again near term or at delivery.

The IgG status of seropositive mothers is confirmed indirectly using the new sandwich ELISA IgM test. All mothers with positive latex agglutination results but a negative ELISA IgM assay are considered immunologically protected. Positive IgM mothers are treated and their newborns checked for congenital infections.

Rubella

Although the rubella virus can be isolated from throat cultures, the method is cumbersome and serologic diagnosis is preferred. Included among the available serologic tests are the hemagglutination inhibiting antibody (HAI), complement-fixation assays, single radial hemolysis, immunofluorescence test, RIA, and ELISA methods. The new latex agglutination assay (Rubascan) is promising; it combines the advantages of speed and simplicity with a sensitivity that is comparable to ELISA and HAI. It is anticipated that most laboratories will adopt the latex agglutination method for screening in the near future (Meegan *et al.*, 1982).

The present IgM ELISA (Rubazyme-M†) has demonstrated adequate sensitivity and specificity in our laboratory. This test provides a level of accuracy and sensitivity that is comparable to sucrose density gradients and is very easy to manipulate. The transient appearance of specific IgM and its absence in cases of reactivation make IgM assays useful in the diagnosis of primary infections.

Cytomegalovirus

The isolation of the virus, usually from urine or throat is the most reliable means of diagnosis. Unfortunately laboratories capable of performing such

* Toxotest MT "Eiken", Japan
† Rubazyme-M; Abbot Laboratories, Chicago, USA

cumbersome assays are few. Serologic means of diagnosis, although presumptive remains the only alternative. Serologic diagnosis of primary CMV infections is difficult. Seropositivity in adults is so high that IgG tests are not reliable. Seroconversion measured by sensitive assays, however, have been found to be diagnostic (Reynolds et al., 1979). Various assays, including the indirect immunofluorescence, indirect haemagglutination, ELISA, complement fixation and neutralization tests, all measure antibody concentration at different stages of the infection. The most reliable serologic test is the RIA IgM test which detects 90% of acute infections but not reactivation of latent infection (Griffiths et al., 1982). The indirect IgM ELISA (Enzygnost Cytomegalovirus*) has been used routinely to detect primary infections and is preferred to the indirect immunofluorescence assays which require trained personnel. Absorption tests to remove Rheumatoid factor prior to testing for IgM are mandatory especially in pregnant women and umbilical cord sera where false positivity is high (Meuruman et al., 1978).

Herpes simplex virus

As in the case with CMV, most women are seroreactive for the herpes simplex viruses, and serologic diagnosis is of limited value. However, exfoliative cytology using Papanicolaou staining is a simple and readily available screening device. Unfortunately, the incidence of false-positive and -negative smears may be high and serologic procedures may be necessary. Immunofluorescence and ELISA techniques are more rapid and specific, but they still lack sensitivity. It is anticipated that these technical problems will be solved soon enough to make serologic antenatal screening for herpesviruses generally available. Comparatively rapid clinical decisions during labor or rupture of membranes are required. The present virus isolation on tissue cultures, although adequate for confirmatory diagnosis, is time-consuming. The need for confirmatory IgM tests with high titers comparable to the sensitivity of tissue cultures is anticipated. IgM ELISA plates (Enzygnost Herpes*) currently in use for the diagnosis of acute infections and reactivation of latent infections requires further assessment.

DIAGNOSIS IN THE FETUS OR NEWBORN

The obstetrician depends on maternal history, clinical findings, and serologic tests to establish a conclusive diagnosis. Unfortunately, congenital malformations may be unapparent at birth and maternal history poorly expressed. Differential diagnosis is made difficult by the indistinguishable presentation of signs and symptoms at birth. A great majority of newborns, though normal at birth, may have experienced intrauterine infection with symptoms delayed sometimes until the first decade of life. In those with clinical symptoms cataracts and congenital heart disease are more commonly associated with rubella, jaundice with CMV, and retinopathy, hydrocephaly and cerebral calcification with toxoplasmosis. Most of the diseases overlap with other microbial agents and serologic assays are mandatory for confirmation. Amongst the serologic tests, elevated cord IgM is an indication of intrauterine infection as discussed below.

Cord IgM

In normal pregnancy the fetus begins to synthesize IgM by around 20 weeks' gestation. By the 30th week, fetal serum levels may have reached 13% of maternal levels. At birth, about 20% of maternal IgM is achieved and there is a very rapid rise to 90% of mean normal adult levels (50–200 mg/100 ml) by 18 months. Infants born into germ-free incubators do not show IgM elevation until they leave the protected environment. Low levels of IgM up to 20 mg/100 ml may usually be demonstrated in cord blood. In response to intrauterine infections, however, such as *Toxoplasma gondii*, rubella virus, or *Treponema pallidum*, fetal IgM synthesis rises to unusually high levels.

Although the prevalence of elevated cord IgM is low in most European countries and the United States, it is high in developing countries. Sever (1969) reported prevalence of 0.8% elevated IgM in Caucasians in USA whereas Stiehm (1975) found 5% cord IgM elevation in low socioeconomic groups (presumably non-Caucasian) in the United States. Values as high as 40% (Lechtig, 1970) and 31% (Logie, 1973) have been reported for Guatemala and Gambia respectively. In a study of 1884 cord samples in Saudi Arabia, a 16.3% elevated IgM was reported (Basalamah and Serebour, 1981). Although the clinical significance of elevated cord IgM in a low-risk population is questionable, it has been shown to be of value in the diagnosis of perinatal infection in high-risk populations (Blankenship *et al.*, 1969). The availability of RIA and ELISA techniques for specific IgM has made it possible to diagnose intrauterine infections on cord blood. Early treatment in such cases may change the whole clinical course of the disease.

PREVENTION OF MATERNOFETAL TRANSMISSION OF INFECTION

The 40 weeks' gestational period is accompanied by emotional, physiological and psychological changes in the pregnant mother. All aspects of effective prevention must begin at the preconceptual period. In adjusting herself to pregnancy, the mother may need to acquire certain habits, paramount of which must be cleanliness, avoidance of contacts with sources of infections, and immunization if possible.

The risk of toxoplasmosis can be minimized by hygienic procedures, such as avoiding handling raw meat, washing fruits and vegetables before consumption, preventing the access of flies and cockroaches to foods and most importantly, avoiding contact with materials that are potentially contaminated with cat feces. The rubella vaccination program in European countries in which a high degree of herd immunity is induced in prepubertal children has been very successful. There has been a dramatic reduction of congenital rubella from 15,000 cases in 1969 to 2000 cases in 1981 (Horstmann, 1982). Although such programs have not been implemented in developing countries, a very high percentage of women have protective antibodies by the time they reach adolescence. The few who remain susceptible can be identified during antenatal screening. In our obstetric practice, susceptible women are placed on contraceptives soon after parturition and then given active immunization postpartum. In seronegative transfused patients it is advisable to delay immunization since acquired passive antibody may prevent an immunizing infection with the virus (Watt and McGucken, 1980).

Unfortunately the apparent success of rubella immunization programs has not been imitated with CMV infection. There is still no available method for prevention of CMV. Some live attenuated vaccines have been found immunogenic in adult volunteers (Elek and Stern, 1974; Plotkin, et al., 1976), but their efficacy and specificity are yet to be proven. Neonatal herpes infection is usually acquired during labor, but ascending infections also occur. Reactivation of latent infection in the face of a rather high exposure rate is possible. At present there are no known ways of controlling reactivation of chronic mucocutaneous herpes infection. The mortality in infants with neonatal herpes may be as high as 50%. The survivors may be left with permanent damage if untreated (Nahmias et al., 1975). Therefore, women with active genital lesion may require a caesarean section to avoid fetal involvement. In the immediate neonatal period, transmission of infection through contact can be minimized through careful handwashing and personal hygiene. The prevention of transmission of other microbes such as hepatitis A and B, varicella-zoster, influenza and measles viruses and enteroviruses may be found in the use of specific immunoglobulin for passive immunization or the use of attenuated vaccines. The efficacy for most of these vaccines depends how closely they resemble the real virus.

Pregnant women may be advised to avoid crowded public places during periods of community-wide influenza outbreaks. Pregnant women exposed to measles should receive immune serum globulin.

Most enteroviral infections are acquired by the fecal–oral route. Handwashing after handling infants and children with acute upper respiratory illnesses is mandatory.

The above procedures provide a general outline of preventive measures. Specific recommendations may depend on the microbial agent involved, and appropriate references must be consulted.

CONCLUSION

Maternofetal transmission of infection remains a worldwide problem with a great socioeconomic impact. The wide range of pathogens are involved and the two separate hosts of mother and fetus with their different susceptibilities makes the outcome of infection wide and varied. Diagnosis of such conditions is difficult. Maternal history, routine antenatal screening, and close observation of the outcome of pregnancy may help in early diagnosis and possible curative measures. The ultimate goal must be prevention, since the sequelae of the disease cannot be remedied.

References

Basalamah, A. H. and Serebour, E. F. (1981) Toxoplasmosis in Pregnancy: A survey of 1000 pregnant Saudis and Non-Saudis attending King Abdulaziz University Hospital in Jeddah. *Saudi Med. J.*, **2**, 125

Birkelande, S. A. and Kristoffersen, I. (1977). Cellular immunity in pregnancy: blast transformation and rosette formation of maternal T and B lymphocytes. A cross section analysis. *Clin. Exp. Immunol.*, **30**, 408

Blankenship, W. J., Cassidy, G., Gardner, S. D. *et al.* (1969). Serum gamma-M globulin responses in acute neonatal infections and their diagnostic significance. *J. Pediatr.*, **75**, 1271

Cockburn, W. C. (1969). World aspects of the epidemiology of Rubella, *Am. J. Dis. Child.*, **118**, 112

Desmonts, G. and Couvreur, J. (1974). Congenital Toxoplasmosis: a prospective study of 378 pregnancies. *New. Engl. J. Med.*, **290**, 1110

Dowdle, F. R., Ferreira, W., De Salles Gomes, L. F. *et al.* (1970). WHO collaborative study on the sero epidemiology of Rubella in Caribbean and Middle and South American populations in 1968. *Bull. WHO*, **42**, 419

Eilard, T. and Stannegard, O. (1974). Rubella reinfection in pregnancy followed by transmission to the fetus. *J. Infect. Dis.*, **129**, 594

Elek, S. D. and Stern, H. (1974). Development of a vaccine against mental retardation caused by cytomegalovirus infection in utero. *Lancet*, **1**, 1

Enzygnost Cytomegalovirus, Behring, Germany

Enzygnost Herpes, Behring, Germany

Forsgren, M., Carlstrom, G. and Strangert, K. (1979). Congenital rubella after maternal reinfection. *Scand. J. Infect. Dis.*, **11**, 81

Gehrz, R. C., Christianson, W. R., Linner, K. M. *et al.* (1981). A longitudinal analysis of lymphocyte proliferative responses to mitogens and antigens during human pregnancy. *Am. J. Obstet. Gynecol.*, **140**, 665

Gregg, N. M. (1941). Congenital cataract following German measles in the mother. *Trans. Ophthalmol. Soc. Aust.*, **3**, 35

Griffiths, P. D., Stagno, S. and Pass, R. F. *et al.* (1982). Cytomegalovirus infection during pregnancy: specific IgM antibodies as a marker of recent primary infection. *J. Infect. Dis.*, **145**, 647

Hanshaw, J. B. and Dudgeon, J. A. (1978). Congenital cytomegalovirus, *Viral Diseases of the Fetus and Newborn*. (Philadelphia: W. B. Saunders)

Horstmann, D. M. (1979). Rubella: the challenge of its control, *J. Infect. Dis.*, **123**, 649

Horstmann, D. M. (1982). Rubella. In *Clin. Obstet. Gynecol.*, **25** (3), 585 (Harper & Row)

Kantorovic, R. A., Volodina, N. I. and Telesevskaja, E. A. (1979). Congenital rubella in the USSR. *Bull. WHO*, **57**, 145

Kaye, M. D. and Jones, W. R. (1971). Effect of hCG on *in vitro* lymphocyte transformation. *Am. J. Obstet. Gynecol.*, **109**, 1024

MacDonald, H. and Tobin, J. O'H. (1978). Congenital cytomegalovirus infection: a collaborative study on epidemiological, clinical, and laboratory findings. *Dev. Med. Child. Neurol.*, **20**, 471

Meegan, J. M., Evans, B. K. and Horstmann, D. M. (1982). Comparison of latex agglutination test with the hemagglutination-inhibition test, enzyme linked immunosorbent assay, and neutralization test for detection of antibodies to rubella. *J. Clin. Microbiol.*, **16**, 644

Meurman, O. *et al. Lancet*, **2**, 685

Murgita, R. A. (1976). The immunosuppressive role of alpha-feto protein during pregnancy. *Scand. J. Immunol.*, **5**, 1003

Nahmias, A. J. (1971). Perinatal infections associated with toxoplasma and rubella, cytomegalo- and herpes viruses. *Pediatr. Res.*, **5**, 405

Nahmias, A. J., Visintine, A. M., Reimer, C. B. *et al.* (1975). Herpes simplex virus infection of the fetus and newborn. *Prog. Clin. Biol. Res.*, **3**, 63

Odelola, H. A. (1978). Rubella haemagglutination inhibiting antibodies in females of child bearing age in Western Nigeria. *J. Hygie. Epidemiol., Microbiol. Immunol.*, **22**, 190

Olding, L. B. and Oldstone, M. B. A. (1974). Lymphocytes from human newborns abrogate mitoses of their mother's lymphocytes. *Nature*, **249**, 161

Olding, L. B. and Oldstone, M. B. A. (1976). Thymus-derived peripheral lymphocytes from human newborns inhibit division of their mother's lymphocytes. *J. Immunol.*, **116**, 682

Ovary, Z. (1974). The structure of antibody molecules as related to transplacental passage. In Centaro, A. and Narretti, N. (eds.). *Immunology in Obstetrics and Gynecology*, p. 231 (Amsterdam: Elsevier)

Plotkins, A., Farquhar, J. and Hornberger, E. (1976). Clinical trials of immunization with the Towne 125 strain of human cytomegalovirus. *J. Infect. Dis.*, **134**, 470

Rawls, W. E., Melnick, J. L. and Bradstreet, C. M. P. *et al.* (1967). WHO collaborative study on the seroepidemiology of Rubella, *Bull. WHO*, **37**, 79

Reynolds, D. W., Stagno, S. and Alford, C. A. (1979). Laboratory diagnosis of cytomegalovirus infections. In Lennette, E. H. and Schmidt, N. J. (eds). *Diagnostic Procedures for Viral Rickettsial and Chlamydial Infection*, p. 399 (Washington; DC: American Public Health Association)

Rola-Pleszczynski, M., Frenjel, L. D., Fucillo, D. A. *et al.* (1977). Specific impairment of cell-mediated immunity in mothers of infants with congenital infection due to cytomegalovirus. *J. Infect. Dis.*, **135**, 386

Schoenbaum, S. L., Hyde, J. N., Bartoshesky, L. *et al.* (1976). Benefit-cost analysis of rubella vaccination policy. *N. Engl. J. Med.*, **294**, 306

Schopfer, K., Laube, E. and Kreck, U. (1978). Congenital cytomegalovirus infection in newborn infants of mothers infected before pregnancy. *Arch. Dis. Child.*, **53**, 536

Sever, J. L., Hardy, J. B., Korones, S. B. *et al.* (1969). Cord immunoglobulins in a middle class Caucasian population. *J. Pediatr.*, **75**, 1224

Stagno, S., Reynolds, D. W., Huang, E. S. *et al.* (1977). Congenital cytomegalovirus infection: occurrence in an immune population. *N. Engl. J. Med.*, **296**, 1254

Stagno, S., Pass, R. F., Dworsky, M. E. *et al.* (1982). Maternal cytomegalovirus infection and perinatal transmission. In Pitkin, R. M. and Scott, J. R. (eds.). *Clin. Obstet. Gynecol.*, **25**, 585

Stiehm, E. R. (1975). Fetal defense mechanisms. *Am. J. Dis. Child.*, **129**, 438

Thong, Y. H., Steele, R. W., Vincent, M. M. *et al.* (1973). Impaired *in vitro* cell-mediated immunity to rubella virus during pregnancy. *N. Engl. J. Med.*, **289**, 604

Toivanen, P. and Granberg, C. (1980). Mother/child mixed lymphocyte reaction: is it depressed? *Immunol. Today.* October, 1980, 76

Watt, R. W. and McGucken, R. B. (1980). Failure of rubella immunization after blood transfusion: birth of a congenitally infected infant. *Br. Med. J.*, **281**, 977

Wilson, C. B. and Remington, J. S. (1980). What can be done to prevent congenital toxoplasmosis? *Am. J. Obstet. Gynecol.*, **138**, 357

17
Contraceptive usage and pelvic infection in women

L. G. KEITH, G. S. BERGER and E. R. BROWN

INTRODUCTION

Although it is widely recognized that sexually transmitted diseases (STDs) are a major international health problem, a connection between the use of a specific contraceptive method and the occurrence of genital tract infection often goes unrecognized. The bulk of STDs in industrialized nations no longer are caused by the traditional or 'major' venereal diseases – syphilis, gonorrhea, chancroid, lymphogranuloma venereum and granuloma inguinale. Sexually active women in the United States presently stand a far greater chance of contracting a so-called 'minor' STD, such as herpes (HSV), chlamydia, ureaplasm, trichomoniasis, hepatitis B, and condyloma acuminata.

According to Hansfield (1982) STDs are inherently 'sexist'. Not only are many STDs more difficult to diagnose among women, but their complications are more frequent and often more serious than in men. Pelvic inflammatory disease (PID) represents a complication of genital tract infections unique to the female. Although, like females, males may acquire upper tract infections resulting in infertility, females must also contend with recurrent infection, ectopic pregnancy, and chronic pelvic pain, often requiring major surgery.

The accurate differentiation of PID from other intra-abdominal conditions has troubled physicians for decades. In 1928, Farr and Findlay noted a diagnostic error rate (over-diagnosis) of 30% in a series of more than 500 patients operated upon with this preoperative diagnosis. Four decades later, Jacobsen and Westrøm (1969) observed a similar rate of over-diagnosis (35%) in a series of patients who underwent laparoscopy for a preoperative diagnosis of acute salpingitis.

Error in the other direction (under-diagnosis) tends to occur in the office setting where the diagnosis of PID often is not considered until its symptoms are extensive. This is not surprising considering that most physicians obtain their training in the diagnosis of PID in hospitals where patients present with severe symptoms of disease. In terms of numbers, however, patients who are acutely ill from PID represent 'the tip of the iceberg'. Sweet has proposed rather strict criteria for the diagnosis of PID, which are listed below (Sweet, 1981). All patients should have the following findings:

(1) history of lower abdominal pain;
(2) lower abdominal tenderness;
(3) cervical motion tenderness; and
(4) adnexal tenderness.

In addition, one of the following laboratory findings should be present:

(1) fever;
(2) leukocytosis;
(3) elevated ESR;
(4) inflammatory adnexal mass on sonography; or
(5) culdocentesis revealing bacteria and white blood cells in the peritoneal fluid.

It is worth noting that even among laparoscopically proven cases of PID, however, less than one-third of the patients had elevated sedimentation rates, leukocytosis or fever (Handsfield, 1982).

In addition to mistreatment due to faulty diagnosis, PID is often inadequately treated, especially during initial episodes before symptomatology becomes clear. Even though many patients may be prescribed oral antibiotics when they have low-grade fever and no obvious pelvic mass, subsequent hospitalization and the institution of intravenous therapy may be required at a more advanced stage in the disease to attenuate a possibly life-threatening situation such as occurs following the rupture of a tubo-ovarian abscess. Some authorities, in particular those working in Scandinavia, recommend that all patients with PID be hospitalized to receive parenteral antibiotic therapy (Weström and Mårdh, 1983). Because of the prevalence of the disease, this suggestion has not been judged as practical in the USA for a variety of reasons, mostly economic.

Definitions

Pelvic infection in the female consists of a number of conditions caused by a variety of microbiologic agents (Table 1). A simple classification distinguishes between infections of the lower genital tract and infections of the upper genital tract. Lower genital tract infections (LGTI) include those of the Bartholin's glands, urethra, Skene's ducts, vagina and cervix. Upper genital tract infections (UGTI) include those of the endometrium, myometrium, parametrium, fallopian tubes, ovaries and the adjacent connective tissue structures, including the lymphatics and the blood supply.

In clinical practice, the term PID is used imprecisely as a 'wastebasket' term. The use of more precise anatomic and etiologic terminology would assist in clarifying the nature of the infection. Examples of more specific diagnoses include terms such as gonococcal or chlamydial salpingitis, streptococcal endoparametritis, etc.

246

Table 1 Etiologic classification of presently known agents causing STDs*

Bacteria	
Neisseria gonorrhoeae	Viruses
Chlamydia trachomatis	Herpes simplex
Treponema pallidum	Hepatitis A
Ureaplasma urealyticum	Hepatitis B
Mycoplasma hominis	Cytomegalovirus
Haemophilus ducreyi	Genital wart
Calymmatobacterium granulomatis	Molluscum contagiosum
Shigella spp.	Protozoa
Campylobacter fetus	*Trichomonas vaginalis*
Gardnerella vaginalis	*Entamoeba histolytica*
Streptococcus, group B	*Giardia lamblia*
	Ectoparasites
	Phthirus pubis (crab louse)
	Sarcoptes scabiei (scabies mite)

* Handsfield (1982)

Incidence

Although estimates exist (Jones *et al.*, 1980; St. John *et al.*, 1981a,b), the full extent to which pelvic infection exists in the United States is unknown. Clinical experience indicates that few sexually active women pass through their reproductive years (15–45) without at least one episode of lower genital tract infection. It is not known with certainty what proportion of women have recurrent LGTI and/or what percentage of LGTI are followed by UGTI. According to the National Ambulatory Medical Care Survey (St. John *et al.*, 1981b), there were approximately 2 million patient visits annually for PID between 1973 and 1977 at the offices of private physicians. During the same time an additional 700,000 visits were made annually for PID to public clinics and hospital emergency rooms (Curran, 1980). Between 1970 and 1975 slightly more than 200,000 hospitalizations for PID occurred annually (Jones *et al.*, 1980). The direct and indirect costs of providing care for these women are great, approaching 1 billion dollars per year (Curran, 1980).

Medical consequences of pelvic infection

The sequelae of pelvic infection can be serious and frequently require additional medical or surgical care subsequent to the initial infection. Weström (1975) noted a greater than six-fold increase in the risk of ectopic pregnancy and a four-fold increase in the rate of chronic pelvic pain among women with laparoscopically confirmed PID followed for 6–14 years compared to a group of women who did not have PID. Infertility after one, two or three episodes of acute PID was observed in 13%, 36%, and 75% of the patients, respectively (Weström, 1975). When women who did not desire to become pregnant were excluded from consideration, only 69% of the women who had had acute PID achieved a subsequent pregnancy compared to 96% of the control group. In more recent years these same investigators noted an infertility rate of 22%

among women with one episode of laparoscopically verified PID and 46% after subsequent episodes of PID (Svensson *et al.*, 1983). These women had been followed from 2.5 to 7.5 years after laparoscopic diagnosis of PID.

The problem of involuntary infertility arising secondary to PID has become a major concern for gynecologists everywhere (Population Reports, 1979). Even when therapy is available it is lengthy and costly. Cost-effectiveness studies indicate that an average of 10–20 office visits are required, and the total cost of treatment for infertility may be in excess of $10,000 (Population Reports, 1979; Belsey, 1983). Despite these costs, not all treated women will have their fertility restored.

CAUSATIVE AGENTS OF INFECTION

General comments

The female genital tract possesses unique characteristics suitable for the growth of particular microorganisms. Several distinct microenvironments exist; these include the vaginal squamous epithelium, the cervical columnar epithelium and the endocervical glandular crypts. These environments are all conducive to the growth of aerobic, anaerobic and microaerophilic organisms. Specific organisms may exist either as a part of the normal flora or as pathogens. Each specific anatomic site possesses slightly different characteristics that relate to microbial growth, and each site may harbor a microbial population which differs from the others. These differences are influenced by changes in the tissue substrate upon which the organisms grow. These occur regularly throughout the menstrual cycle, during gestation, and as a woman passes from the reproductive years into the climacterium. As the tissue substrate changes, so does the microbial flora that lives on or in it. Thus, the substrate and its flora represent an ecosystem in miniature (Larsen, 1984).

The tissue substrate on which specific organisms thrive results from a genetically determined rate of maturation of cells from the basal layers to the luminal surface of the genital tract in the presence of host specific tissue fluids (Larsen, 1984). Whatever the genetic background of the woman, a variety of exogenous factors influence the microbial composition of the specific niches within the generative tract. External factors include the use of tampons, douching, the presence of microorganisms in the ejaculate of the partner(s) of those women who are sexually active, the timing of coitus relative to the menstrual cycle, the frequency of coital activity and the number of sexual partners, to cite but a few.

The interactions between the microorganisms of a given 'niche' in the female generative tract influence the make-up of the microbial flora that reside there. Various microorganisms compete with one another for space and nutrients available within a given niche. In the vagina, for example, it is widely held that the acid production by certain organisms (*Lactobacillus* in particular) renders that area less hospitable to the presence of other bacteria. This same acidity, however, favors the growth of certain other organisms such as *Bacteroides*.

As the onset of menses approaches, the population of bacteria changes qualitatively as well as quantitatively. The latter change is probably more important than the former in terms of the possible mechanism of onset of PID as it relates to menses. According to Bartlett *et al.* (1977) there is a 100-fold decrease in concentrations of facultative bacteria in the immediate premenstrual week compared to the first week after the onset of menses. The net effect of such changes is to drastically raise the proportions of anaerobes present at or about the time of menses. The observation of Monif (1982) that tampon use further reduces the oxygen available in the area of the vaginal vault and cervix is particularly relevant here. The use of tampons at a time when the anaerobic bacterial population is proportionately increased may be inappropriate, and may contribute to the onset of UGTI.

Microorganisms well adapted to growth in a particular microenvironment such as the vagina, endocervix, etc., tend to fill that site to maximal capacity. Any alteration in the microenvironment changes the ability of specific bacteria to exist in that site (Larsen, 1984). In particular, the hormonal changes of the menstrual cycle exert a profound background change, almost like a continuously moving cyclorama at the back of a theatrical stage, upon which other changes are superimposed (De Osma, 1980). A frequently cited example of dramatic differences related to hormonal status is the inability of *N. gonorrhoeae* to invade the cornified epithelium of the estrogen-stimulated sexually mature vagina. In contrast, gonococcal vaginitis occurs in prepubertal girls.

The female genital tract is particularly susceptible to transient contamination with organisms from the external environment. These organisms interact with the resident bacterial population by competing for space or nutrients. This is the case with so-called 'non-specific' vaginitis caused by *Gardnerella vaginalis*. According to Spiegel *et al.* (1980) the presence of this organism is accompanied by an abnormal over-growth of anaerobic organisms which are not extraordinary for their presence but extraordinary for their abundance. It has also been shown that patients with trichomoniasis have a larger number of anaerobic organisms than individuals without trichomoniasis (Lindner *et al.*, 1978). Although topical agents often are prescribed as a part of the therapy of such infections, even the use of povidone–iodine has a short-lived effect and the bacterial flora returns to the pretreatment milieu within 30–120 minutes (Monif *et al.*, 1980).

Description of organisms

Gynecologic literature for the last several decades has implicated *Neisseria gonorrhoeae* as a major cause of UGTI. In addition, various yeasts such as cryptococcus and candida, as well as *Gardnerella vaginalis*, have long been thought to be major causes of LGTI. More recent work, however, indicates that these explanations represent an oversimplification of the facts (Eschenbach *et al.*, 1975).

With regard to UGTI, *Chlamydia trachomatis*, *Mycoplasma hominis* and a variety of other aerobic and anaerobic microorganisms are causal in the majority of cases. Current data indicate that chlamydial infection is more prevalent than gonococcal infection in the United States as well as other Western countries

(Holmes *et al.*, 1975; Schachter *et al.*, 1975). With the exception of *N. gonorrhoeae* infections, it is not clear what proportion of LGTI progress to UGTI. At least 10-17% of women with cervical gonorrhea subsequently develop acute clinical PID (Hager and Wiesner, 1977). In some countries (USA, England and Wales) the rates of gonorrhea infections parallel the rates of PID (Jones *et al.*, 1980; Rendtorff *et al.*, 1977; Adler, 1980). In other countries (Sweden), a recent decline in the prevalence of gonorrhea has not been accompanied by a decline in the rate of PID (Westrøm, 1980).

Since 1970 a variety of bacteriologic studies have demonstrated an increasing diversity in the flora of the cervix and/or vagina. For example, in 1973 Gorbach *et al.* isolated 14 groups of anaerobic species or groups of species from 30 asymptomatic patients. In 1975, Ohm and Galask named 23 anaerobic species or groups of species in a series of 100 patients about to undergo hysterectomy. Whereas Gorbach *et al.* averaged 1.5 anaerobes per culture, Ohm and Galask reported 2.4 anaerobic species per culture. By 1977 Bartlett *et al.* named 40 anaerobic species or groups of species from a study of 52 specimens taken from 22 healthy adult women. An average of 3.8 anaerobes were found per specimen. An evaluation of contemporary medical literature indicates that it is not uncommon to isolate 10 or more aerobic and anaerobic species simultaneously, with an average of four to six from the vagina or cervix of a given woman (Larsen, 1984).

The mere presence of potentially pathogenic species does not in itself imply the presence of clinical disease. Many 'nonpathogens', for example *E. coli*, may become pathogenic given the proper circumstances. The actual quantity of the specific bacteria is of great importance in its ability to override the intrinsic host defense mechanisms. Although bacterial quantitation studies are not generally performed as one of the means by which the cause of the onset of PID is determined, they should be. The available data on healthy individuals are of interest. Bartlett *et al.* (1977) found a mean bacterial count of $10^{8.1}$ aerobic colony-forming units per gram of vaginal material and $10^{9.1}$ anaerobic colony-forming units per gram of vaginal material. In the majority of specimens, anaerobic species quantitatively outnumbered aerobic species (Bartlett *et al.*, 1977).

CONTRACEPTIVE METHODS

Risk factors

Table 2 lists major risk factors for PID that have been well described in the literature (Keith and Berger, 1984). Among the risk factors that have been evaluated to date, contraceptive methods have received major attention only in the past decade. Except for the IUD, all contraceptive methods, including sterilization of the female protect against the development of PID (Keith and Berger, 1984). If IUD users are compared to a group of non-contraceptive users with a similar risk of exposure to sexually transmitted diseases, then IUD users probably do not have any higher risks of acquiring PID (Keith and Berger, 1984).

Table 2 Risk factors associated with PID

Age
Race
Parity
Marital status
Education
Age at first intercourse
Number of sexual partners
Prior pelvic infection
Present cervical infection
Prior abortion
Current IUD use

Specific contraceptives

Condoms

Condoms have been known to protect against venereal disease since the time of Casanova. Quantitation of the degree of protection, however, has been difficult to obtain. Most studies involve retrospective interviews as the principal source of obtaining information about the efficacy of disease prevention. In addition, condom studies have almost invariably focused on the ability of the condom to prevent transmission of disease from the woman to the man. In this regard the condom has a strong protective effect against gonorrhea or syphilis – a relative risk of 0.1 among regular and correct users compared with non-users (Barlow, 1977). For those who use condoms irregularly or incorrectly, the protective effect is far less – a relative risk of 0.8 (Barlow, 1977). Although not strictly comparable because condom use was considered along with diaphragm and foam use, cervical gonorrhea was about one-fifth as common in women whose partners used condoms as in Pill or IUD users in a study at a Louisiana family planning clinic (Keith *et al.*, 1976).

Two studies of military personnel corroborate the protective effect of the condom. In Hart's study of Australian soldiers, no individual who regularly used a condom acquired venereal disease, whereas 35% who did not always use a condom had one or more episodes of venereal disease (Hart, 1974). In Hooper's study of American servicemen, a similar trend was noted (Hooper *et al.*,1973). McCormack reported that women whose partners use condoms were less likely to be infected with *C. trachomatis* or the herpes simplex virus than women whose sexual partners did not use condoms (McCormack, 1982).

Spermicides

The literature delineating the protective effect of spermicide contraception alone against the development of pelvic infection is scanty. The best evidence for the protective effect of vaginal spermicides against specific venereal infections comes from *in vitro* tests of the growth characteristics of *N. gonorrhoeae*, *T. pallidum*, *T. vaginalis* and herpes-simplex II (Jackson *et al.*, 1981). Some spermicidal preparations are more potent than others in inhibiting the growth of these organisms *in vitro*; these differences are possibly due to the wetting agents used in their bases (Population Reports, 1979). The only product to date associated with significantly lower rates of gonorrheal infection when consistently used in clinical studies is Conceptrol Cream. After 6 months of use, however, the protective effect disappeared due, in the opinion of the authors, to inconsistent use by the study population (Cutler *et al.*, 1977). The ability of vaginal contraceptive preparations to inhibit the growth of *T. vaginalis* suggests clinical importance in light of recent evidence that *T. vaginalis* may be a vector for transmission of other microorganisms to the upper genital tract in the development of PID (Keith *et al.*, 1983). A similar statement regarding clinical importance may be made with respect to the viricidal activity of surfactants such as nonoxynol-9 on the envelope of herpes-simplex virus (Asculai *et al.*, 1978).

Barrier methods

The protective effect of condoms and diaphragms alone was evaluated *vis-à-vis* the effect of spermicides in one study (Kelaghan *et al.*, 1982). Both condoms and diaphragms had a protective effect (relative risk of 0.6 and 0.4, respectively) compared to women using no contraception.

Oral contraceptives

No other contraceptive method has been studied as extensively, or for so long a period of time, as oral contraceptive hormones. During the 1960s reports were focused on the prevalence of vaginal infections among oral contraceptive users compared to non-users of oral contraceptives. Some studies found that oral contraceptive use significantly increased the risk of vaginal infections; others found that it did not or that the increase was not statistically significant (Population Reports, 1982). Even among major prospective studies there was no agreement. For example, the Royal College Study reported slightly higher risks of vaginal infections for oral contraceptive users than for non-users, but the Oxford/FPA and Walnut Creek studies found no difference (Population Reports, 1982).

In recent years emphasis has shifted to the possible protective role of oral contraceptives against the occurrence of PID. There now seems little doubt that the user of oral contraceptives has approximately half the risk of developing PID relative to women using no contraceptive method. The protective effect of current oral contraceptive use has been described for women using them for more than 12 months (Rubin *et al.*, 1982). Other studies which have documented a protective effect of oral contraceptives have not looked at duration of use (Senanayake and Kramer, 1980). According to Rubin *et al.* (1982) an estimated 50,000 initial cases of PID are prevented annually by oral contraceptive use and 12,500 hospital admissions are thereby averted.

The mechanism by which oral contraceptives protect against PID is not entirely clear. At least five possibilities have been suggested. These include: (1) hindrance of movement of bacteria from the vagina to the uterus by changing the biochemical nature of cervical mucus and by reducing menstrual flow; (2)

reduction in the strength and frequency of normal uterine contractions; (3) inhibition of the growth of bacteria at the level of the fallopian tube; (4) prevention of pregnancy and abortion, both of which provide opportunity for infection postoperatively.

Intrauterine devices

The IUD has been the most extensively studied contraceptive method in terms of an increased risk of acquiring PID (Keith and Berger, 1984; Edelman *et al.*, 1982). The magnitude of this risk has varied from study to study; a range of relative risk estimates from 1.5 to 5.5 has been cited (Senanayake and Kramer, 1980). At present it would appear that there are two components to the risk of PID related to IUD use. The first is the risk of infection resulting from the insertion procedure *per se*, and the second is the risk of infection associated with continued use of the IUD.

The risk of PID associated with IUD insertion probably results from transmission of bacteria from the lower genital tract (endocervix) into the upper tract (uterine cavity). The studies of Mishell *et al.* (1966) demonstrated contamination of the uterine cavities of women following IUD insertion. Several weeks after IUD insertion, however, Mishell *et al.* were unable to isolate bacteria, implying that the host mechanisms were able to re-establish the endometrial cavity as a sterile environment. More recent observations by Sparks *et al.* (1980) suggest that bacteria may also be isolated from uteri of asymptomatic women not using IUDs. It should be noted, however, that some of the studies cited by Sparks *et al.* (1980) may represent false-positive results based on sampling methodology since these relied on transcervical cultures; the cultures in Mishell's study were performed on uteri immediately after hysterectomy.

With regard to the continued use of IUDs, the question of whether the IUD tail places women at higher risk of PID remains unanswered. Four of the five published studies that have compared tailed and tailless IUDs found no increased risk of PID to users of tailed IUD (Edelman *et al.*, 1979). A presently ongoing study of 1100 women randomly assigned a copper-T IUD with or without a tail found no significant difference in PID rates among the two groups of women when they were followed for up to 1 year (Cole, 1984).

Since 1975, the question of the type of tail string and its relationship to the onset of PID has been a matter of wide discussion. In the past, several IUDs used tails constructed from a bundle of fine filaments (multifilament tails). These IUDs included the Antigon-F, Birnberg Bow, Dalkon Shield, Latex Leaf and Majzlin Spring. None of these IUDs is available commercially today. An evaluation of the PID rates obtained from studies of different types of IUDs did not attribute higher PID rates to IUDs with the multifilament tail (Edelman, unpublished data, 1984).

Major clinical concerns about the construction of the IUD tail began in 1975 with the publication of a paper by Tatum *et al.* (1975). The inference of Tatum *et al.* that the multifilament tail 'wicked' bacteria has never been substantiated *in vivo* although bacteria appear to migrate along the external surface of monofilament as well as multifilament IUD tails (Purrier *et al.*, 1979; Sparks *et al.*, 1981). Since one of these studies (Sparks *et al.*, 1981) contained a small number of subjects, all of whom required surgery for the treatment of a gynecologic condition, the results may not be representative of the condition found in asymptomatic IUD users. Whether bacteria are present on the outside or the inside of an IUD tail appears to have no correlation to the presence of clinical infection. Both Tatum (Tatum *et al.*, 1975) and Bank and Williamson (1983) who later examined an additional series of Dalkon Shield tail strings noted that the IUDs in their studies had been removed from asymptomatic women.

Contraceptive sterilization

Women who use sterilization as their method of contraception are at a reduced risk of pelvic infection compared with women using no contraception (Hajj, 1978). The mechanism of protection apparently results from limitation of access of portions of the tube to pathogenic organisms from the endometrium. This is true whether ascent is by direct extension or by piggybacking to sperm or trichomonads. According to Eschenbach *et al.* (1977) limited access is of particular importance at the time of ovulation and menstruation when a greater susceptibility to infection may exist. Another important explanation for the protective effect of sterilization lies in the fact that sterilized women most commonly are in demographic subgroups known to have lower risks of PID, i.e., married women and women over 30 years of age.

Non-contraceptors as a comparison group

It has already been noted that most contraceptive users receive some protection against upper genital tract infection from the contraceptive method *per se*. The only exception to this statement is the IUD. At present, questions exist regarding the magnitude of the risk of PID associated with IUD use, the underlying basis of this risk and whether this risk remains past the post-insertional period.

It is appropriate to question whether non-contracepting women (including women using rhythm, coitus interruptus or natural family planning methods) should be utilized as a comparison group for IUD users. The group of non-contracepting women include the following subgroups, all of whom are likely to have different risks of acquiring PID based upon their sexual practices and exposures to sexually transmitted pathogens:

(1) sexually inactive women;
(2) currently married, sexually active women desiring pregnancy;
(3) unmarried, sexually active women not desiring pregnancy.

A thorough discussion of the reasons why this large group of women may be an inappropriate comparison group has been presented elsewhere (Keith and Berger, 1984). An example of the confounding influence of the inclusion of the non-user of contraception is found in the study of Lee *et al.* (1983). When sexually inactive, amenorrheic, sterile and recently delivered women are excluded from consideration, it is found that the relative risk of PID to IUD users of less than 5 months duration is 3.1 when compared to women using no contraceptive methods. This risk falls to 1.1 for women who had their IUDs for over 4 months (Lee *et al.*, 1983). This finding does not agree with the general opinion that IUD use is associated with an increased risk of PID at any time following insertion. The inclusion of non-contraceptors who may have different patterns of sexual activity that place them at a lower risk of PID suggests that the estimated relative risk value may be an overestimate of the true value, at least in this case. A similar point of view has been set forth by other workers (Luukkainen *et al.*, 1979), who suggest that the higher rate of PID among IUD users in case–control studies may only reflect the risk of infection which accompanies insertion.

THE CLINICAL IMPLICATION OF THE SELECTION OF THE CONTRACEPTIVE METHOD

Two major concerns regarding the use of any contraceptive method are its safety and efficacy. In the past two decades it has become abundantly clear that modern contraceptive methods are efficacious; that is, when used properly and regularly they prevent conception. The question of safety is not so clear. The question must always be posed, 'Do the benefits outweigh the risks?' In addition to the risks posed by the contraceptive method, clinicians must consider

Table 3 Simplified model of annual mortality associated with pregnancy and reversible contraception in developed countries (per 100,000 fertile women at risk[a])*

Contraceptive method and user status	Maternal death rate[b]	Number of method-related deaths[c]
None: under 35	12	0
35 and over	22	0
OCs: nonsmoker under 35	0.6	1
smoker under 35	0.6	10
nonsmoker 35 and over	1.1	15
smoker 35 and over	1.1	48
IUDs: under 35	1	1
35 and over	1.8	2
Condoms: under 35	2.8	0
35 and over	5.6	0

[a] Women sterilized or in lactational amenorrhea not included.
[b] Maternal death rates in developed countries are estimated at 20/100,000 live births for women under age 35 and 60/100,000 live births for women age 35 and over (Tietze and Lewit, 1979).
[c] Method-related deaths based on Royal College of General Practitioners (1981) for OCs and Tietze and Lewit (1979) for IUDs and condoms.
* Adapted from Population Reports (1982).

the risks of pregnancy *per se* and its associated complications. Table 3 shows a comparison of pregnancy- and contraceptive-related morbidity and mortality data.

More recently concerns have been expressed about the protective effects of specific contraceptive methods with regard to their ability to prevent upper genital tract infection. As set forth above, the IUD differs from other contraceptive methods in that it affords no protection against UGTI. At the time of ovulation, when cervical mucus is most receptive, there is no barrier to the entrance of sperm and/or bacteria to the upper genital tract as would be the case if the woman were using oral contraceptives (no ovulatory mucus), barrier methods (ascent blocked), or sterilization (tubes inaccessible). Thus, the higher risk of PID to IUD users frequently quoted in the literature may not indicate a truly higher risk inherent in the IUD itself but simply reflect the lower risk of PID to women in comparison groups (Keith and Berger, 1984).

Improvements in microbiology in the past decade have provided laboratory evidence to support the widely held clinical impression that PID is almost always a sexually derived disease. Unfortunately, those specific aspects of sexual activity that place a woman at a higher risk of PID have been inadequately studied. Clearly, microorganisms are transmitted to the lower genital tract during coitus by direct contact and/or via the ejaculatory fluids. These organisms are added to those already present in the vagina and cervix. Some, but not all, LGTIs progress to an UGTI. The risk of this taking place depends upon numerous interrelated factors. Among these are the type of sexual activity, the frequency of sexual contact, the number of sexual partners and the presence or absence of genital tract infection in the partners, and the number of partners of the sexual partner and whether these individuals were infected. Little effort has been made to date to determine either the relative importance of these factors or the interrelationships between them. Most studies have been concerned with demographic risk factors for acquiring PID.

Subsequent research on the relationship between contraceptive utilization and pelvic inflammatory disease will have to be directed toward these issues if further understanding is to be gained about their role in the etiology of PID.

References

Adler, M. W. (1980). Trends for gonorrhea and pelvic inflammatory disease in England and Wales and for gonorrhea in a defined population. *Am. J. Obstet. Gynecol.*, **138,** 901

Asculai, S. S., Weis, M. T., Rancourt, M. W. *et al.* (1978). Inactivation of herpes simplex viruses by nonionic surfactants. *Antimicrob. Agents Chemother.*, **13,** 686

Bank, H. L. and Williamson, H. O. (1983). Scanning electron microscopy of Dalkon shield tails. *Fertil. Steril.*, **40,** 334

Barlow, D. (1977). The condom and gonorrhoea. *Lancet*, **2,** 811

Bartlett, J. G., Onderdonk, A. B., Drude, E. *et al.* (1977). Quantitative bacteriology of the vaginal flora. *J. Infect. Dis.*, **136,** 271

Belsey, M. A. (1983). Epidemiologic aspects of infertility. In: Holmes, K. K. and Mårdh, P.-A. (eds) *International Perspectives on Neglected Sexually Transmitted Diseases*, p. 269. (Washington: Hemisphere Publishing)

Cole, L. (1984). Family health international: Research Triangle Park, North Carolina. Unpublished data

Curran, J. W. (1980). Economic consequences of pelvic inflammatory diseases in the United States. *Am. J. Obstet. Gynecol.*, **138,** 848

Cutler, J. C., Singh, B., Carpenter, U. *et al.* (1977). Vaginal contraceptives as prophylaxis against gonorrhea and other sexually transmissible diseases. *Adv. Plan. Parent.*, **12,** 45

De Osma, G. (1980). *Mariano Fortuny: His Life and Work*, p. 58. (New York: Rizzoli)

Edelman, D. A., Berger, G. S. and Keith, L. G. (1979). *Intrauterine Devices and their Complications.* (Boston: G. K. Hall)

Edelman, D. A., Berger, G. S. and Keith, L. (1982). The use of IUDs and their relationship to pelvic inflammatory disease: A review of epidemiologic and clinical studies. In Leventhal,

J. M. (ed.) *Current Problems in Obstetrics and Gynecology*, vol. 6. (Chicago: Yearbook Medical Publishers)

Eschenbach, D. A., Buchanan, T. M., Pollock, H. M. *et al.* (1975). Polymicrobial etiology of acute pelvic inflammatory disease. *N. Engl. J. Med.*, **293**, 166

Eschenbach, D. A., Harnish, J. P. and Holmes, K. K. (1977). Pathogenesis of acute pelvic inflammatory disease: Role of contraception and other risk factors. *Am. J. Obstet. Gynecol.*, **128**, 838

Farr, C. E. and Findlay, R. T. (1928). Salpingitis: A detailed analysis based on the study of 545 cases – January 1914 to December 1927, inclusive. *Surg. Gynecol. Obstet.*, **49**, 647

Gorbach, S., Menda, K., Thadepalli, H. *et al.* (1973). Anaerobic microflora of the cervix in healthy women. *Am. J. Obstet. Gynecol.*, **117**, 1053

Hager, W. D. and Wiesner, P. J. (1977). Selected epidemiologic aspects of acute salpingitis: A review. *J. Reprod. Med.*, **19**, 47

Hajj, S. M. (1978). Does sterilization prevent pelvic infection? *J. Reprod. Med.*, **20**, 289

Handsfield, H. (1982). Sexually transmitted diseases. *Hosp. Prac.*, **xxx**, 99

Hart, G. (1974). Factors influencing venereal infection in a war environment. *Br. J. Vener. Dis.*, **50**, 68

Holmes, K. K., Handsfield, H. H., Wang, S. P. *et al.* (1975). Etiology of nongonococcal urethritis. *N. Engl. J. Med.*, **292**, 1199

Hooper, R. R., Harrison, W. D., Campbell, A. F. *et al.* (1973). *Cohort Study of Venereal Disease: Prophylaxis.* Presented at the convention of the American Public Health Association, San Francisco

Jackson, M. A., Berger, G. S. and Keith, L. G. (1981). *Vaginal Contraception.* (Boston: G. K. Hall)

Jacobsen, L. and Weström, L. (1969). Objectivized diagnosis of acute pelvic inflammatory disease. *Am. J. Obstet. Gynecol.*, **105**, 1088

Jones, O. G., Zaidi, A. A. and St. John, R. K. (1980). Frequency and distribution of salpingitis and pelvic inflammatory disease in short-stay hospitals in the United States. *Am. J. Obstet. Gynecol.*, **138**, 905

Keith, L. and Berger, G. S. (1984). The etiology of pelvic inflammatory disease. In Zatuchni, G. I. (ed.) *Research Frontiers in Fertility Regulation* PARFR vol. 3. (Chicago: Northwestern University)

Keith, L., Berger, G. S., Edelman, D. A. *et al.* (1983). On the causation of pelvic inflammatory disease. *Am. J. Obstet. Gynecol.*, **149**, 215

Keith, L., Berger, G. S. and Moss, W. (1976). Cervical gonorrhea in women using different methods of contraception. *J. Am. Vener. Dis. Assoc.*, **3**, 17

Kelaghan, J., Rubin, G. L. and Ory, H. W. *et al.* (1982). Barrier-method contraceptives and pelvic inflammatory disease. *J. Am. Med. Assoc.*, **248**, 184

Larsen, B. (1984). Normal genital microflora. In: Keith, L. G., Berger, G. S. and Edelman, D. A. (eds) *Infections in Reproductive Health*, Vol. 1. (Lancaster: MTP Press)

Lee, N. C., Rubin, G. L., Ory, H. W. *et al.* (1983). Type of intrauterine device and the risk of pelvic inflammatory disease. *Obstet. Gynecol.*, **62**, 1

Lindner, J. G. E. M., Plantema, F. H. F. and Hoogkamp-Korstanje, A. A. (1978). Quantitative studies of the vaginal flora of healthy women and of obstetric and gynaecologic patients. *J. Med. Microbiol.*, **11**, 233

Luukkainen, T., Nielson, N. C., Nygren, K. G. *et al.* (1979). Nulliparous women, IUD and pelvic infection. *Ann. Clin. Res.*, **11**, 121

McCormack, W. M. (1982). Sexually transmitted diseases: women as victims. *J. Am. Med. Assoc.*, **248**, 117

Mishell, D. R., Bell, J. H., Good, R. G. *et al.* (1966). The intrauterine device: A bacteriologic study of the endometrial cavity. *Am. J. Obstet. Gynecol.*, **96**, 119

Monif, G. R. G. (1982). Tampons and toxic shock syndrome. *Fem. Patient*, **7**, 42

Monif, G. R. G., Thompson, J. L., Stephens, H. D. *et al.* (1980). Quantitative and qualitative effects of povidone-iodine liquid and gel on the aerobic and anaerobic flora of the female genital tract. *Am. J. Obstet. Gynecol.*, **137**, 432

Ohm, M. J. and Galask, R. P. (1975). Bacterial flora of the cervix from 100 prehysterectomy patients. *Am. J. Obstet. Gynecol.*, **122**, 683

Population Reports (1979). *Barrier Methods. Spermicides: Simplicity and Safety are Major Assets, series H, no. 5*, p. H-78. (Baltimore: Johns Hopkins University)

Population Reports (1982). *Oral Contraceptives. Oral Contraceptives in the 1980s, series A, no. 6*, p. A-189. (Baltimore: Johns Hopkins University)

Population Reports (1983). *Issues in World Health. Infertility and Sexually Transmitted Disease: A Public Health Challenge, series L, no. 4*, p. L-113. (Baltimore: Johns Hopkins University)

Purrier, B. G. A., Sparks, R. A., Watt, P. J. *et al.* (1979). In vitro study of the possible role of the intrauterine contraceptive device tail in ascending infection of the genital tract. *Br. J. Obstet. Gynecol.*, **86**, 374

Rendtorff, R. C., Packer, H., Glassco, S. *et al.* (1977). The impact of urban community hospital surveillance for gonorrhoea on the infection rate and complications in the female: A progress report. *Br. J. Vener. Dis.*, **53**, 364

Royal College of General Practitioners' oral contraception study (1981). Further analyses of mortality in oral contraceptive users. *Lancet*, **1**, 541

Rubin, G. L., Ory, H. W. and Layde, P. M. (1982). Oral contraceptives and pelvic inflammatory disease. *Am. J. Obstet. Gynecol.*, **144**, 630

Schachter, J., Hanna, L., Hill, E. C. *et al.* (1975). Are chlamydial infections the most prevalent venereal disease? *J. Am. Med. Assoc.*, **231**, 1252

Sennayake, P. and Kramer, D. G. (1980). Contraception and the etiology of pelvic inflammatory disease: new perspectives. *Am. J. Obstet. Gynecol.*, **138**, 852

Sparks, R. A., Purrier, B. G. A., Watt, P. J. *et al.* (1980). Bacteriology of the uterus in relation to IUDs and their appendages. In: Hafez, E. S. E. and van Os, W. A. A. (eds) *IUD Pathology and Management*, p. 129. (Boston: G. K. Hall)

Sparks, R. A., Purrier, B. G. A., Watt, P. J. *et al.* (1981). Bacteriological colonisation of uterine cavity: role of tailed intrauterine contraceptive device. *Br. Med. J.*, **282**, 1189

Spiegel, C. A., Amsel, R., Eschenbach, D. *et al.* (1980). Anaerobic bacteria in non-specific vaginitis. *N. Engl. J. Med.*, **303**, 601

St. John, R. K., Blount, J. and Jones, O. (1981a). Pelvic inflammatory disease in the United States: incidence and trends in private practice. *Sex. Transm. Dis.*, **8**, 56

St. John, R. K., Jones, O. G., Blount, J. H. *et al.* (1981b). Pelvic inflammatory disease in the United States: epidemiology and trends among hospitalized women. *Sex. Transm. Dis.*, **8**, 62

Svensson, L., Mårdh, P.-A. and Westrøm, L. (1983). Infertility after acute salpingitis with special reference to *Chlamydia trachomatis. Fertil. Steril.*, **40**, 322

Sweet, R. L. (1981). Pelvic inflammatory disease: etiology, diagnosis, and treatment. *Sex. Transm. Dis. Suppl.*, **8**, 308

Tatum, H. J., Schmidt, F. H., Phillips, D. *et al.* (1975). The Dalkon shield controversy: Structural and bacteriological studies of IUD tails. *J. Am. Med. Assoc.*, **231**, 711

Tietze, C. and Lewit, S. (1979). Life risks associated with reversible methods of fertility regulation. *Int. J. Gynaecol. Obstet.*, **16**, 456

Westrøm, L. (1975). Effect of acute pelvic inflammatory disease on fertility. *Am. J. Obstet. Gynecol.*, **121**, 707

Westrøm, L. (1980). Incidence, prevalence, and trends of acute pelvic inflammatory disease and its consequences in industrialized countries. *Am. J. Obstet. Gynecol.*, **138**, 880

Westrøm, L. and Mårdh, P.-A. (1983). Pelvic inflammatory disease: Epidemiology diagnosis, clinical manifestations, and sequelae. In: Holmes, K. K. and Mårdh, P.-A. (eds) *International Perspectives on Neglected Sexually Transmitted Diseases*, p. 235. (Washington: Hemisphere Publishing)

18
Barrier methods of contraception as prophylaxis against venereal diseases

T. A. CHAPEL

INTRODUCTION

The pandemic of gonorrhea, nongonococcal urethritis (NGU), and of other sexually transmitted diseases (STDs), plus the frequency and severity of their potential complications, in women particularly, have rekindled interest in venereal disease prophylaxis. Preventive methods to control venereal disease include restricting sexual activity and mechanical, local, and systemic prophylaxis (Darrow and Wiesner, 1975). Due to the lack of controlled studies on prophylactic methods in humans, the effectiveness of various techniques remains controversial.

Barrier contraceptives are the most readily available means to reduce the incidence of STDs. Unfortunately, barrier methods, including the condom and the diaphragm, have fallen into disfavor among wide segments of the population, many people preferring the more modern and convenient oral contraceptives and intrauterine devices. In the United States the advantages of barrier contraceptives in the control of venereal disease have not been widely advertised, and the public continues to hold misconceptions that contribute to the underutilization of these methods.

Penile sheaths and mechanical barriers to the cervix have been used as contraceptive devices for centuries. Recent studies document that these methods minimize the transmission of numerous venereal pathogens. The history of the development of the condom and the diaphragm, the measure of prophylaxis afforded by these methods, and the potential application of the barrier contraceptive methods in the control of venereal disease are discussed in this chapter.

HISTORICAL BACKGROUND

The condom

The earliest penile sheaths were used by primitive people as amulets to promote fertility, as badges of rank or status, and for protection against venereal and tropical disease and insect bites (Himes, 1963). The early Chinese made penile sheaths of oiled silk paper, and in imperial Rome animal bladders were used on the penis to protect men from contracting venereal infection (Finch and Green, 1963).

In the 16th century Fallopius, the noted Italian anatomist and early authority on syphilis, described a linen sheath that was designed to cover the glans penis (Himes, 1963). The device was held onto the glans by the foreskin. Fallopius extolled the prophylactic virtues of the sheath, claiming that no venereal infections were observed in over 1100 men who had used it. From Fallopius's time forward, the caeces of many animals were used as penile sheaths. Houses of prostitution used the penile sheath in the 18th century and perhaps even in an earlier period. The word condom, however, does not appear in the literature before 1680 (Finch and Green, 1963).

The discovery of the process of vulcanization of rubber in 1844 revolutionized the condom by allowing the production of inexpensive products that could be used instead of the membranous sheath. The efficacy of the rubber sheath was ultimately eclipsed by the latex condom. Improved technology in latex manufacturing provided thinner, more durable products. The addition of semi-dry silicone lubricants decreased the probability of tearing the condoms and sealed foil packages enhanced its shelf life.

In the United States there were no quality control programs for condoms prior to 1938. The Food and Drug Administration has estimated that approximately 75% of the condoms produced before 1938 were defective and that 1 in 150–300 broke during usage. The first formal regulatory program was introduced in 1949 and revised in 1957 (Free and Alexander, 1976). This Act strictly limited defects, and by 1968 the tolerance for defective condoms had been reduced to 0.25% (Shenefelt, 1981).

Public acceptance of the condom varies from country to country. In the United States the Comstock Act of 1873 declared contraception and information related to contraception obscene and illegal (Shenefelt, 1981). Thereafter, condoms were sold only as prophylactics against venereal disease, and condom use was commonly linked to prostitution and promiscuity. In the United Kingdom and Sweden, however, the use of the condom as a contraceptive method was kept separate from its function as a prophylactic.

The diaphragm

From ancient times, prostitutes of Japan and China applied disks of oiled paper to the cervix to prevent conception (Himes, 1963). German–Hungarian women applied disks made of melted beeswax 1 cm in thickness and aproximately 5–10 cm in diameter onto the cervical os (Himes, 1963) to prevent conception. The beeswax would soften at body temperature, and in effect, form a cervical cap.

Dr. C. Hasse of Germany, under the pseudonym of W. P. J. Mensinga, is credited with the invention of the modern diaphragm (Hafez, 1980). The original device was a vulcanized rubber cup attached to a circular spring that occluded the upper vagina and cervix. Before the end of the 19th century, women all over Europe were using the Mensinga diaphragm. Today, the most widely used diaphragms are the coil spring, flat spring, and the arcing spring – all modifications of the original Mensinga diaphragm. Spermicidal chemicals are usually used with the diaphragm, and these agents enhance the device's contraceptive properties.

EFFECTIVENESS OF BARRIER CONTRACEPTIVES IN PREVENTING VENEREAL DISEASE

The value of the diaphragm as a prophylactic against sexually transmissible diseases has not been adequately studied. *Chlamydia trachomatis* and *Neisseria gonorrhoeae* primarily infect the endocervix, and it is reasonable that a diaphragm should provide protection against infections with these organisms. Moreover, spermicidal agents that are designed to be used in conjunction with the diaphragm have *in vitro* activity against the gonococcus and certain other venereal pathogens, thereby enhancing the protective effect of the diaphragm (Singh *et al.*, 1972). It is difficult, under these circumstances, to separate the effect of the diaphragm and the spermicidal agents used with it.

The prophylactic effects of the condom have been better studied, but experts disagree as to the measure of protection afforded by its regular use. Some venereologists assert that the condom is valueless, while others contend that use of the condom throughout coitus significantly reduces the risk of venereal infection. Objections to the condom as a prophylactic have been published by Fiumara (1971). He contends that the usefulness of the condom is seriously compromised by foreplay, imperfections of the condom, the technique of using it, and the fact that the condom does not cover the base of the penis or the thighs. Other venereologists argue that modern production techniques and quality control programs have eliminated almost all structural defects from condoms (Hinman, 1976; Felman, 1979). They also contend that, although some venereal diseases can be spread by contact with extragenital mucous membranes, the bulk of sexually transmitted diseases among heterosexuals are passed by genital to genital contact making nonintromissive foreplay an uncommon method of disease transmission.

Most investigations have shown that the condom exerts a protective effect against venereal disease when used regularly and correctly. Studies of patients seen at sexually transmissible disease clinics in Belfast (Pemberton *et al.*, 1972) and London (Barlow, 1977) found that those who had no sexually transmissible disease were more likely to have used condoms than those with gonorrhea or syphilis. The relative risk of having gonorrhea or syphilis was about 0.4, or less than half as great for men who used condoms regularly than for men who did not use condoms or used them irregularly or incorrectly.

In France, Siboulet (1972) studied the effectiveness of the condom as a prophylactic in a group of young men between the ages of 16 and 22. Men who used condoms and men who did not, as well as the female sexual partners of both groups, were examined for sexually transmitted diseases. Among 302 women who were sexual contacts of men who used condoms regularly, Siboulet found 142 women with gonorrhea and 160 women with trichomoniasis. Only two of these men developed gonorrhea, and only six contracted trichomoniasis. The control group consisted of 480 men who did not use condoms; the female sexual partners of these men had 465 episodes of gonorrhea and 160 of *Trichomonas vaginalis*. Gonorrhea and trichomoniasis were found in 89 and 164 of the male controls, respectively.

Studies in health facilities in the United States also have shown a reduction in venereal disease in patients using barrier contraceptive techniques. An investigation of 2019 women attending a Louisiana family planning clinic found that women who used a diaphragm or whose partners used condoms had cervical gonorrhea about one-fifth as often as users of oral contraception and intrauterine devices (Keith *et al.*, 1976). Moreover, Darrow (1973), using data from a clinic for sexually transmissible diseases, found lower rates of infection with gonorrhea that were statistically significant for men who always used condoms as compared to men who occasionally or never used condoms.

Retrospective and prospective studies of military personnel have shown a protective effect for the condom. In World War I, the American Army was able to effect a dramatic reduction in the gonorrhea rate by supplying condoms and enforcing their use; the effectiveness of the condom was confirmed in World War II (Anon, 1971). More recently, Hart (1974) interviewed 400 Australian soldiers returning home after 12 months of duty in Vietnam. The men were asked about sexual exposures while in Vietnam, about any episodes of venereal disease, and about their use of condoms or other means of prophylaxis. Sexual intercourse during their tour of duty was acknowledged by 246 soldiers, and 55 (22.4%) reported having used a condom on all occasions of coitus. No individual who regularly used a condom acquired venereal disease, but 34.6% of those who did not always use a condom had one or more episodes of venereal disease. This difference was found to be statistically significant.

Hooper *et al.* (1973) reported a prospective study involving personnel aboard a US aircraft carrier whose crew members were granted a 4-day liberty in the Philippines. Study entrants were examined for signs of urethritis, and they were cultured for *N. gonorrhoeae* before they went on liberty and again upon their return. At the end of the liberty the men were questioned about the number of sexual exposures they had had and whether or not they had used condoms. Seventy-one (6.9%) of the 1024 crew members studied acquired gonococcal urethritis during the liberty and 34 (3.3%) acquired NGU. None of the 29 crewmen who always used condoms acquired either disease: however, the difference in rates of infection for each group was not statistically significant. Protection from agents responsible for NGU was also reported by McCormack *et al.* (1973), who found that men who use condoms are significantly less likely to have urethral colonization with genital mycoplasmas. Moreover, McCormack (1982) suggests that women whose partners use condoms are less likely to be infected with *C. trachomatis*. However, Barlow (1977) and Pemberton *et al.* (1972) found no significant difference in the frequency of nongonococcal urethritis among men who used condoms and men who did not use condoms, but the reasons for this finding were not clear.

There is some controversy regarding the prophylactic benefit of the condom for sexually transmitted viral diseases. The small size of viruses has led some researchers to speculate that these agents may pass through the pores of the condom. Condoms, however, are airtight and watertight, and since gas and water molecules are approximately 1000 times smaller than the herpes simplex virus, the passage of these organisms through the pores of the condom is unlikely. In addition, what meager data exist supports the barrier effectiveness of the condom. In the London study, Barlow (1977) found herpes genitalis more than twice as often in noncondom users. *In vitro* studies suggest that intact condoms are impenetrable barriers to the herpes simplex virus. A condom filled with nutrient broth that had been inoculated with herpes simplex virus was suspended in nutrient medium. The virus was viable for over 24 hours within the condom, but none was recovered from samples of outside medium. Another experiment was designed to test the durability of the condom to frictional stresses simulating those experienced during coitus. A condom inoculated with an herpesvirus was fastened around a plunger of a syringe. The plunger was reinserted into the barrel of the syringe, and a nutrient medium was aspirated and expelled 50 times, but no virus was recovered from the medium.

BARRIER CONTRACEPTION AND PELVIC INFLAMMATORY DISEASE

Pelvic inflammatory disease (PID) may be caused by *N. gonorrhoeae, C. trachomatis, M. hominis*, or a mixture of aerobic and anaerobic microorganisms that are often included in the normal vaginal flora. The relative contribution of each of these agents to PID varies from area to area.

Toth *et al.* (1982) have shown that some and perhaps all organisms responsible for salpingitis are transmitted by attaching to sperm and being carried through the cervix. Condoms and diaphragms prevent sperm and, therefore, the organisms producing PID from reaching the cervix. The *in vivo* prophylactic value of barrier contraceptives was shown in a study involving 306 women with PID and 1175 controls (Kelaghan *et al.*, 1982). Women using barrier contraception were 0.6 times as likely to develop PID as women using no contraceptive methods. The relative risk of PID for women whose sexual partners used condoms was 0.6, for users of diaphragms was 0.4, and for users of a spermicide was 0.7.

THE CONDOM AND CERVICAL CANCER

Several studies have shown that the use of a condom prevents and possibly ameliorates abnormalities of cervical cells. Certain sexually transmissible agents including the herpesvirus, appear to promote dysplastic and neoplastic changes of the cervix (Fish *et al.*, 1982; Richardson and Lyon, 1981). In a case-controlled study, Harris *et al.* (1980) has shown that use of the condom or diaphragm decreased the risk of developing cervical atypia but that the risk increased with duration of oral contraceptive use. Moreover, a study by Richardson and Lyon (1981) suggests that the use of barrier methods helps to reverse atypia in patients who used no other treatment.

CONTROL OF VENEREAL DISEASE USING BARRIER METHODS OF CONTRACEPTION

The potential for reducing venereal disease with the use of barrier methods of contraception is substantial. According to one model, a prophylactic method that is only 50% effective in preventing the transmission of *N. gonorrhoeae* and that is used during coitus by only 25% of the population at risk would reduce the prevalence of gonorrhea by about 80% in 1 year (Lee *et al.*, 1972). It is unrealistic to assume that the reduction of disease achieved in real life would equal the reduction predicted in a theoretical model, but a significant impact could certainly be anticipated.

Mathematical models of the epidemiology of gonorrhea in the United States have suggested that there is a core population of approximately $\frac{1}{2}$ million people with a high prevalence of gonorrhea (May 1981). Each infective individual in the core population will, on average, infect more than one susceptible individual, while newly infected individuals outside of the core group infect less than one new contact. At equilibrium, these two rates combine to produce an overall average of one new infectee for each current infection. Programs designed to control venereal disease using preventive measures must be directed at this core population, but unfortunately these individuals have little enthusiasm for using barrier methods of prophylaxis. Darrow (1973) reported that, while 29.5% of patients attending a clinic for sexually transmissible diseases in the United States occasionally used condoms, only 1.8% used them consistently. Moreover, when clinic patients were offered free prophylactics for future use, 73% declined. Similar findings have been reported elsewhere in the world. For example, Pemberton *et al.* (1972) found that only 11.6% of patients at a Belfast venereal disease clinic used condoms; in Sweden, Juhlin (1968) found that a condom was used by 44% of individuals who had one sexual partner but by only 15% of those who had multiple partners.

A US program designed to prevent VD by encouraging use of barrier methods of contraception has received almost no support. Shenefelt (1981) points out that an ironic indication of health values in the United States is that cigarettes, which are known to cause significant diseases, are prominently advertised on billboards and in popular magazines, while condoms, which prevent disease and unwanted pregnancy, are considered unsuitable for such display.

In Sweden the Sex Research Institute undertook a program in 1970 to improve the image of the condom (Hinman, 1976). Advertising displays popularized the use of the condom and made the product trendy. In 2 years, sales of condoms rose 50% and gonorrhea concomitantly decreased by 20%. For unknown reasons, however, the prevalence of gonorrhea began to rise again in 1975 (Wallin, 1978). Nonetheless, the Swedish experience suggests that barrier methods of contraception can reduce the prevalence of some sexually transmissible pathogens. The promotion of the condom and diaphragm should be included as an integral part of programs for the control of venereal disease, and multifaceted approaches should be adopted to increase their use.

References

Anon (1971). The condom as a venereal disease preventive: *Medical Lett. Drugs Therapeutics*, **13**, 108

Anon (1982). Update on condoms: products, protection, promotion. *Population Reports*, Series H, **6**, 121

Barlow, D. (1977). The condom and gonorrhea. *Lancet*, **2**, 811

Darrow, W. W. (1973). Innovative health behavior. *Thesis*, Emory University, Atlanta

Darrow, W. W. and Wiesner, P. J. (1975). Personal prophylaxis for venereal diseases. *J. Am. Med. Assoc.*, **233**, 444

Felman, Y. M. (1979). A plea for the condom, especially for teenagers. *J. Am. Med. Assoc.*, **241**, 2517

Finch, B. E. and Green, H. (1963). *Contraception Through the Ages*, p. 48. (Springfield: Charles C. Thomas)

Fish, E. N., Tobin, S. M., Cooter, N. B. E. *et al.* (1982). Update on the relation of herpes virus hominis type 2 to carcinoma of the cervix. *Obstet. Gynecol.*, **59**, 220

Fiumara, N. J. (1971). Effectiveness of condoms in preventing VD. *N. Engl. J. Med.*, **285**, 972

Free, M. J. and Alexander, N. J. (1976). Male contraception without prescription. *Publ. Hlth. Rep.*, **91**, 437

Hafez, E. S. E. (1980). *Human Reproduction Conception and Contraception*, 2nd edn, p. 768. (Hagerstown: Harper & Row)

Harris, R. W. C., Brinton, L. A., Cowdell, R. H. *et al.* (1980). Characteristics of women with dysplasia or carcinoma in situ of the cervix uteri. *Br. J. Cancer.*, **42**, 359

Hart, G. (1974). Factors influencing venereal infection in a war environment. *Br. J. Vener. Dis.*, **50**, 68

Himes, N. E. (1963). *Medical History of Contraception*, p. 186. (New York: Gamut Press)

Hinman, A. R. (1976). The condom as prophylactic. *Bull. N. Y. Acad. Med.*, **52**, 1004

Hooper, R. R., Harrison, W. D., Campbell, A. F. *et al.* (1973). Cohort study of venereal disease: Prophylaxis. Convention of the American Public Health Association, San Francisco

Juhlin, L. (1968). Factors influencing the spread of gonorrhea. II. Sexual behavior at different ages. *Acta Derm. Venereol.*, **48**, 82

Keith, L. G., Berger, G. S. and Moss, W. (1976). Cervical gonorrhea in women using different methods of contraception. *J. Am. Vener. Dis. Assoc.*, **3**, 17

Kelaghan, J., Rubin, G. L., Ory, H. W. *et al.* (1982). Barrier-method contraceptives and pelvic inflammatory disease. *J. Am. Med. Assoc.*, **248**, 184

Lee, T. Y., Utidijian, H., Singh, B. *et al.* (1972). Potential impact of chemical prophylaxis on the incidence of gonorrhea. *Br. J. Vener. Dis.*, **48**, 376

May, R. M. (1981). The transmission and control of gonorrhea. *Nature*, **291**, 376

McCormack, W. M. (1982). Sexually transmitted diseases: Women as victims. *J. Am. Med. Assoc.*, **248**, 177

McCormack, W. M., Lee, Y. H. and Zinner, S. H. (1973). Sexual experience and urethral colonization with genital mycoplasmas: A study in normal men. *Ann. Intern. Med.*, **78**, 696

Pemberton, J., McCann, J. S., Mahoney, J. D. H. *et al.* (1972). Socio-medical characteristics of patients attending a V.D. clinic and the circumstances of infection. *Br. J. Vener. Dis.*, **48**, 391

Richardson, A. C. and Lyon, J. B. (1981). The effect of condom use on squamous cell cervical intraepithelial neoplasia. *Am. J. Obstet. Gynecol.*, **140**, 909

Shenefelt, P. D. (1981). The condom as contraceptive and prophylactic: an appraisal. *Wisc. Med. J.*, **80**, 19

Siboulet, A. (1972). Maladies sexuelles transmissibles: Intéret des traitements prophylactiques. *Proph. Sanit. Mor.*, **44**, 155

Singh, B., Cutler, J. C. and Utidjian, H. M. D. (1972). Studies on the development of a vaginal preparation providing both prophylaxis against venereal disease and other genital infections and contraception. II. Effect in vitro of vaginal contraceptive and non-contraceptive preparations on Treponema pallidum and Neisseria gonorrhoeae. *Br. J. Vener. Dis.*, **48**, 57

Toth, A., O'Leary, W. M. and Ledger, W. (1982). Evidence for microbial transfer by spermatozoa. *Obstet. Gynecol.*, **59,** 556

Wallin, J. (1978). Sexually transmitted diseases: the present situation in Sweden. *Br. J. Vener. dis.*, **54,** 24

19
Cytologic manifestations of infections in the female genital tract

B. F. ATKINSON and V. A. LIVOLSI

This chapter will discuss the morphologic effects of infectious agents on cytologic smears obtained from the female genital tract. First, the general effects of infection will be described; then the specific effects of the following microorganisms will be considered: bacteria, *Chlamydia*, *Actinomyces*, trichomonads, parasites, fungi, and viruses. The clinical significance of these cytologic changes will also be mentioned, specifically as they relate to systemic diseases and to the development of neoplasia.

GENERAL EFFECTS

The cytologic changes associated with infection may also be found in patients with a variety of other conditions, such as trauma, prolapse, cervical polyps, etc. Patten (1973) has classified these inflammatory alterations into three types: protection, destruction, and regeneration. Protective mechanisms include keratinization of the squamous epithelium (hyperkeratosis and parakeratosis) and squamous metaplasia of the endocervix. Cytologically, keratinization is recognized by the presence of hypereosinophilic superficial cells and anucleate squames. By themselves, these changes are benign. Squamous metaplasia occurs almost universally as a result of repair of endocervical eversion. Squamous metaplasia *per se* does not imply specific inflammation nor infection (Bibbo *et al.*, 1971, 1974; Patten, 1973).

The destructive type of inflammatory alteration (Bibbo *et al.*, 1971, 1974; Patten, 1973), is characterized by cytolysis, karyorrhexis, nuclear enlargement, binucleation, and the presence of nuclear chromocentres. Such changes are found in infection and in traumatic lesions; a marked inflammatory cell reaction often is present.

The third inflammatory reaction, regeneration (and repair) (Patten, 1973), is characterized cytologically by sheets of epithelial cells showing eosinophilic cytoplasm, a moderate degree of anisocytosis, changes in nuclear chromatin pattern, and the formation of chromocenters or nucleoli. Mitoses may also be present. This general configuration may be confused with neoplastic processes

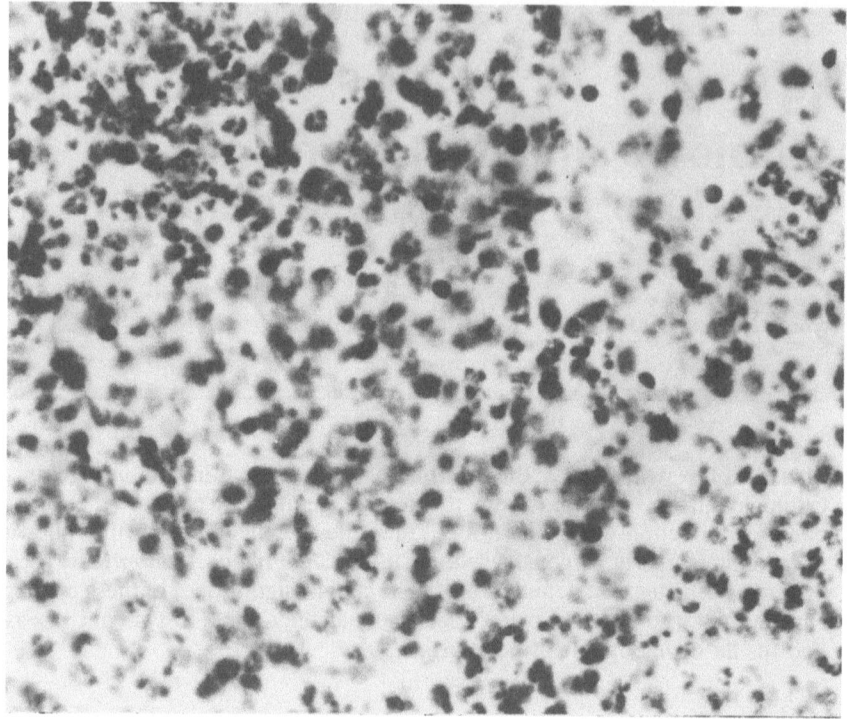

Fig. 1. Marked inflammation. This smear shows a marked acute inflammatory infiltrate which is obscuring all cellular detail. Sometimes with this degree of inflammation it is not possible to exclude the diagnosis of dysplasia or carcinoma. In this instance it is necessary to treat the patient for a specific inflammatory agent if one has been identified or give nonspecific treatment for vaginitis and then repeat the smear. (Papanicolaou stain, ×225)

(Fig. 1), but reparative anaplasia or atypia is distinguished from cancer by the fact that neither tumor diathesis nor necrosis is present, nuclear chromatin remains regular, and the atypical cells are found in groups rather than singly (Patten, 1973).

Since bacteria are a normal component of the cervical and vaginal milieu, their presence on cytologic smears does not alone imply infection (Bibbo *et al.*, 1974). A mixed bacterial picture including rods and/or cocci (aerobes and anaerobes), is a normal finding in asymptomatic adults, especially in the absence of cytologic changes in the squamous epithelium (Bibbo *et al.*, 1974). When an inflammatory cell reaction or epithelial cell changes are encountered, however, infection must be suspected. Microorganisms that evoke a predominantly inflammatory reaction include bacteria (bacilli and cocci) as well as trichomonads. Nonspecific epithelial alterations may accompany this reaction. Inflammatory changes in the epithelium generally include cytologic vacuolization, perinuclear haloes, irregularities of cell shape, and staining alterations. Nuclear changes includes prominent nucleoli, vacuolization, chromatin clumping, and karyorrhexis. Specific organisms that induce specific epithelial cytologic changes are *Chlamydia*, herpesvirus, and human papilloma virus.

In an acute infection the inflammatory reaction is characterized by the presence of numerous polymorphonuclear leukocytes, debris, and abundant microorganisms.

Since polymorphonuclear leukocytes constitute a normal finding in premenstrual as well as menstrual smears and in smears of the cervical mucus plug (Koss, 1979), their presence alone does not reflect infection. The large numbers of bacteria and leukocytes, along with their metabolic byproducts, alter the pH and produce staining changes in the epithelial cells. Cytoplasmic eosinophilia results (Bibbo *et al.*, 1974).

The inflammatory response may be influenced by a woman's hormonal status. In premenopausal women the numbers of parabasal cells are increased and these cells may demonstrate enlarged nuclei and nucleoli. In postmenopaual women, on the other hand, the inflammatory process may be characterized by hyperkeratosis. Endocervical cells may also be affected and contain large nuclei with conspicuous nucleoli. Multinucleation and mitoses may also be seen.

In chronic cervicitis, parakeratosis and hyperkeratosis of the squamous epithelium may be found with or without infection. Rarely is follicular cervicitis found. On histologic preparation, numerous lymphocytes with germinal centers are reflected in a mixture of histiocytes and lymphocytes of varying degrees of maturity. Plasma cell cervicitis is a related disorder in which plasma cells infiltrate the cervical stroma. In and of themselves, plasma cells do not reflect any specific infection (Bibbo *et al.*, 1974).

SPECIFIC INFECTIONS

Gram-positive cocci

Many variants of this bacterium can be seen in cervico-vaginal smears. Identification of specific organisms requires culture. Pyogenic infections may be produced by *Staphylococcus* and *Streptococcus* (Bibbo *et al.*, 1974). Often mixed infections occur, especially in the presence of *Trichomonas* (Bibbo *et al.*, 1974).

Gram-negative cocci

A diagnosis of *Neisseria* gonococcus infection cannot be made cytologically with certainty. Other Gram-negative cocci (e.g., *Mima* sp.) resemble the intracellular diplococcus. When Gram-negative diplococci are observed adherent to or within squamous cells or leukocytes, the clinician should be alerted to the possibility of gonorrhea; appropriate microbiologic cultures must be obtained for definitive diagnosis, however (Koss, 1979).

Lactobacillus vaginalis (Doderlein bacillus, *Bacillus vaginalis*) refers to a large group of normal inhabitants of the lower genital tract. The frequency of occurrence of *Bacillus vaginalis* is difficult to estimate and prevalence data are dependent upon the population studied; as many as 50% of women harbor this organism at some time in their lives (Bibbo *et al.*, 1974). *Lactobacillus vaginalis* is more commonly found in diabetics (Bibbo *et al.*, 1974; Koss, 1979). The presence of these organisms lowers vaginal pH, and the resultant acidity acts to prohibit growth of other organisms. This bacillus is more predominant in circumstances where intermediate cells prevail; that is, during the late luteal phase of the cycle, during pregnancy and early postmenopause. In smears taken from these women, cellular debris, free nuclei, mucus, and numerous bacteria are seen (Bibbo *et al.*, 1974); the slender, basophilic rods are present

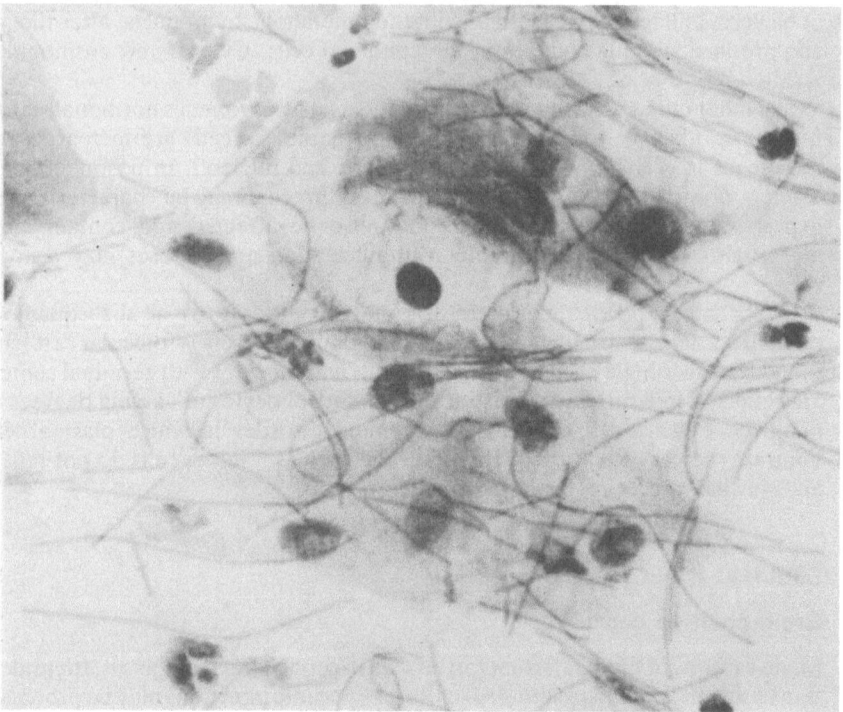

Fig. 2. *Lactobacillus.* Long filamentous rods are seen overlying squamous cells. There is a relatively clean background to this smear. (Papanicolaou stain, ×576)

on the cell surfaces and in the background (Fig. 2). Smears dominated by this organism are characterized by isolated nuclei of intermediate cells reflecting cytolysis.

Gardnerella (Hemophilus or Corynebacterium) vaginalis

This Gram-negative rod is found in about 5% of premenopausal women in whom it causes vaginitis and cervicitis (Hume, 1983). The characteristic cytologic picture is one of sparse leukocytes, an absence of Doderlein bacilli, a lack of cytolysis, the presence of small, dark blue staining rods, and the identification of *clue cells* (Bibbo *et al.*, 1974). The latter, though not specific

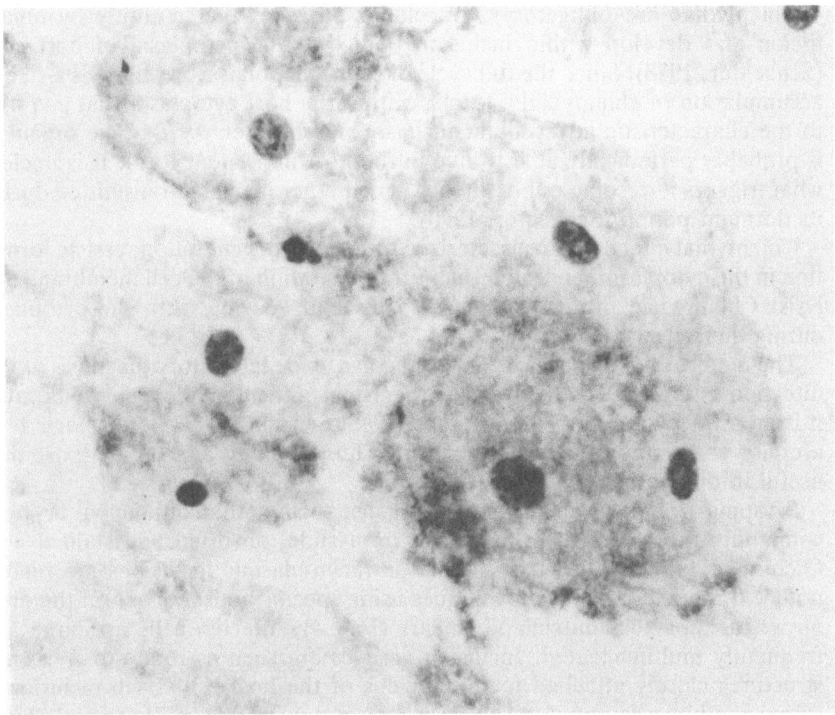

Fig. 3. *Hemophilus*. Superficial squamous cells are seen with small bacteria clinging to the cellular cytoplasm (clue cells). The bacteria are also visible in the background of the smear. (Papanicolaou stain, ×576)

for the presence of *G. vaginalis*, are distinctive. The organisms adhere to the surface of epithelial cells (Fig. 3) producing the characteristic peppered surface which is aptly termed the *clue cell* (Bibbo *et al.*, 1974).

Leptothrix vaginalis

This long, filamentous organism is commonly found in conjunction with *Trichomonas* (Bibbo *et al.*, 1974; Koss, 1979); it is not a cause of infection. Present in pre- and postmenopausal women, these rods do not form spores, as do fungi and yeasts.

Mycoplasma

Mycoplasma have been isolated in individuals whose smears show numerous leukocytes, coccoid bacteria, and squamous cells. The significance of positive *Mycoplasma* culture has not yet been assessed; it is found more commonly in women with venereal disease (92%) than in asymptomatic women (30%) (McCormack, *et al.*, 1973). No known cytologic changes are attributable to this organism.

Chlamydiae are obligatory intracellular parasites that multiply by binary fission and develop within inclusion bodies in the cytoplasm of host cells (Schachter, 1978). Since the full cycle of reproduction is slow, there is a steady accumulation of chlamydial particles within the host cytoplasm that give rise to the characteristic intracellular inclusions (Schachter, 1978). The organism is probably periodically able to live in the host in a latent form. It is unclear what triggers it to come out of latency, or whether it can be transmitted during its dormant period (Schachter, 1978).

Chlamydial infection is characterized by cellular degeneration, vesicle formation in the cytoplasm, and subsequent fragmentation of the cell membrane and lysis. Chlamydiae probably release toxins and enzymes into the cytoplasm during their growth.

The medical significance of *Chlamydia* has made laboratory diagnosis of this infection essential. Isolation of the organism is difficult and expensive because it is an intracellular parasite (Holmes, 1983; Schachter, 1978). Serologic tests are also costly and difficult to perform. Thus cytologic smears are extremely useful in diagnosing chlamydial infection.

Scraping from suspected infected organs, such as the conjunctiva or more commonly the cervix, can be spread on a slide, air-dried and stained with Giemsa or iodine. The characteristic intracytoplasmic inclusions are readily noted. Immunfluorescence techniques using specific antisera confirm the diagnosis. In Papanicolaou-stained smears (Fig. 4), infected cells are large and frequently multinucleated. Inclusion vesicles are seen as round-to-crescentic structures closely attached to the nucleus of the host cell. Each inclusion is surrounded by a faint halo. The inclusions vary in size from $25\,m\mu$ to $1\text{-}2\,\mu$ in diameter. By staining smears with an immunoperoxidase technique using specific antisera, Gupta *et al.* (1979) have shown that such inclusions indeed represent *Chlamydia*.

The finding of *Actinomyces* organisms in smears of women with IUDs *in situ* has been reported in recent years (Gupta *et al.*, 1976, 1978; Spence *et al.*, 1978). Most studies show a correlation with the type of IUD used (affected women more often wear plastic rather than copper IUDs (Duguid *et al.*, 1980; Hager *et al.*, 1979)) and with duration of use (usually 2 years or more) (Duguid *et al.*, 1980). The presence of this organism in the absence of an IUD is rare, although Christ and Haja (1978) have reported *Actinomyces* in women with other vaginal foreign bodies such as the pessary.

The organisms, identified as *Actinomyces israelii*, are readily detectable in cervico-vaginal smears, although it is important to recognize that colonization of the cervix and vagina by *Actinomyces* does not imply infection (Duguid *et al.*, 1980; Hager *et al.*, 1979). Most women whose smears are positive for *Actinomyces* are asymptomatic (Hager *et al.*, 1979), with the possible exception of some IUD wearers who are more likely to have abdominal pain, painful menses, and dyspareunia.

Cytologic smears with *Actinomyces* show background inflammatory changes and occasional epithelial atypias, purportedly related to IUD use (Duguid *et al.*, 1980). *A. israelii* appear as clumps of basophilic debris amidst neutrophils and histiocytes. High-power magnification discloses branching, filamentous structures staining blue or brown with Papanicolaou stain (Fig. 5) (Gupta *et*

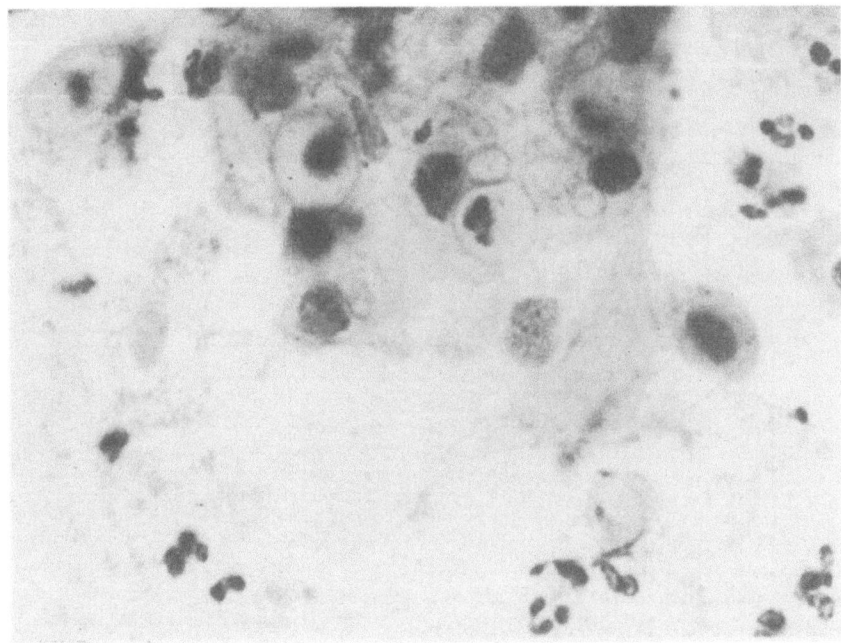

a

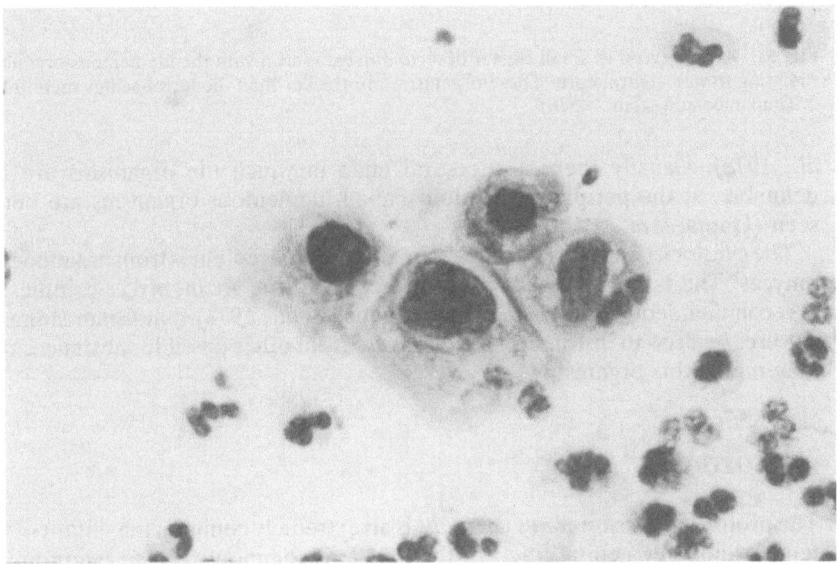

b

Fig. 4(a). *Chlamydia.* Intracellular vacuoles of *Chlamydia* are seen. (Papanicolaou stains, ×225). **(b)** In this cell cluster is it possible to see the numerous vacuoles containing the small organisms which are seen as single dots that would appear to be red. (Papanicolaou stain, ×576)

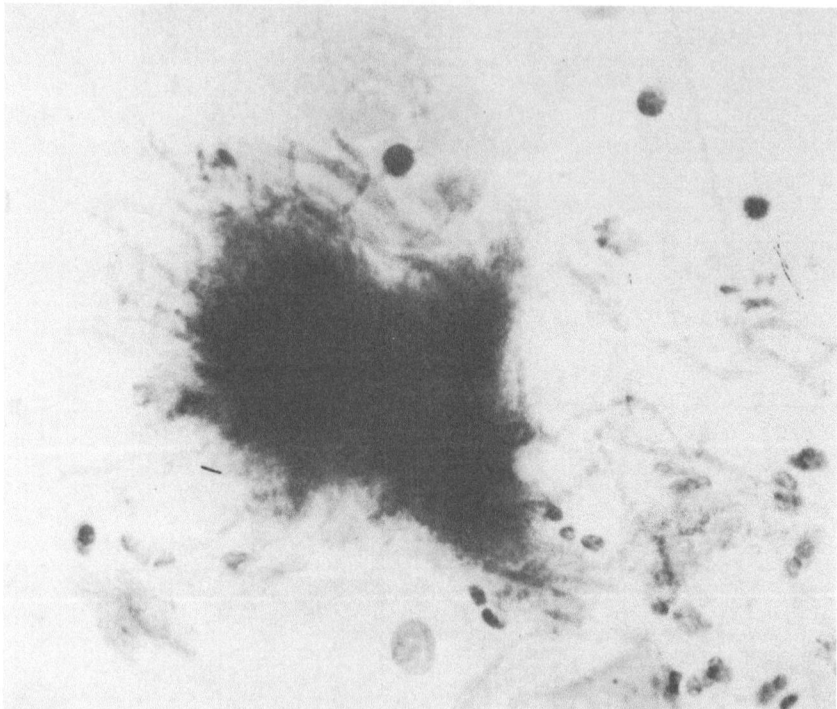

Fig. 5. *Actinomyces*. A small cluster of *Actinomyces* is seen with the filamentous organisms radiating from a central core. These organisms are thicker than the lactobacillus seen in Fig. 2. (Papanicolaou stain, ×576)

al., 1978). Usually there is a central mass in which the organisms are not definable; at the periphery the club-shaped filamentous organisms are better seen (Gupta *et al.*, 1978).

The cytologist must differentiate true *Actinomyces* colonies from pseudoactinomyces. The latter are easily misinterpreted as true *Actinomyces* colonies. It is recommended (Gupta *et al.*, 1978; Spence *et al.*, 1978) that Gram stains or cultures be used to distinguish *Actinomyces* from other possible substances that may mimic this organism.

PROTOZOA

The protozoan *Trichomonas vaginalis* is an extremely common inhabitant of the female and male genital tract. In the female it commonly causes symptomatic vaginitis. The cellular atypias associated with the inflammatory effects of this organism as well as its coexistence with cervical carcinoma and its antecedent lesions (Koss and Wolinska, 1959; Naguib *et al.*, 1966) make the recognition of *T. vaginalis* of great diagnostic importance. *T. vaginalis* is a protozoon which has no cyst state; it occurs only in the trophozoite stage. Its size may vary from

5 to 30 μ; the four anterior flagellae are not viable on a cytologic smear. Cytologically, the organism appears pear-shaped with pale blue-green cytoplasm. The nucleus is small, round-to-oval, and slightly basophilic (Naib, 1976). To make a positive identification it is essential to find the nucleus in some of the organisms since cytoplasmic fragments, mucus or other debris, can mimic its staining characteristics (Ziabrowski and Naylor, 1976), particularly in atrophic and cytolytic smears. The organisms may also have reddish-brown cytoplasmic granules which aid in their identification; however, only nuclear identification is confirmatory (Naib, 1976).

The presence of trichomonads in a totally noninflammatory Papanicolaou

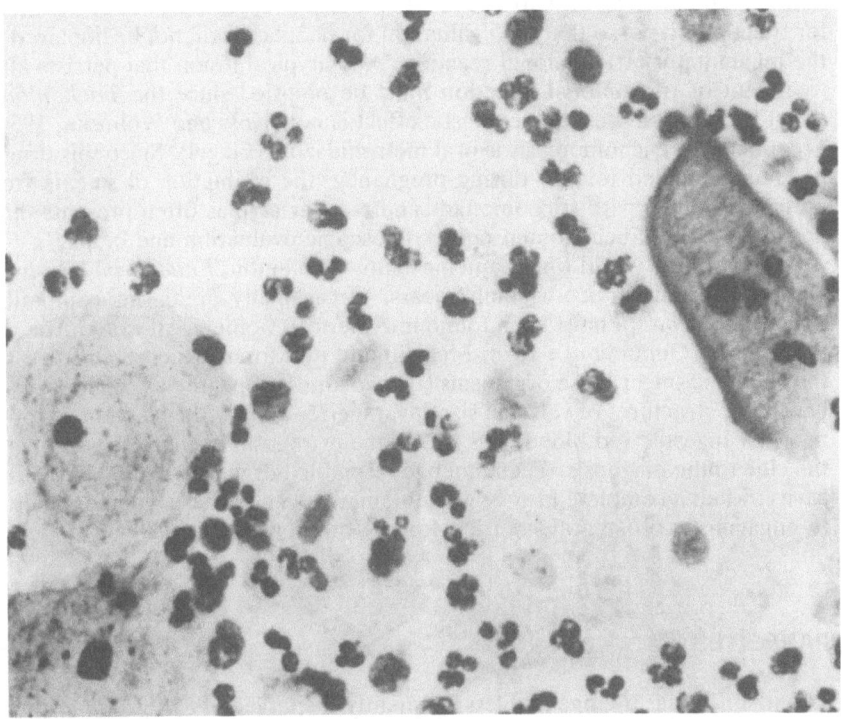

Fig. 6. *Trichomonas.* Two small oval structures are trichomonads seen in the center of the specimen. The nucleus is identified within each of these organisms. Numerous polymorphonuclear leukocytes are present and the smear has a dirty background. (Papanicolaou stain, ×576)

smear indicates an asymptomatic infestation (Fig. 6). Changes in vaginal pH or hormonal status permit the organism to invade the tissue, leading to nonspecific inflammatory reactions including congestion, edema, polymorphonuclear leukocytosis and a lymphocytic response. Epithelial cell degeneration may also occur (Koss and Wolinska, 1959). These cellular changes are commonly called the *Trichomonas* effect (Figs 7, 8 and 9) and include: squamous cell degeneration with loss of cytoplasmic margins (the cytoplasm may appear eosinophilic or orangophilic); small perinuclear haloes around slightly enlarged but pale nuclei; collections of polymorphonuclear leukocytes in clusters of organisms over epithelial cells (85% accuracy as an indicator of the presence of *Trichomonas*); an inflammatory background with necrosis, leukocytes, and coccoid bacterial debris (Naib, 1976).

More marked epithelial atypias can occur concomitantly and mimic the cellular change of intraepithelial or invasive neoplasia. Cells involved in these latter reactions (Fig. 10) show nuclear enlargement and hyperchromasia, cytoplasmic orangophilia, and cellular degeneration (Koss and Wolinska, 1959). Since trichomonads may coexist with invasive carcinoma (the necrotic environment of tumor may enhance the growth of the trichomonads), caution is required when interpreting smears with a high degree of atypia in the presence of trichomonads. The best approach is to request a repeat smear after treatment for trichomoniasis, so that the evaluation for neoplasia will not be impaired by the inflammatory trichomonal reaction. Any atypical lesion that persists after treatment of trichomonal infection must be biopsied since the *Trichomonas* effect is reversible but the neoplastic effect is not (Koss and Wolinska, 1959). Treatment for trichomoniasis is oral metronidazole (Flagyl). Since this drug is not recommended for use during pregnancy, the evaluation of smears from pregnant women with trichomonads and cellular atypias often presents diagnostic difficulty. Such women need colposcopic evaluation and biopsy.

In areas of the world where amebic colitis is common, *Entamoeba histolytica* may be seen in cervico-vaginal smears. Occasionally organisms compatible with *Entamoeba* sp. have been found in American women. All wore intrauterine devices (Gupta *et al.*, 1978; McNeill and de Moraes-Ruehsen, 1978). On the cytologic smear these organisms (trophozoites) appeared as round-to-oval, basophilic structures of variable size (average 15–20 μ) with an eccentric round nucleus. Ingested red blood cells within the cytoplasm of these cells provided the clue to the diagnosis. The amoebae resembled organisms found in the oral cavity; when a complete history was obtained, some of these women admitted to engaging in orogenital sex (de Moraes-Ruehsen *et al.*, 1980).

PARASITES

In endemic areas the ova and less frequently the larvae of *Schistosoma* sp. can be seen in cervico-vaginal smears (Coelho *et al.*, 1979). Occasionally eggs are also seen in smears containing neoplastic cells (Coelho *et al.*, 1979). The schistosomes dwell in mesenteric and hemorrhoidal vessels from where they gain access to pelvic and genital vasculature to parasitize the female reproductive organs. Identification of the parasites is based on recognition of the ova in cervical and vaginal smears (Coelho *et al.*, 1979). In cytologic material stained with the Papanicolaou stain, ova of *Schistosoma* sp. display a semitranslucent shell with a spine. The latter is located at one end of *S. hematobium* (found in the Orient), and on the lateral aspect of the ovum in *S. mansoni*. Often these ova have degenerated and their identification is difficult (Coelho *et al.*, 1979).

In developed countries, on the other hand, parasites are rarely seen in cervico-vaginal smears. The one important exception is *Enterobius vermicularis* which occasionally is found in smears of children with perianal pinworm infestation and associated vaginitis (Koss, 1979). These ova measure about 50 μ, stain yellow, and show a partly folded thick membrane or shell.

FUNGI

Candida is a saphrophytic, yeast-like organism of the family Cryptococcaceae. It exists predominantly as a round, unicellular, blastophore yeast which reproduces by budding. Buds may adhere and coalesce to form long chains or pseudohyphae. Organisms may be round, oval or oblong and measure about 3–5 μ in diameter. They usually stain a pinkish color on the cytologic smear. To make a diagnosis of *Candida* sp. it is necessary to see both pseudohyphae and budding blastosphores (Fig. 11). To confirm identification of the species *C. albicans*, it is necessary to culture the organism. If only the yeast form is seen, the organism may be *Torulopsis glabrata*, a small budding yeast also present in the female genital tract. This organism has a small capsular halo and no pseudohyphae (Koss, 1979). *Geotrichum* is a common filamentous fungus with true hyphae occasionally present in smears. It does not exist in a yeast form and its true hyphae are larger than the pseudohyphae of *Candida* (Koss, 1979).

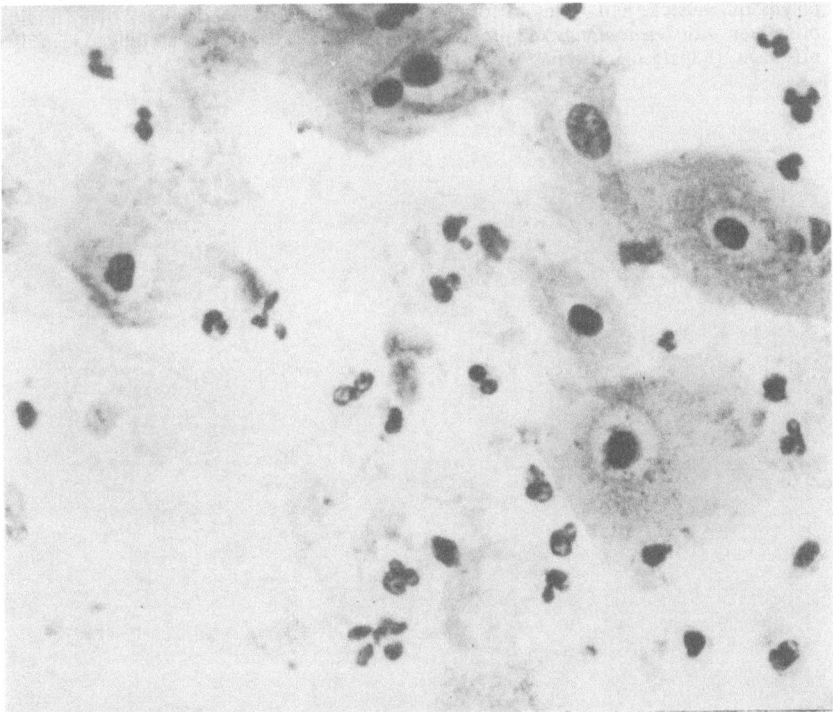

Fig. 7. *Trichomonas* and *Trichomonas* effect. Several trichomonads appear in the center of the specimen, but most striking is the cellular effect on the squamous cells. Each squamous cell has a distinct perinuclear halo; many cells have frayed cytoplasmic margins and loss of cytoplasmic detail. Again, the background of the smear is quite dirty. (Papanicolaou stain, ×576)

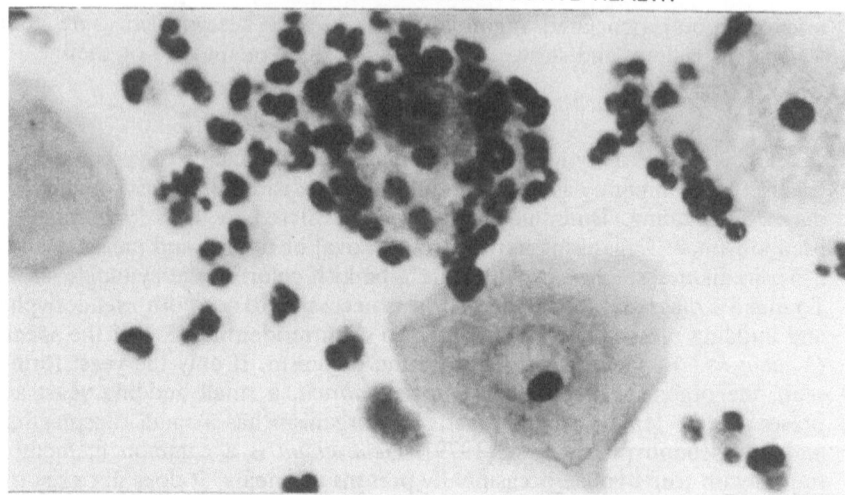

Fig. 8. *Trichomonas* effect. *Trichomonas* are seen in the center at the bottom of the picture. Several cells have perinuclear haloes. The squamous cell in the center is overlaid with polymorphonuclear leukocytes to form a ball-like structure or "bee-bee". This finding is often seen with *Trichomonas* and provides a clue to search the smear carefully to identify the organism. (Papanicolaou stain, ×576)

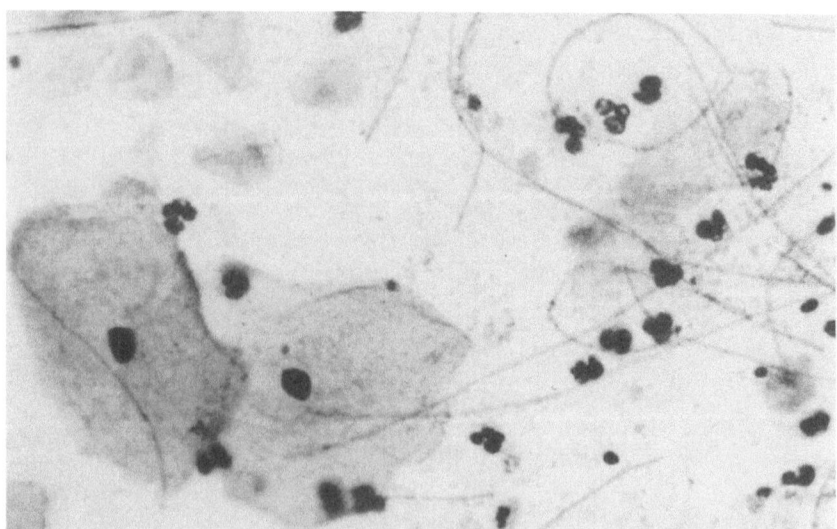

Fig. 9. *Trichomonas* and *Lactobacillus*. This smear again shows *Trichomonas* organisms with numerous lactobacilli present. The latter are quite commonly seen with *Trichomonas*. When lactobacilli are seen against a dirty background such as this, in contrast to the clean background in Fig. 2, it is important to search for the *Trichomonas* organism. Notice that the nuclei of several organisms are clearly visible. (Papanicolaou stain, ×576)

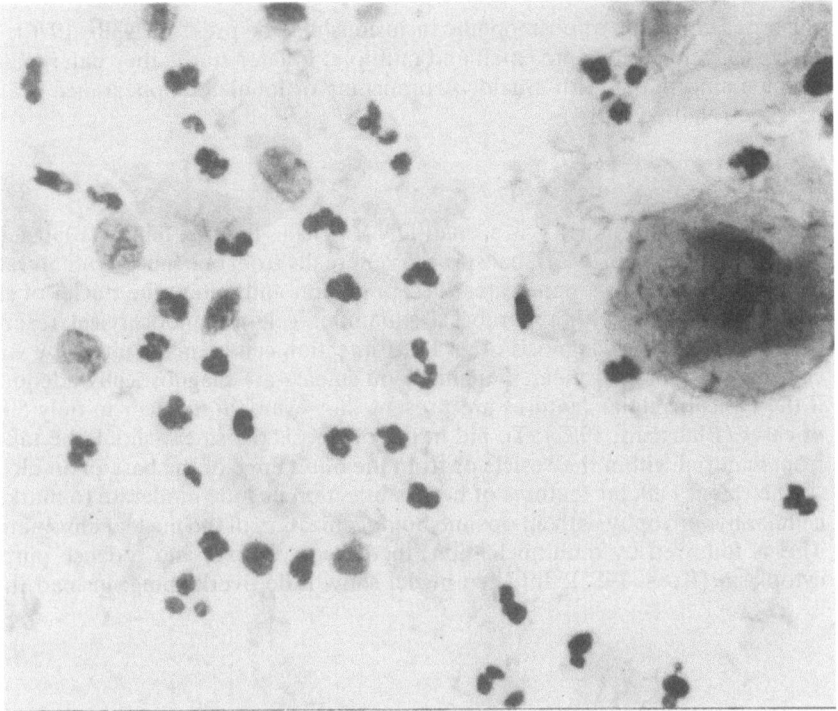

Fig. 10. Cytolytic effect. In a cytolytic smear, as seen near the end of a menstrual cycle, or in an atrophic smear, it is fairly common to have fragments of intermediate or parabasal cell cytoplasm which mimic the *Trichomonas* organism. In such smears it is not possible to identify distinct nuclei in these cytoplasmic fragments. (Papanicolaou stain, ×576)

No specific cellular or histologic findings are noted in candidal vaginitis. An acute inflammatory infiltrate may be present but rarely is epithelial atypia found since the organism does not penetrate the mucosa (Blaustein, 1982).

VIRUSES

Cytomegalovirus

Although evidence of cytomegalovirus (CMV) infection can be demonstrated in up to 80% of women (Vesterinen *et al.*, 1975), the presence of typical CMV-infected cells on cervico-vaginal smears is unusual. CMV preferentially infects the endocervical cells *in vitro* (Vesterinen *et al.*, 1975). An infected cell is hypertrophic, has one large nucleus, and scant dark cytoplasm. The nucleolus is red and large, usually half the diameter of the entire nucleus. A distinct halo is seen around the inclusion; the residual chromatin is precipitated adjacent to the nuclear membrane (Naib, 1976).

Adenovirus

Adenovirus is rarely identifiable in cells present in a cervical smear (Naib, 1976). Infected cells are usually basal endocervical cells present singly or in clusters. Basophilic or eosinophilic inclusions may be present (Naib, 1976). In early stages inclusions are small and multiple; in later stages they enlarge and become amorphous with a halo. A branching or lobulated appearance is also possible (Naib, 1976).

HSV

Herpes simplex virus HSV is a small DNA virus in the pox family (Blaustein, 1982; Lennette *et al.*, 1974) that spreads venereally from one mucous membrane to another. The virus penetrates the epithelium and enters the nuclei of the proliferating cells, either parabasal squamous cells or endocervical reserve cells (Naib, 1976). Diagnosis of an HSV infection can be made either by viral cultures or cytologic smear. Papanicolaou smears are diagnostically adequate if the typical cellular features are present; however, these occur in only 50% of cases (Blaustein, 1982). To aid in the diagnosis the smear should be taken from material within the vesicle or from the outer edge of the base of an ulcer.

The classic cellular features of herpes infection include moderate to marked cellular hypertrophy with an opaque homogenization of the nuclear chromatin. This is followed by multinucleation, increased cell size, and a dense purple cytoplasm (Koss, 1982). Infected nuclei show little overlapping; instead they

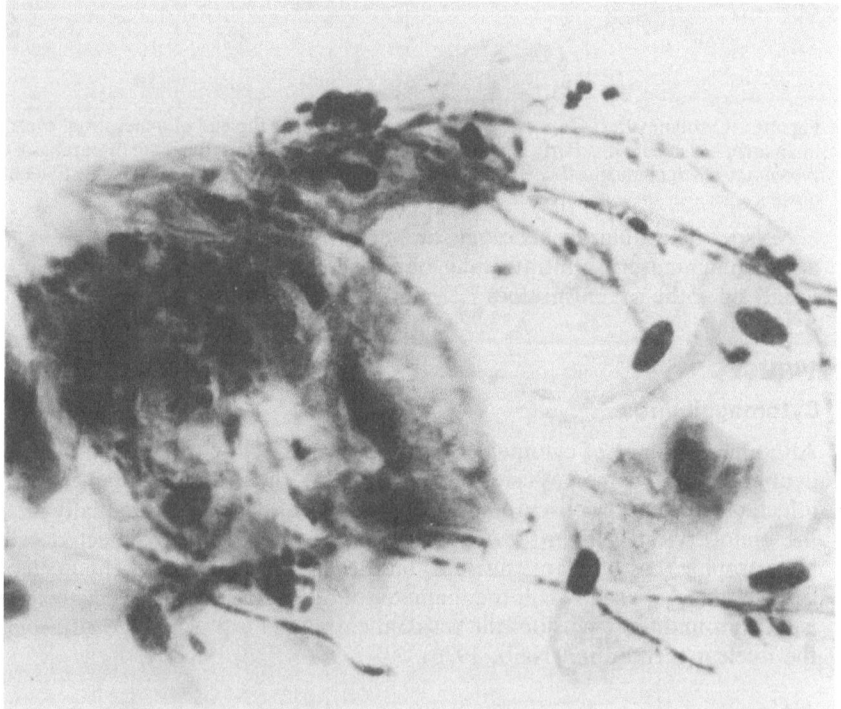

Fig. 11. *Candida. Candida* organisms in both the oval yeast form and the pseudohyphal form. Yeast forms are attached and budding from the pseudohyphal filament. (Papanicolaou stain, ×576)

mold to each other. During the late stages of infection viral particles may condense in the center of the nucleus. This is reflected in a large red inclusion surrounded by an equally large halo (Koss, 1979; Naib, 1976). The chromatin lies on the margin against the nuclear membrane. Viral inclusions may be seen in both primary and secondary herpes (Fig. 12) (Koss, 1979). Because the clinical picture is so characteristic, biopsy is rarely needed. Histologic examination reveals multinucleated cells and a very marked inflammatory infiltrate.

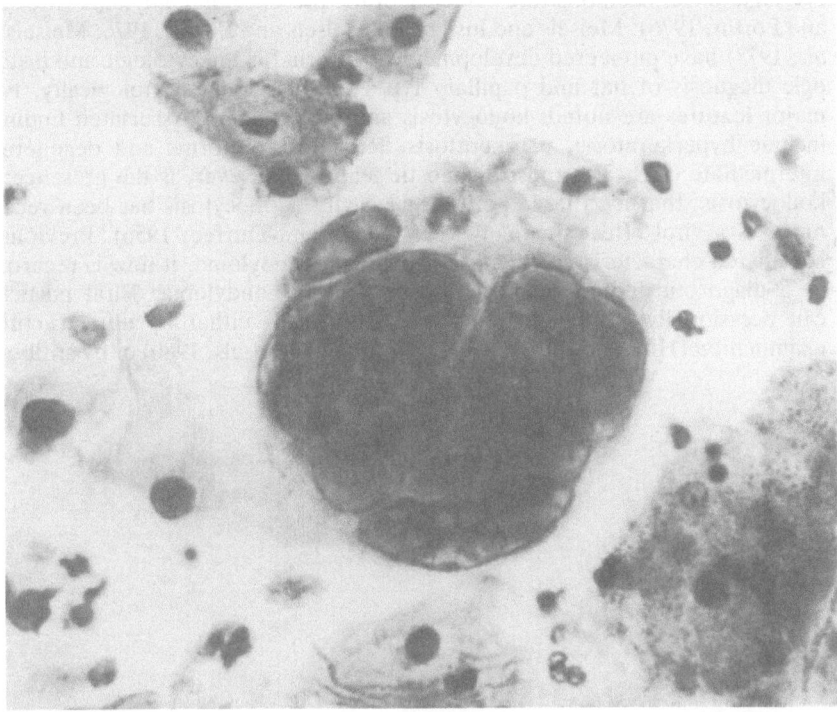

Fig. 12. Herpes cytopathic effect. Cells in the center of this smear are markedly enlarged and contain numerous nuclei with prominent nuclear molding and an amorphous granular nuclear chromatin pattern. (Papanicolaou stain, ×230)

HPV

The human papilloma virus (HPV) is a small DNA virus of the papovavirus group which exists in at least 18 related viral types (zur Hausen, 1982). Skin and genital warts or condyloma acuminata are caused by different types of HPV (zur Hausen, 1982). Recently, portions of the viral genome of HPV type 16 have been found in 12 of 20 cervical squamous cancers (zur Hausen, 1982). This finding has encouraged further investigations into the relationship of this virus in the development of cervical tumors.

Genital warts have been recognized since ancient times. Confusion existed about the mode of spread and the relationship to skin warts until Oriel studied a group of patients with genital warts in a London venereal disease clinic (Oriel, 1971). This study documented the venereal spread of condyloma separate and distinct from other venereal diseases and bearing no relationship to skin warts.

In women, condyloma lesions usually begin in the posterior introitus but may also be present on the labia minora and majora. They also occur on the lower vagina, urethra, perineum, anus and cervix (Oriel, 1971); however, only 6% of all females affected with condyloma were thought to have them on the cervix (Oriel, 1971). Recently, it has been shown that as many as 1% of all cytologic smears demonstrate evidence of the presence of condyloma (Meisels and Fortin, 1976). Meisels and his group (Meisels and Fortin, 1976; Meisels *et al.*, 1977) have pioneered development of criteria for the cytologic and histologic diagnosis of flat and papillary types of condyloma. Cytologically, two major features are noted: koilocytosis and dyskeratosis. Associated findings include hyperkeratosis, parakeratosis, large bizarre forms and degenerate intermediate cells. The most diagnostic feature, however, is the presence of koilocytosis; that is, a large perinuclear cavity. Koilocytosis has been recognized as a viral effect for many years (Koss and Durfee, 1956). Previously considered characteristically only for papillary condyloma, it now is regarded as a diagnostic feature in both flat and raised condyloma. Viral particles can occasionally be detected in koilocytotic cells either by ultrastructural examination (Hills and Laverty, 1979; Morin and Meisels, 1980) or by antibody

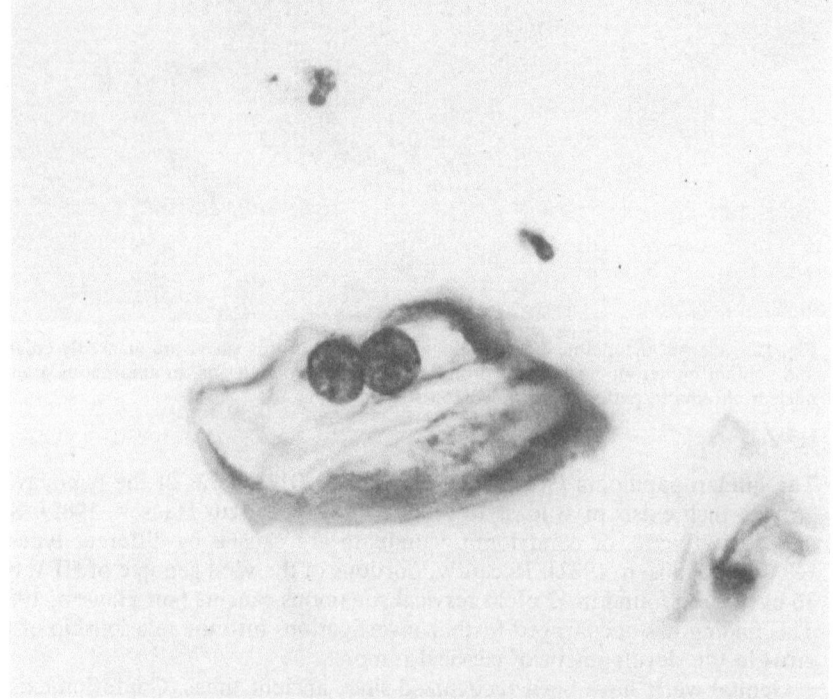

Fig. 13. Koilocytosis from condyloma. This binucleate cell has a distinct cytoplasmic rim with the two nuclei within a very large clear vacuole. A cell with such a large cavity around the nucleus is called a koilocyte. (Papanicolaou stain, ×576)

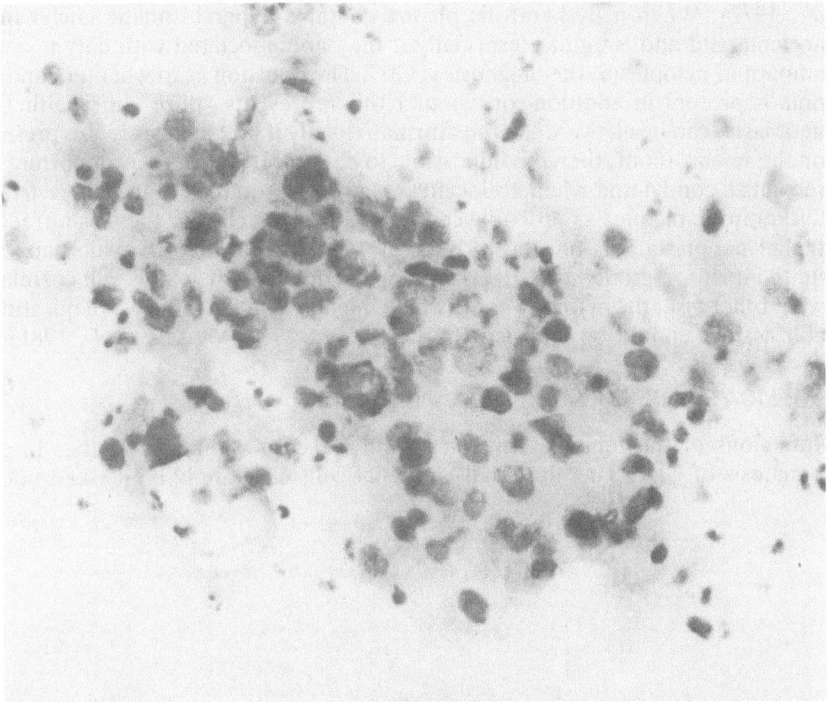

Fig. 14. Dyskeratosis of condyloma. This plaque-like arrangement of squamous cells is the typical surface layer from a condylomatous epithelium. This plaque would stain orange; the cells would have a variety of nuclear sizes, shapes and staining characteristics. (Papanicolaou stain, ×230)

localization (Kurman *et al.*, 1981; Morin *et al.*, 1981). The koilocytotic cell is present in approximately 50% of smears from cases diagnosed by biopsy as having condyloma (Ludwig *et al.*, 1981; Meisels *et al.*, 1977). Since this cell type may not be present on the surface of the lesion, it is not always demonstrable on cytologic smear.

The most common surface reaction of condyloma is abnormal nuclear maturation associated with an inappropriate keratinization, called dyskeratosis (Figs 13 and 14). The dyskeratotic cells usually are in clusters and contain hyperchromatic and irregular nuclei. Within these clusters or plaques a variety of nuclear degenerative changes can also be observed. The cytoplasm is often hyperkeratinized, seen as yellow-to-orange, although bright red or polychromatic cytoplasm can also be noted (Meisels and Fortin, 1976). Dyskeratosis is suggestive of condyloma but similar changes are present in a variety of conditions which lead to hyperkeratosis, including chronic trauma caused by prolapse or a pessary. Since the surface of a keratinized cervical carcinoma may also display dyskeratosis, a biopsy must be performed in doubtful cases. The major diagnostic dilemma in evaluating condyloma is distinguishing this lesion from cervical intraepithelial neoplasia (CIN) (Fig. 15). Since the two conditions often coexist, the cytologist faces a dilemma (Ludwig *et al.*, 1981; Meisels *et al.*, 1977). When a dyskeratotic plaque contains hyperchromatic nuclei that are enlarged and irregular, especially if they are associated with only a small amount of cytoplasm, the diagnosis is CIN. The question as to whether condyloma is present in addition, or whether this represents "pure" intraepithelial neoplasia, can be answered in the affirmative only if koilocytosis is also present on the smear. If not, then it is impossible to be sure. It is extremely important to recognize condyloma when koilocytosis is present and to recognize *degenerate* dyskeratotic plaques as probable condyloma and not classify them as intraepithelial neoplasia. If only those dyskeratotic cells and plaques which appear quite intact are graded as CIN, then biopsy and cytology results will correlate well; otherwise, the cytology grade will be higher than the biopsy. All questionable lesions should be biopsied (Ludwig *et al.*, 1981; Meisels *et al.*, 1981).

IMPLICATIONS FOR CERVICAL NEOPLASIA

Infections of the female genital tract may lead to several difficulties in the diagnosis of CIN. The abnormal epithelial cells can simply be masked under

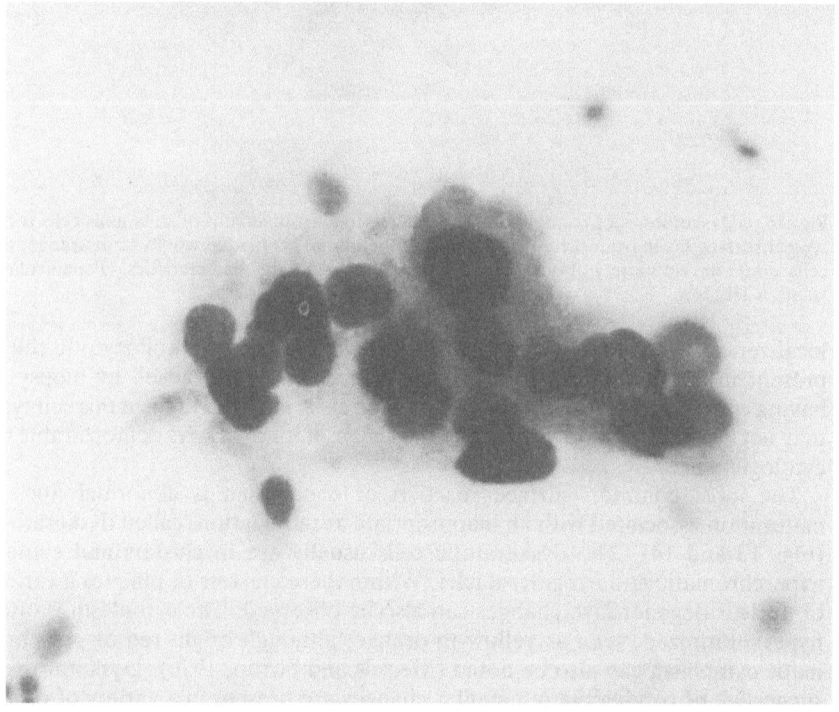

Fig. 15. Plaque of cells representing either a dyskeratosis of condyloma or cervical intraepithelial neoplasia. This plaque has orange cytoplasm and very dense hyperchromatic nuclei which are too large for the amount of cytoplasm present. This type of plaque may represent the surface dyskeratosis of condyloma as in Fig. 14. When the nuclei are this hyperchromatic and irregular, and there is such scant cytoplasm, it possibly represents true cervical intraepithelial neoplasia. It may be necessary to examine the patient colposcopically and take a biopsy of such lesions to determine their significance. (Papanicolaou stain, ×576)

a marked inflammatory infiltrate. If the smear is so inflamed that the squamous and endocervical components cannot be evaluated, then the inflammation must be treated and the smear repeated. In other instances the inflammatory effect on the squamous cells, i.e. the enlarged slightly hyperchromatic nuclei of *Trichomonas* effect, can be misinterpreted as mild dysplasia or CIN. Care should always be taken not to overdiagnose a smear once a specific infectious agent is identified.

Specific infections may exist contemporaneously with CIN and/or invasive carcinoma and yet be unrelated. *Trichomonas*, for instance, is fairly common in patients with invasive cervical carcinoma, probably because the necrotic tissue debris presents a favourable environment for the organism's growth. Other infections are associated metasynchronously with cervical carcinoma, particularly HSV–2.

Recent studies have demonstrated genetic sequences that hybridize with two types of HPV (HPV–6 and HPV–11) in lesions of CIN. A different HPV genetic sequence, HPV–16, hybridizes with many cases of cervical squamous carcincoma (zur Hausen, 1982). This may mean that a different HPV virus is associated with invasive tumors. While this is an extremely exciting finding because it links at least one type of papilloma virus to cervical carcinoma, it is not evidence of causation.

Zur Hausen has postulated that HPV virus may act as a promoter for cervical cancer while another agent, possibly the herpes simplex virus, acts as the tumor initiator (zur Hausen, 1982). Hybridization studies have shown herpes virus DNA genome in cervical dysplasia and carcinomas (McDougal *et al.*, 1980). What relationships exist between HPV and HSV and cervical carcinoma await prospective epidemiologic, serologic, and biochemical studies. This area of research promises to provide clues to some of the etiologic factors in the development of neoplasia.

References

Bibbo, M., Harris, M. J. and Wied, G. L. (1974). Microbiology of the female genital tract. In: Wied, G. L., Koss, L. G. and Reagan, J. W. (eds.), *Compendium of Diagnostic Cytology*. (Chicago: Tutorials of Cytology)

Bibbo, M., Keebler, C. M. and Wied, G. L. (1971). The cytologic diagnosis of tissue repair in the female genital tract. *Acta Cytol.*, **15**, 133

Blaustein A. (ed.) (1982). *Pathology of the Female Genital Tract*, 2nd edn (New York: Springer)

Christ, M. L. and Haja, J. (1978). Cytologic changes associated with vaginal pessary use, with special reference to the presence of actinomyces. *Acta Cytol.*, **22**, 146

Coelho, L. H. M. R., Carvalho, G. and Carvalho, J. M. (1979). Carcinoma *in situ* and invasive squamous cell carcinoma associated with schistosomiasis of the uterine cervix. *Acta Cytol.*, **23**, 45

de Moraes-Ruehsen, M., McNeill, R. E., Frost, J. K. *et al.* (1980). Amebae resembling Entamoeba gingivalis in the genital tract of IUD users. *Acta Cytol.*, **24**, 413

Duguid, H. L. D., Parratt, J. and Traynor, R. (1980). Actinomyces-like organisms in cervical smears from women using intrauterine contraceptive devices. *Br. Med. J.*, **281**, 534

Gupta, P. K., Burroughs, F., Luff, R. D. *et al.* (1978). Epithelial atypias associated with intrauterine contraceptive devices (IUD). *Acta Cytol.*, **22**, 286

Gupta, P. K., Hollander, D. H. and Frost, J. K. (1976). Actinomyces in cervicovaginal smears: An association with IUD usage. *Acta Cytol.*, **20**, 295

Gupta, P. K., Lee, E. F., Erozan, Y. S. *et al.* (1979). Cytologic investigation in Chlamydia infections. *Acta Cytol.*, **23**, 315

Hager, W. D., Douglas, B., Majmuder, B. *et al.* (1979). Pelvic colonization with Actinomyces in women using intrauterine contraceptive devices. *Am. J. Obstet. Gynecol.*, **135**, 680

Hills, E. and Laverty, C. R. (1979). Electron microscopic detection of papilloma virus particles in selected koilocytotic cells in a routine cervical smear. *Acta Cytol.*, **23**, 53

Holmes, K. K. (1983). The *Chlamydia* epidemic. *J. Am. Med. Assoc.*, **245**, 1718

Hume, J. C. (1981). Trichomoniasis, Candidiasis, and Gardnerella vaginalis vaginitis as sexually transmitted diseases. *Dermatol. Clin.*, **1**, 137

Koss, L. G. (1979). *Diagnostic Cytopathology and its Histopathologic Basis.* (Philadelphia: J. B. Lippincott)

Koss, L. G. and Durfee, G. R. (1956). Unusual patterns of squamous epithelium of the uterine cervix: Cytologic and pathologic study of koilocytotic atypia. *Ann. N.Y. Acad. Sci.*, **63**, 1245

Koss, L. G. and Wolinska, W. H. (1959). Trichomonas vaginalis cervictis and its relationship to cervical cancer: A histocytological study. *Cancer.*, **12**, 1171

Kurman, R., Shah, K., Lancaster, W. *et al.* (1981). Immunoperoxidase localization of papillomavirus antigens in cervical dysplasia and vulvar condylomas. *Am. J. Obstet. Gynecol.*, **140**, 931

Lennette, E. H., Spaulding, E. H. and Truant, J. P. (eds). (1974). *Manual of Clinical Microbiology.* (Washington: American Society for Microbiology)

Ludwig, M., Lowell, D. and LiVolsi, V. A. (1981). Cervical condylomatous atypia and its relationship to cervical neoplasia. *Am. J. Clin. Pathol.*, **76**, 255

McCormack, W. M., Braun, P., Lee, Y. H. *et al.* (1973). The genital mycoplasmas. *N. Engl. J. Med.*, **288**, 78

McDougall, J. K., Galloway, D. A. and Fenoglio, L. M. (1980). Cervix cancer: Detection of herpes simplex virus DNA in cells undergoing neoplastic change. *Int. J. Cancer*, **25**, 1

McNeill, R. E. and de Moraes-Ruehsen, M. (1978). Ameba trophozoites in cervicovaginal smear of a patient using an intrauterine device. *Acta Cytol.*, **22**, 91

Meisels, A. and Fortin, R. (1976). Condylomatous lesions of the cervix and vagina. I. Cytologic patterns. *Acta Cytol.*, **20**, 505

Meisels, A., Fortin, R. and Roy, M. (1977). Condylomatous lesions of the cervix. II. Cytologic, colposcopic and histopathologic study. *Acta Cytol.*, **21**, 379

Meisels, A., Roy, M., Fortier, M. *et al.* (1981). Human papillomavirus infection of the cervix: the atypical condyloma. *Acta Cytol.*, **25**, 7

Morin, C., Braun, L., Casas-Cordero, M. *et al.* (1981). Confirmation of the papillomavirus etiology of condylomatous cervix lesions by the peroxidase–antiperoxidase technique. *J. Natl. Cancer Inst.*, **66**, 835

Morin, C. and Meisels, A. (1980). Human papilloma virus infection of the uterine cervix. *Acta Cytol.*, **24**, 82

Naguib, S. M., Cornstock, G. W. and Davis, H. J. (1966). Epidemiologic study of trichomoniasis in normal women. *J. Am. Col. Obstet, Gynecol.*, **27**, 607

Naib, Z. M. (1976). *Exfoliative Cytology.* (Boston: Little, Brown)

Oriel, J. D. (1971). Natural history of genital warts. *Br. J. Vener. Dis.*, **47**, 1

Patten, S. F. (1973). Benign proliferative reactions of the uterine cervix. In: Wied, G. L., Koss, L. G. and Reagan, J. W. (Eds). *Compendium on Diagnostic Cytology.* (Chicago: Tutorials of Cytology)

Schachter, J. (1978). Chlamydial infections. *N. Engl. J. Med.*, **298**, 428

Spence, M. R., Gupta, P. K., Frost, J. K *et al.* (1978). Cytologic detection and clinical significance of Actinomyces israelii in women employing intrauterine contraceptive devices. *Am. J. Obstet. Gynecol.*, **131**, 295

Tack, K. J., Peterson, P. K., Rasp, F. L. *et al.* (1980). Isolation of Chlamydia trachomatis from the lower respiratory tract of adults. *Lancet*, **1**, 116

Vesterinen, E., Leinikki, P. and Saksela, E. (1975). Cytopathogenecity of cytomegalovirus to human ecto- and endocervical epithelial cells in vitro. *Acta Cytol.*, **19**, 473

Witwer, M. W., Farmer, M. F., Wand, J. S. *et al.* (1977). Extensive actinomycosis associated with an intrauterine contraceptive device. *Am. J. Obstet. Cytol.*, **128**, 913

Wolner-Hanssen, P., Savensson, L. and Westrøm, L. (1982). Isolation of *Chlamydia trachom-*

atis from the liver capsule in Fitz-Hugh–Curtis syndrome. *N. Engl. J. Med.*, **306,** 113

Ziabrowski, T. A. and Naylor, B. (1976). Cyanophilic bodies in cervico-vaginal smears. *Acta Cytol.*, **20,** 340

zur Hausen, H. (1982). Human genital cancer: synergism between two virus infections or synergism between a virus infection and initiating events. *Lancet*, **2,** 1370

20
Preoperative and intraoperative antibiotics in reducing the incidence of infections

M. GALBRAITH and D. H. GREMILLION

INTRODUCTION

Historical perspective

The use of perioperative antimicrobials for minimizing the incidence of postoperative surgical infection has been a subject of active controversy for decades. Since the publication of the initial clinical trial in 1938, a plethora of studies involving thousands of patients and dozens of antibiotics has attempted to establish the efficacy of this practice. Many of these trials, however, suffered from design flaws that rendered the results equivocal and, occasionally, uninterpretable.

The wide number of variables that affect the surgical patient during and preceding hospitalization make it difficult for the clinical investigator to standardize important aspects of the study population. Many facets of the preoperative, intraoperative and postoperative environments may be controlled. Much investigation has centered on identifying those facets that most critically impact on the results of clinical trials. Unfortunately many investigations were conducted concurrently with, or consecutively to, the earlier antibiotic prophylaxis trials. Therefore, some studies became obsolete as subsequent data revealed that factors such as the placement of surgical drains or the preoperative preparation of the incision site affected the incidence of postoperative wound infections (Cruse and Foord, 1973). Those prophylaxis studies that neglected to control these factors became suspect. Among 157 English-language papers reviewed through July 1977, 29 various antimicrobial agents alone or in combination were evaluated. Amazingly, 11% of these studies neglected to indicate when the agent had been administered in relation to the surgery, and in 10% the agent used was not specified. Thirty-four percent omitted the dosage of the drug, and 42% the duration of antibiotic administration (Berger *et al.*, 1978).

A review of the obstetric and gynecologic English-language literature on antimicrobial prophylaxis, which encompassed the period January 1960 to August 1976, identified only 11 acceptable studies (Chodak and Plaut, 1978). All of these acceptable trials appeared after 1970. Many investigators have identified 1968 as a demarcation point before which studies addressing the issue of surgical antibiotic prophylaxis are difficult to interpret because of the changes in patient care, hospital flora, and antibiotic potencies that occurred during the 1970s (Hirschmann and Inui, 1980). Medical advances notwithstanding, most early surgical investigations of prophylactic antibiotics remain difficult to evaluate because of errors in their design.

Developing standards

Several authorities have already reviewed the clinical trials of antimicrobial prophylaxis in multiple surgical procedures (Chodak and Plaut, 1977; Berger *et al.*, 1978; Hirschmann and Inui, 1980) and in obstetric and gynecologic surgery (Chodak and Plaut, 1978; Hirschmann and Inui, 1980; Berger *et al.*, 1980). They generally required that the following standards be applied in the conduct of clinical studies to ensure the validity of the data.

(1) Human subjects. While animal studies are necessary during the development of an antimicrobial agent, data obtained from nonhuman models cannot always be extrapolated to the human patient.

(2) Randomization. Randomly assigning subjects to treatment and control groups prevents investigator bias from skewing the study population, i.e. from subconsciously assigning certain patients to specific treatment groups.

(3) Prospective design. Prospective studies avoid the many errors inherent in the retrospective study, most notably the failure to recall accurately conditions or problems that may have a bearing on the study results.

(4) Adequate controls. A control population with similar demographic data must concurrently serve as a reference against which the efficacy of a new technique or drug may be assessed. Patients should be assigned to this cohort through a randomization technique, with the control population receiving either a placebo or a standard form of therapy. Historical controls are inadequate for studying antimicrobial prophylaxis, because of the various changes that have occurred in medical personnel and practices over the course of years.

(5) Double-blind design. Concealing the treatment that a specific subject is to receive from both the subject and the evaluating physician creates a double-blind study, minimizing the participants' subjective responses.

(6) Criteria for inclusion in the study group. The investigator must state the specific requirements for inclusion into the study cohort. He should also establish disqualifying factors. Failure to describe these criteria prevents those evaluating the study design from ascertaining the homogeneity of the patient population. For example, in reviewing a population undergoing cesarean section it is important to know whether the group included women in labor and whether it excluded elective repeat procedures.

(7) Criteria for assessing outcome. Quantitative definitions for such conditions as wound infection, fever, etc., should be established. Nebulous terms such as febrile morbidity cannot supplant objective, measurable standards. Furthermore, the investigator should clearly state the criteria that in his opinion will determine the success of the clinical trial, i.e. a lower incidence of postoperative wound infections or a shorter hospitalization.

(8) Standard protocols for multi-institutional studies. Whenever more than one group of investigators is involved, a standard protocol must be followed by all parties to ensure the homogeneity of the study population and the application of therapeutic interventions.

(9) Limitation on multiple exclusions. Investigators excluding more than 20–25% of the study population from final analysis may bias their data by selecting for factors which were initially not considered in the study design.

(10) Statistical analysis. The application of statistical methods to the analysis of the data, or at least the presentation of data, in a format that allows statistical analysis is necessary to ensure the validity of the study.

(11) Underlying diseases. The criteria for admission to the clinical trial should specify which underlying medical conditions would exclude a patient from participating in the study since it is recognized that certain disease states may predispose to postoperative complications.

Clinical trials of prophylactic antibiotics that apply all of the preceding criteria are rare. Studies that incorporate most of these standards do exist, however, and have provided adequate data on the efficacy of antimicrobial prophylaxis in obstetric and gynecologic surgery. Nonetheless, inconsistencies in study design continue to create difficulties in comparing the results of different investigators, difficulties that are often due to dissimilar criteria for evaluating the outcome of a study. Inconsistencies in definitions of postoperative infections and in the surgical procedure itself further complicate the direct comparison of data from one study to another. Some authors choose to report only wound infections, while others include postoperative infections at other sites, e.g. pneumonia or cystitis. The method of reporting wound infections also varies. Thus it is often difficult to compare the data from a study which separates major from minor wound infections with data from one that does not, since the morbidity from a wound infection can range from local inflammation to bacteremia with dehiscence.

In all of these matters the specific conditions under which the study was conducted should be stated along with the author's results in order to allow for an accurate assessment of the therapeutic method and its outcome. The presence of postoperative drains can also bias a study's results and omission of such information precludes a fair interpretation of the data. The total antibiotic regimen in both control and prophylaxis groups, preoperatively and postoperatively, should be indicated. A cohort harboring a subpopulation that received preoperative antimicrobial therapy for pelvic inflammatory disease or bronchitis can skew the clinical trial's outcome. Likewise, a large number of patients receiving therapy for postoperative urinary tract infections can influence the incidence of wound infections.

291

Having addressed the inadequacies found in clinical trial designs and the inconsistencies present in published definitions of wound infections and methods of selected study populations, we can now turn to the issue of what constitutes the true efficacy of antimicrobial prophylaxis. The National Research Council's Ad Hoc Committee of the Committee on Trauma published a classification of surgical wounds and their acceptable infection rates in 1964 (Table 1) (NRC, 1964). A subsequent study of over 20,000 surgical wounds

Table 1 Surgical categories by infection risk

Category	Definition	Risk of infection	
I.	Clean	Nontraumatic, elective, no drains, primary closure, sterile technique	<5%[a]
II.	Clean–contaminated	Same as I, plus GI, GU, or respiratory tract entry or minor break in sterile technique	10%[b]
III.	Contaminated	Fresh trauma, GI spillage, entry of an infected focus, or major break in sterile technique	20%[c]
IV.	Dirty	Traumatic wounds with necrotic tissue, foreign body, delayed treatment, or fecal contamination	30%[c]

[a] AB prophylaxis indicated only when consequences potentially severe
[b] AB prophylaxis usually indicated
[c] AB treatment, not prophylaxis, given

found infection rates using this classification to be 1.8%, 8.9%, 21.5%, and 38.3% respectively (Cruse and Foord, 1973). An infection rate of 2.1% was reported for clean gynecologic surgery, including abdominal hysterectomies. The overall infection rate for all gynecologic surgery was 2.7%; the authors, however, excluded vaginal operations from their survey.

With an anticipated wound infection rate of 10% for vaginal hysterectomies and 2% for abdominal hysterectomies performed without antibiotic prophylaxis, the administration of any prophylactic antimicrobial agent must be associated with a lower incidence of wound infections in order to be judged truly efficacious. Other criteria also exist to evaluate the effectiveness of these agents. Febrile morbidity, defined as a temperature exceeding 38 °C on two occasions separated by 6 hours after the initial 24-hour postoperative period, may serve as a standard in the absence of obvious wound infections. Decreased postoperative febrile morbidity in the group receiving prophylactic antibiotics is frequently employed as a criterion of efficacy. The data usually include a statistically analyzed difference in the mean postoperative temperature, the number of patients with a postoperative temperature above 38 °C, or the number of postoperative temperature-free patient days between the study groups.

Although comparisons of these parameters may achieve statistical significance, their clinical importance may be less apparent. Other relevant criteria are needed. For example, a documented decrease in the number of days of postoperative hospitalization in the treated population reflects the value of the prophylactic agent. At the same time complications associated with administration of the prophylactic antibiotic must also be evaluated. Untoward reactions may contribute to postoperative morbidity, prolonged hospitalization and even mortality. Omission of such information from any data analysis precludes a thorough assessment of postoperative complications.

These criteria not only directly assess the benefits of a particular method on the patient's physical condition, but also indirectly examine certain financial aspects of therapy. Fewer wound infections require less antibiotics and shorter hospitalizations, thereby reducing costs. With the increasing emphasis on health care cost containment, documentation of a financial benefit may become an important aspect in judging the value of prophylactic antibiotic regimens. In one recent study using prophylactic cefazolin, a saving of $492.00 per patient undergoing abdominal hysterectomy was realized (Shapiro *et al.*, 1983).

The final evaluation of a clinical trial relies upon the collective application of the aforementioned criteria. Study designs vary and certain of these criteria may be compromised; their glaring violation or omission, however, renders the results suspect. Unfortunately, this sanction applies to many of the early published studies of surgical antibiotic prophylaxis.

Antibiotic pharmacokinetics

Following intravenous (IV) or intramuscular (IM) administration, antibiotic serum levels peak within minutes. Specific pharmacokinetic characteristics such as (IM) absorption rate, tissue distribution, and rate and route of elimination ultimately determine the antibiotic's concentration in interstitial fluid. As a dynamic equilibrium between the tissue and the plasma is attained, the plasma level of most antibiotics declines exponentially. The initial rate of decline depends on the affinity of antibiotic for tissue; subsequent elimination depends on metabolism and excretion.

Shortly after administration of an antibiotic, interstitial fluid levels of the medication rapidly rise, then plateau and gradually decline. This interstitial fluid level usually persists for 1 or 2 hours after the serum level has become negligible. Differential tissue perfusion rates further alter the distribution of the antibiotic. Renal, hepatic, and cardiac perfusion exceed that of skin, muscle, and fat, resulting in interstitial fluid levels in the former which closely parallel the serum level. Soft tissue requires a longer time to accumulate antibiotic concentrations.

Only the free, nonprotein-bound fraction of antibiotic present in the blood stream is pharmacologically active. The activity of an antibiotic is directly related to the amount of free antibiotic available. Binding of an agent by plasma proteins limits the amount of drug available for tissue distribution, since cell membranes are impermeable to the large protein molecules. Ionic forces can also prevent passage of an ionized antibiotic across a cell's lipid membrane. Consequently, during its distribution phase the level of free antibiotic in the plasma must exceed the inhibitory concentration for the target organism, since the interstitial fluid level wll be lower than the plasma level. Intracellular proteins may also bind the antibiotic as it passes through the tissue, further decreasing the amount available to combat the infection.

Multiple investigations measuring tissue levels of antibiotics have produced inconsistent results. Overall, higher serum levels of free antibiotic result in higher free antibiotic levels in tissue. The lag between peak serum levels and peak tissue levels of antibiotic is reported to be about 60 minutes or more, but this figure varies (Neu, 1977).

Among the cephalosporins, the degree of protein binding varies from 15% with cephradine to 86% with cefazolin. Most of the cephalosporins show a protein-binding rate of approximately 70%, while antistaphylococcal penicillins usually have a rate that exceeds 90%. Aminoglycosides are not significantly protein bound.

The percentage of plasma protein binding does not directly reflect the percentage of distribution of the antibiotic within the body. Although cephradine has five times the amount of unbound drug as cefazolin, cefazolin is administered less frequently and at a lower dosage. Other factors affect a drug's performance, including hepatic metabolism and renal excretion and reabsorption, which control the antibiotic's serum half-life. Each element becomes important in evaluating an agent's appropriateness for antimicrobial prophylactic efficacy.

Systemic antibiotics have been found to be ineffective in suppressing primary staphylococcal tissue infection if administered more than 3 hours after tissue inoculation occurs (Burke, 1961). This observation, along with other earlier work by Burke, provides the foundation for administering prophylactic antibiotics preoperatively. Burke (1961) stresses the importance of local tissue defense mechanisms acting within the initial 3 hours of contamination. This critical time interval determines the magnitude of the inflammation or infection that will develop over the following hours. After 3 hours, antibiotics will have no effect in suppressing pre-existing infection.

These data strongly indicate that in order for antimicrobial agents to be effective they must penetrate into the tissues in adequate concentrations preceding as well as during the initial 3–4 hours of bacterial contamination. Since contamination theoretically begins at the moment of incision, any effective prophylactic antibiotic must be temporally administered so that adequate preoperative tissue levels are achieved. After this, the medication must remain in the tissues during the initial 3 hours of possible wound contamination. Clinical data have demonstrated a decreasing efficacy of prophylactic antibiotics in abdominal or vaginal hysterectomy as the procedure's length approached 3 hours (Shapiro et al., 1982).

The prophylactic antibiotic must be administered at least 1 hour prior to the operation to allow the attainment of protective tissue levels. Subsequent doses protect against bacterial contamination that may occur after the moment of incision. Most investigators prefer to administer a preoperative dose followed by two postoperative doses at divided intervals within the first 24 hours. Prolonged postoperative courses of prophylactic antibiotics offer no further protective value over regimens administered on the day of surgery (Ledger et al., 1975). Unfortunately, this concept is not well appreciated and approximately 80% of patients received prophylactic antibiotics for 48 hours or longer in a review of several hospitals (Shapiro et al., 1979).

MICROBIOLOGICAL ASPECTS

Microbial flora

The presence of a specific organism on the skin or in the female genital tract does not of itself guarantee that the organism will cause an infection. The potential for infection by that organism exists if local mechanisms of host defense at that specific site falter. The organisms that commonly reside on the skin and in the female genital tract are only potentially pathogenic based on normal patterns of colonization. A review of surgical wound cultures from various procedures, including traumatic injuries and gastrointestinal surgeries, shows that *Staphylococcus aureus* is the most frequently isolated organism. *S. epidermidis* and *Corynebacterium* species (diphtheroids) are the next most frequent isolates. *Streptococcus*, *Escherichia coli*, and enterococci are found even less frequently but with equal prevalences. *Bacteroides fragilis* was isolated only one-tenth as often as *S. aureus* (Moellering *et al.*, 1977). While the presence of *S. aureus* in a wound indicates a pathogenic process, this assumption is seldom true for *S. epidermidis* and the corynebacteria, which are commonly encountered skin flora. One must therefore examine the normal flora of the skin and the female genital tract, and especially the potential pathogens, when selecting an appropriate prophylactic antibiotic for obstetric and gynecologic surgical procedures.

Various groups of organisms inhabit the skin of the normal host, including staphylococci, streptococci, anaerobic Gram-positive cocci, and corynebacteria, as well as *Bacillus* and *Neisseria* species, mycobacteria, fungi, and yeasts. The Gram-negative bacilli are not usually a part of the normal skin flora, although they colonize the skin immediately adjacent to the genitourinary and gastrointestinal tract orifices. They also appear on the skin of patients after prolonged hospitalization, as these organisms constitute a significant percentage of the hospital flora. Specific pathogens inhabiting the skin include *S. aureus*, beta-hemolytic and viridans group *Streptococcus*, and enterococci. The corynebacteria and coagulase-negative *Staphylococcus* species (*S. epidermidis*), although frequently encountered on the skin, are less virulent and seldom have clinical significance as pathogens.

Defining the flora of the normal female genital tract is more difficult. The results of vaginal cultures are often cited to represent this region, although they normally isolate greater quantities and varieties of organisms than are found in the endocervix. Because parturition, surgery, invasive carcinoma of the cervix, and estrogens all can act to alter the resident vaginal flora (Larsen and Galask, 1980), various patient populations may harbor different types and amounts of organisms.

The vaginal flora contains aerobic and anaerobic, Gram-positive and Gram-negative cocci and bacilli which form a dynamic, interrelated system. Mycoplasmas, Chlamydiae, mycobacteria, and yeasts coexist in this environment. *Corynebacterium* and *Lactobacillus* species are most frequently isolated from vaginal cultures. Quantitatively, the lactobacilli are the most abundant of any genus. Fortunately, their pathogenicity is minimal. Among the Gram-positive aerobic cocci, the group B streptococci, *Streptococcus agalactiae*, and the enterococci are frequently encountered organisms, along with group A beta-hemolytic streptococci and the viridans streptococci. Of these, the latter are usually pathogenic.

The role of the enterococcus as a pathogen in wound infections remains controversial, as it is often isolated from mixed aerobic and anaerobic infections. This organism clearly has demonstrated its pathogenicity at other sites ranging from heart to lungs to bladder.

S. agalactiae primarily infects neonates and does not have a significant role as a wound pathogen. Staphylococci also colonize the vagina, with *S. epidermidis* being isolated routinely. *S. aureus* infrequently inhabits this region. Aerobic Gram-negative bacilli are uncommon denizens of the vagina compared to the aerobic Gram-positive bacilli and the anaerobic organisms. The predominant enteric pathogen is *E. coli*, both as a colonizer of the vagina and as a pathogen.

Anaerobes other than the lactobacilli abound in the vagina with *Peptococcus*, *Peptostreptococcus*, and *Bacteroides* species among the more common isolates. *B. melaninogenicus* is isolated more frequently than *B. fragilis* both from the vagina and from female genital tract infections, from which it is isolated 16% and 10% of the time, respectively (Chow *et al.*, 1975). It is important to remember that as laboratory techniques have improved over the years, other *Bacteroides* species have also been identified as pathogens in pelvic infections.

These aforementioned organisms comprise the normal flora of most healthy women; however, variations in the quantities and occasionally the types of organisms do occur under specific circumstances. For example, pregnancy alters the vaginal flora primarily by decreasing the anaerobic population (Goplerud *et al.*, 1976) and increasing the aerobic lactobacilli and yeast populations. These observations do not imply that the gravid patient is free of other potential pathogens in her vagina, but illustrates the variable frequency of isolation of certain bacteria. On the third postpartum day after a vaginal delivery, the anaerobic organisms transiently increase in numbers and variety so that a return to predelivery rates of isolation is seen by the sixth postpartum week (Goplerud *et al.*, 1976).

Comparisons of cultures obtained from premenopausal and postmenopausal women reveal no statistically significant differences in the mean number of aerobes and anaerobes isolated per patient (Osborne *et al.*, 1979). Postmenopausal women treated with estrogens have a greater frequency of *Lactobacillus* species, while postmenopausal women not receiving estrogens have a higher rate of anaerobic bacteria (Larsen and Galask, 1980).

Prolonged ruptured membranes increase the risk of myometrial contamination and subsequent infection. Aerobic and anaerobic streptococci predominate among isolates obtained from amniotic fluid obtained at the time of cesarean section in women whose membranes were ruptured over 6 hours (Gilstrap and Cunningham, 1979). *E. coli* and *Bacteroides* species were present 21% and 23% of the time, respectively.

The presence of a malignancy also modifies the vaginal flora. Women with invasive carcinoma of the cervix have less frequent isolation of *Lactobacillus* species and *S. epidermidis*, while *E. coli* and *Clostridium perfringens* occur more frequently (Larsen and Galask, 1980). The clinical importance of this change remains undetermined.

Surgery of the female genital tract appears to alter the vaginal flora. In patients not receiving antibiotics, postoperative cultures following vaginal hysterectomy revealed an increase in the isolation of group D streptococci, *E. coli*, *Klebsiella pneumoniae*, and *B. fragilis* and a concomitant decrease in lactobacilli, corynebacteria, and *S. epidermidis* (Ohm and Galask, 1975; Grossman and Adams, 1979). Similar findings occurred in women undergoing total abdominal hysterectomy (Ohm and Galask, 1976; Grossman and Adams, 1979), although *K. pneumoniae* was less prominent and *Proteus mirabilis* more so in this cohort. Alterations in the vaginal flora such as described here may be an epiphenomenon secondary to increased colonization of the vagina by hospital flora. Postoperative cultures were obtained in these studies no sooner than 5 days following surgery – an adequate period for colonization to occur. Unfortunately, no study included a suitably matched control group of demographically matched women hospitalized for a similar duration but not undergoing genital tract surgery.

An altered vaginal flora in the postoperative period does not affect the choice of a preoperative prophylactic antibiotic, but it does provide assistance in selecting therapy for a postoperative pelvic infection. The actual effect of a prophylactic antibiotic on the vaginal flora is related to the duration of prophylaxis. Among women undergoing vaginal or abdominal hysterectomy, those receiving 5 days of cephalosporin therapy, combined (IM) cephaloridine and oral cephalexin, had increased isolation of cephalosporin-resistant organisms, primarily aerobic Gram-negative bacilli and especially *Pseudomonas aeruginosa*, than did the placebo-matched control population (Ohm and Galask, 1975, 1976). In a similar group of women receiving either IV penicillin G, cefazolin, or placebo over 2 days, there was no difference in vaginal flora among the three cohorts and no recovery of *Pseudomonas* organisms (Grossman and Adams, 1979).

In summary, the quantitative majority of organisms inhabiting the skin and vagina are nonpathogenic for most women. The population of pathogenic bacteria, irrespective of their decreased numbers of actual colonies isolated, remains the primary source of wound infections. These organisms include *S. aureus*, streptococci, *E. coli*, and *Bacteroides*.

Antimicrobial agents

General comments

An effective prophylactic antibiotic should act against the pathogens most likely to invade the operative site, but it need not act against every potential pathogen. Incisions of the vaginal mucosa create an opportunity for *S. aureus* and other Gram-positive cocci, as well as *E. coli* and *Bacteroides* species, to foster infection. These organisms become prime targets for prophylactic antibiotics, and the antimicrobial spectrum of activity should include these pathogens.

The adequacy of the antimicrobial agent also depends on factors such as incidence of adverse reactions, reasonable cost, and good tissue penetration. The shortened courses of currently administered prophylactic antibiotics have minimized the risk of the patient developing a complication of antibiotic therapy. Five-day courses of postoperative prophylactic antibiotics, in addition to showing no increased efficacy, expose the patient to an increased risk of an untoward reaction. Antibiotics limited to the day of surgery greatly reduce the potential for developing an antibiotic-associated colitis, granulocytopenia, or nephropathy. Early clinical trials used cephaloridine, a cephalosporin antibiotic that damaged the proximal renal tubules of certain patients. The usage of cephaloridine was subsequently discontinued as other equally effective and less toxic antibiotics became available.

The cost of an antibiotic is another factor that must be considered. Both the initial drug cost and the administration charges become important when comparing the advantages of one agent over another. The cost of administration becomes especially significant when comparing the various generations of cephalosporin antibiotics.

Finally, tissue penetration must be acceptable to ensure adequate delivery of the antibiotic to the interstitial fluid. The antibiotics currently in use achieve satisfactory levels in the soft tissues with only mild variations among the different groups.

Various classes of antibiotics offer different spectra of antimicrobial activity. Their efficacy in prophylaxis does not guarantee their effectiveness in treating an established infection, nor does their ability to treat an established infection guarantee their usefulness as prophylactic agents. For example, in one institution, 78% of *E. coli* isolates were susceptible to ampicillin (Moellering *et al.* 1977), a figure that may differ at other institutions. This frequency of susceptibility to ampicillin would justify its use prophylactically or empirically while awaiting susceptibility testing of a particular isolate, although another agent, such as gentamicin, would have to be administered if that one *E. coli* in four that is resistant to ampicillin is isolated. Gentamicin is an aminoglycoside antibiotic that is very active against *E. coli*; however, its use as a prophylactic agent is inappropriate because of the risk of developing gentamicin-resistant organisms.

While antibiotic susceptibilities differ somewhat among hospitals, certain patterns of resistance and sensitivity have been sufficiently established to permit generalizations regarding the choice of an antibiotic for a specific organism. Exceptions to this generalization occur and mandate that the physician be familiar with the susceptibility patterns of his own facility.

Penicillin

The penicillins may be categorized into one of three groups: (1) ampicillin and the various forms of penicillin G, (2) the anti-staphylococcal penicillins, and (3) the newer extended-spectrum or anti-pseudomonal penicillins. The resistance of 85% of *S. aureus* organisms to penicillins other than the anti-staphylococcal or penicillinase-resistant penicillins diminishes the usefulness of these agents in its treatment. Penicillin G and ampicillin inhibit the enterococci better than other antibiotics, although they often are combined with an aminoglycoside when treating an enterococcal infection other than a simple cystitis. The penicillinase-resistant penicillins, such as nafcillin, are ineffective against anaerobes and Gram-negative aerobic bacilli. The anti-pseudomonal penicillins, such as ticarcillin, azlocillin, carbenicillin, mezlocillin, and pipericillin, possess varying degrees of activity against specific Gram-negative aerobic and anaerobic bacilli. Unfortunately, they are ineffective against penicillinase-producing staphylococci. These characteristics highlight the strengths and weaknesses of the penicillins in preoperative prophylaxis (Table 2).

Table 2 Acceptability of penicillins for prophylaxis

Organism	Penicillin	Ampicillin	Nafcillin	Ticarcillin
Staphylococcus aureus	−	−	+	−
Group A streptococci	+	+	+	+
Alpha-hemolytic streptococci	+	+	+	+
Enterococci	+	+	−	−
Escherichia coli	−	+	−	+
Anaerobic cocci	+	+	−	+
Bacteroides fragilis	−	−	−	+
Other Bacteroides species	+	+	−	+

Cephalosporins

The cephalosporins usually classify into first-, second-, or third-generation agents. The first-generation cephalosporins are similar and share the same spectrum of antimicrobial activity. Their resistance to beta-lactamases broadens their coverage to include most S. aureus and E. coli organisms; however, B. fragilis remains resistant. Cephalothin is the representative drug for this generation, although cefazolin is frequently used because of its comparatively prolonged half-life.

The second-generation cephalosporins consist of cefoxitin, cefamandole, and cefuroxime, each of which has a different antimicrobial spectrum. Cefoxitin is relatively resistant to the effects of the beta-lactamase-producing bacteria, which explains its activity against S. aureus, certain Gram-negative aerobic bacilli, and several anaerobes, including B. fragilis. Cefamandole shares a similar spectrum but lacks significant activity against B. fragilis. Treatment failures have been reported when this agent was used against apparently susceptible Gram-negative bacilli. Cefuroxime was released in the USA in 1983 after years of clinical experience in Europe. Its spectrum of activity is similar to that of cefoxitin but it also lacks significant activity against B. fragilis.

In comparison to the first- and second-generation agents, the third-generation cephalosporins have increased activity against Gram-negative aerobic bacilli, including some strains of Pseudomonas, but decreased activity against Gram-positive aerobic cocci. Individually, these drugs differ regarding their effectiveness against the Enterobacteriaceae, the Pseudomonadaceae, and the anaerobic bacilli. Antimicrobial susceptibility patterns for one agent cannot be applied to the others. Four of these drugs are currently available: cefoperazone, cefotaxime, ceftazoxime, and moxalactam; other variations remain under investigation.

Cefotaxime has been chosen to represent this class of drugs for prophylactic

Table 3 Acceptability of cephalosporins for prophylaxis

Organism	Cephalothin	Cefoxitin	Cefamandole	Cefotaxime
Staphylococcus aureus	+	+	+	+
Group A streptococci	+	+	+	+
Alpha-hemolytic streptococci	+	+	+	+
Enterococci	−	−	−	−
Escherichia coli	+	+	+	+
Anaerobic cocci	+	+	+	+
Bacteroides fragilis	−	+	−	−
Other Bacteroides species	+	+	+	+

purposes only (Table 3). Actual therapy of an infection secondary to these organisms would require antibiotic sensitivity testing with the caveat that cephalosporins are not the first choice of treatment for any organism. Cephalosporins are uniformly ineffective in treating the enterococci, and enterococcal superinfection has been noted with prolonged moxalactam therapy. Other adverse effects associated with this drug more than the other third-generation cephalosporins are bleeding disorders and the disulfiram reaction. Cefaperazone also has the potential for this latter reaction, which may occur within 72 hours after prior ingestion of alcohol.

Other Agents

The tetracyclines are possible candidates for prophylactic therapy, particularly now that preparations for IV administration are available. The newer modifications of the basic tetracycline molecule, doxycycline and minocycline, possess extended activity against B. fragilis and S. aureus, in the case of the former, and E. coli, in the latter case. The bacteriostatic nature of these agents and the frequency with which resistance is found among these bacteria detract from their clinical usefulness. These agents are also ineffective against the enterococci.

The aminoglycosides are reserved for treatment of serious infections secondary to the Gram-negative aerobic bacilli. Their use as prophylactic agents is actively discouraged to prevent the development of resistant organisms. Clindamycin is effective against B. fragilis and most anaerobes except some Clostridium species. It has no activity against Gram-negative aerobic rods but does provide coverage against nonenterococcal streptococci and many strains of S. aureus. The risk that antibiotic-associated colitis and resistant organisms might develop during clindamycin therapy, as well as its narrow spectrum have minimized its use in prophylaxis. Metronidazole has activity against anaerobes, but it is ineffective against aerobic bacteria. Although a few clinical trials have assessed the efficacy of metronidazole, the data are currently insufficient to advocate its use for prophylaxis; it appears to be as effective as cephalothin (Hamod et al., 1980).

Chloramphenicol is a bacteriostatic drug that is active against most bacteria; however, its association with an idiosyncratic reaction causing aplastic anemia has limited its usage to cases of severe infections in which other agents are inappropriate or in which susceptibility has been demonstrated. Parenteral erythromycin and trimethoprim-sulfamethoxazole are not employed as prophylactic antibiotics but are reserved for treatment of specific infecting organisms. Vancomycin is active against Gram-positive aerobic cocci, including enterococci. Its expense and narrow spectrum make it an unacceptable prophylactic agent except under very special circumstances.

CLINICAL STUDIES

Vaginal hysterectomy

The incidence of febrile morbidity following vaginal hysterectomy has approached 80% in some series, while the rate of pelvic infections has exceeded 60% (Hamod et al., 1982). Other studies have revealed lower, but nonetheless elevated rates of infectious morbidity. Initial analyses of factors that might increase the risk of postoperative fever and infection have suggested that premenopausal women constitute a high-risk group, especially if they had undergone surgery during the secretory phase of their menstrual cycle. Subsequent studies have contested this theory. Surgical factors, such as the quantity of operative blood loss and the necessity of performing a concurrent anterior or posterior repair appear to be unrelated to infectious morbidity (Hamod et al., 1982). Prolonged procedures, however, increase the risk of postoperative infection (Shapiro et al., 1982).

Studies evaluating the efficacy of prophylactic antibiotics in reducing the incidence of postoperative infectious complications have demonstrated that these agents reduce both febrile morbidity and pelvic infection in women undergoing vaginal hysterectomy. Although various studies have utilized differing criteria for defining infectious morbidity and varying types and doses of antibiotics, the results have been similar.

Two groups of studies exist: those employing a single dose or at most 24 hours of prophylactic antibiotics (Table 4), and those using antibiotics for prolonged postoperative courses (Table 5). The latter studies have been selectively presented, primarily for hisorical interest and comparison purposes, since the effectiveness of short-course prophylactic antibiotics in diminishing infectious complications after vaginal hysterectomy has already been established. Of the agents used in the single-day prophylaxis trials, seven were first-generation cephalosporins. The remainder of the studies reviewed dealt with the efficacy of carbenicillin, cefoxitin, and metronidazole, all agents with greater anaerobic activity than the first-generation cephalosporin antibiotics.

During these investigations no single agent emerged as superior to the others to a degree that it could be formally endorsed as the drug of choice for prophylaxis preceding vaginal hysterectomy. Overall, a single dose of cefazolin appears to be adequate prophylaxis; in some cases two subsequent doses at 8-hour intervals may be preferable. The other first-generation parenteral cephalosporins are equally effective and less costly than cefoxitin or metronidazole.

Table 4 Single-day prophylactic antibiotics and vaginal hysterectomy

| | | Incidence of febrile morbidity or infection | |
| | | Placebo (%) | Antibiotics (%) |
Authors	Drug studied		
Ledger et al., 1973	Cephaloridine	60	36
Breeden and Mayo, 1974	Cephaloridine	32	8
Lett et al., 1977	Cephaloridine	49	12
Lett et al., 1977	Cefazolin	49	8
Holman et al., 1978	Cefazolin	36	10
Roberts and Homesley, 1978	Carbenicillin	35	8
Mendelson et al., 1979	Cephradine (one-dose)	86	13
Mendelson et al., 1979	Cephradine (five-dose)	86	0
Mickal et al., 1980	Cefoxitin	30	10
Polk et al., 1980	Cefazolin	31[a]	14[a]
		21[b]	2[b]
Vincelette et al., 1983	Metronidazole	45[a]	44[a]
		22[b]	15[b]

[a] Febrile morbidity
[b] Surgical site infection

Table 5 Multiple-day antibiotics and vaginal hysterectomy

| | | Incidence of febrile morbidity or infection | |
| | | Placebo (%) | Antibiotic (%) |
Authors	Drug studied		
Allen et al., 1972	Cephalothin	50	4
Ohm and Galask, 1975	Cephaloridine/cephalexin	48	0
Jennings, 1978	Cefazolin/cephalexin	75[a]	21[a]
		33[b]	2[b]
Grossman et al., 1979	Cefazolin	67	39
Grossman et al., 1979	Penicillin	67	39

[a] Febrile morbidity
[b] Surgical site infection

Abdominal hysterectomy

The data regarding the efficacy of prophylactic antibiotics in reducing postoperative infections following abdominal hysterectomy are more difficult to interpret than the vaginal hysterectomy trials. Although abdominal hysterectomy is performed approximately twice as frequently as vaginal hysterectomy and the operation itself is considered a risk factor for developing an operative site infection (Shapiro et al., 1982), the incidence of postoperative wound infection associated with it is markedly lower (Amirikia and Evans, 1979) and the need for prophylactic antibiotics clearly less well established.

The clinical trials designed to evaluate a single day or less of prophylaxis (Table 6) have used a variety of antibiotics, including cefazolin, cefoxitin,

Table 6 Single-day prophylactic antibiotics and abdominal hysterectomy

| | | Incidence of febrile morbidity or infection | |
| | | Placebo (%) | Antibiotic (%) |
Authors	Drug studied		
Holman et al., 1978	Cefazolin	71[a]	19[a]
		37[b]	20[b]
Roberts and Homesley, 1979	Carbenicillin	54	4
Polk et al., 1980	Cefazolin	20[c]	14[c]
		21[d]	14[d]
Duff, 1982	Cefoxitin	28	24
Vincelette et al., 1983	Metronidazole	30[c]	28[c]
		13[d]	13[d]

[a] Premenopausal
[b] Postmenopausal
[c] Febrile morbidity
[d] Surgical site infection

carbenicillin, and metronidazole. Only one study (Holman et al., 1978) demonstrated a significant decrease in febrile morbidity and operative site infection primarily in premenopausal patients but also in the postmenopausal group. The other studies did not segregate their patient data to explore this aspect further. The carbenicillin trial had a significant decrease in postoperative urinary tract infections in the treated group, which accounted for its decreased febrile morbidity. The other studies report fewer wound and urinary tract infections but no difference in the incidence of pelvic cellulitis (Polk et al., 1980) or of postoperative infectious complications. The longer courses of therapy (Table 7) demonstrate a decrease in febrile morbidity, but only two (Allen et al., 1972; Jennings, 1978) had significant reductions in wound infections.

The data currently available are ambiguous on the value of prophylactic antibiotics in reducing the rate of postoperative wound infections in women undergoing abdominal hysterectomy. Until new data appear the routine administration of antibiotic prophylaxis to women about to undergo this operation appears unjustified.

Cesarean section

Febrile morbidity following cesarean section ranges from 27% to 85% as compared to 10% for vaginal delivery (Swartz and Grolle, 1981). Numerous investigators have suggested factors that may predispose a woman having a cesarean section to develop an infectious complication. No consistency exists among data regarding the risk of infection for a primary as compared with a repeat section, for ruptured as compared with intact membranes, for general anesthesia, anemia, obesity, multiple vaginal examinations during labor, and the level of surgical skill.

Most studies addressing the significance of febrile morbidity following primary or repeat cesarean section conclude that there is increased morbidity among the primary sections because of the frequently associated prolonged

Table 7 Multiple-day prophylactic antibiotics and abdominal hysterectomy

Authors	Drug studied	Incidence of febrile morbidity or infection	
		Placebo (%)	Antibiotic (%)
Allen et al., 1972	Cephalothin	41	14
Ohm and Galask, 1976	Cephaloridine/cephalexin	39	15
Jennings, 1978	Cefazolin/cephalexin	46[a]	24[a]
		12[b]	0[b]
Grossman et al., 1979	Cefazolin	30	22
Grossman et al., 1979	Penicillin	30	17

[a] Febrile morbidity
[b] Surgical site infection

labor and existence of ruptured membranes (Gibbs et al., 1973). Adequate data exist to implicate prolonged membrane rupture with an increased incidence of postoperative febrile morbidity. Other series report an increased incidence of postoperative endometritis and febrile morbidity in women who have a cesarean section after labor has begun (D'Angelo and Sokol, 1980). Prolonged labor or ruptured membranes usually necessitates internal fetal monitoring, but this practice is not associated with increased frequency or severity of postpartum infections in women undergoing cesarean section (Gibbs et al., 1978). The observation that patients admitted to a teaching service instead of a private service have an increased risk of developing an infectious complication following a cesarean section may be associated with the type of patient likely to be admitted to a teaching service, rather than with the skill of the surgeon in training.

Most studies of the efficacy of prophylactic antibiotics in cesarean sections categorize infectious complications into one of the four following groups: (1) febrile morbidity, (2) endometritis, (3) wound infection, and (4) urinary tract infection. Prophylactic antibiotics have definitely reduced the incidence of the first two, but their effect on the latter two is equivocal. A sampling of the literature reveals several definitions of febrile morbidity, usually consisting of two distinct temperature elevations above a predetermined set point after the first 24 hours. Regardless of the definition utilized, prophylactic antibiotics are effective in decreasing this complication.

Phelan and Pruyn (1979) found a decrease in endometritis and febrile morbidity from 38% in the placebo group to 16% in the treated cohort, using IV cefazolin within 12 hours perioperatively. Cefoxitin also appears effective in this setting, reducing the febrile morbidity from 24% to 6%. Patients hospitalized for longer than 7 days because of infectious morbidity included 26% of the cefoxitin group, 57% of the placebo control, and, interestingly, 66% of a third group receiving cefazolin (Stiver et al., 1983). Both cefazolin and cefoxitin had similar rates of febrile morbidity.

The administration of the antibiotic in cesarean section may be timed to avoid delivering a dose to the newborn child. Although no adverse effects of prophylactic antibiotics on the neonate have been reported, theoretical considerations favor minimizing any potential risk to the newborn. Ampicillin administered immediately after cord clamping is as effective as a preoperative dose of the same drug (Gordon *et al.*, 1979). Other studies have confirmed this finding for ticarcillin and cefoxitin. Irrigation of the uterus with cefamandole may prove to be another effective means of decreasing postpartum infection (Rudd *et al.*, 1982) while avoiding any possibility of affecting the infant; the one existing study must be confirmed with randomized concurrent placebo controls.

Elective abortion

Inadequate data exist to assess the value of prophylactic antibiotics in reducing pelvic infections following elective first-trimester abortions. Danish investigators administered IM penicillin perioperatively and oral pivampicillin postoperatively for 4 days to a group of women undergoing elective first-trimester abortions. Only among those women with prior pelvic inflammatory disease was a significant decrease in infection noted (Sonne-Holm *et al.*, 1981). The other published trial suffers from flaws in the study design.

BACTERIAL ENDOCARDITIS PROPHYLAXIS

The American Heart Association recommends using penicillin and streptomycin primarily for prophylaxis against the alpha-hemolytic streptococci whenever performing a surgical procedure on the genitourinary tract of a patient with valvular heart disease. The incidence of bacteremia associated with such manipulation creates a risk for establishing a nidus of infection on a prosthetic or morphologically altered cardiac valve. The addition of streptomycin provides extended coverage against the enterococci. Ampicillin and gentamicin are acceptable substitutions for penicillin and streptomycin, respectively. In penicillin-allergic patients, vancomycin is recommended (Table 8) (AHA, 1977).

This prophylaxis is not required for a dilatation and curettage (D&C) procedure, the insertion or removal of an intrauterine contraceptive device, the insertion of a urinary tract catheter, performance of a pelvic examination, or an uncomplicated vaginal delivery because the development of endocarditis following these procedures is rare. Endocarditis has occurred following septic abortion and peripartum infections, although treatment of the underlying infection would obviate the need to use additional prophylactic antibiotics. Patients with prosthetic cardiac valves are generally treated extremely conservatively; prophylaxis is recommended for most procedures except routine pelvic examination and urinary catheterization.

Two additional categories of patients pose dilemmas: those with mitral valve prolapse and those with other indwelling prosthetic devices. The necessity for endocarditis prophylaxis in patients with mitral valve prolapse is uncertain at present. The protean manifestations of this condition create a spectrum of risk for developing endocarditis. Many physicians prefer to employ endocarditis prophylaxis in these patients only if a significant degree of mitral regurgitation is manifest. Patients with indwelling prosthetic devices such as vascular grafts

Table 8 American Heart Association recommendations: bacterial endocarditis prophylaxis for genitourinary tract surgery in adults

Penicillin-tolerant	Penicillin-allergic
Aqueous crystalline penicillin G (2 million units, IM or IV) or Ampicillin (1 gram, IM or IV) plus Gentamicin (1.5 mg/kg (80 mg max), IM or IV) or Streptomycin (1 gram, IM) given 30–60 minutes before the procedure and repeated every 8 hours × 2 doses for gentamicin and penicillin/ampicillin or every 12 hours × 2 doses for streptomycin and penicillin/ampicillin	Vancomycin (1 gram, IV given over 30–60 minutes) plus Streptomycin (1 gram, IM) given 3–60 minutes before the procedure. A second dose may be necessary in 12 hours for prolonged procedures

should be treated as if they have a prosthetic cardiac valve. Those patients without vascular prostheses but with ventriculoperitoneal shunts, prosthetic joints, or other indwelling artificial devices are not at increased risk for endocarditis, although the risk of infection at the prosthetic site may be increased. There are inadequate data to recommend prophylactic antibiotics in these patients; each case must be addressed individually.

CONCLUSIONS

Multiple clinical trials have appeared in the literature promoting the efficacy of prophylactic antibiotics for various surgical procedures. Many of these studies are flawed because of their original study design. Any physician assessing these trials must be familiar with the components of a well-designed study.

The Gram-positive aerobic cocci, particularly *S. aureus*, and the Gram-negative anaerobic bacilli, primarily *B. fragilis*, are the major pathogens encountered in the female genital tract. *E. coli* (a Gram-negative aerobic rod), the streptococci, and other anaerobic bacteria also frequently cause postoperative infections following vaginal hysterectomy or cesarean section. Prophylactic antibiotics should have activity against most, but not necessarily all, of these organisms.

The cephalosporins have emerged as the prophylactic agents of choice after appropriate clinical investigations. Their ease of administration, low incidence of side-effects, and broad spectrum of activity make them ideal. Cefazolin, with its longer half-life and higher tissue levels, has emerged the leading first-generation agent. Notwithstanding their extended aerobic and anaerobic spectra, the second- and third-generation cephalosporins have never been shown to be superior to first-generation agents for perioperative prophylaxis in obstetric and gynecologic surgery.

PREOPERATIVE AND INTRAOPERATIVE ANTIBIOTICS

The perioperative administration of prophylactic antibiotics reduces the incidence of febrile morbidity and operative site infections following vaginal hysterectomy. Routine use in the perioperative period is recommended. Whether future studies of newer antibiotics can be conducted with an untreated control group remains doubtful. This recommendation does not extend to abdominal hysterectomy where the results of various investigations have not shown an unequivocal benefit from prophylactic antibiotics. Further research is needed in this area.

Prophylactic antibiotics reduced the incidence of endometritis and febrile morbidity following cesarean section. Patients on teaching services in active labor should receive antibiotic coverage. This may be administered as a single dose given preoperatively or immediately after clamping the umbilical cord. Women undergoing primary section or with prolonged membrane rupture should also be considered for therapy. Administration of these agents to women having an elective repeat section is optional.

Antibiotics are not routinely recommended for women having an elective first-trimester abortion. They may prove beneficial, however, if the woman has a history of prior pelvic inflammatory disease.

The views expressed are solely those of the authors and not those of the United States Air Force or the Department of Defense.

References

AHA, Committee on Rheumatic Fever and Bacterial Endocarditis of the Council on Cardiovascular Disease in the Young (1977). Prevention of bacterial endocarditis. *Circulation*, **56**, 139A

Allen, J. L., Rampone, J. F. and Wheeless, C. R. (1972). Use of a prophylactic antibiotic in elective major gynecologic operations. *Obstet. Gynecol.*, **39**, 218

Amirikia, H. and Evans, T. N. (1979). Ten-year review of hysterectomies: Trends, indications, and risks. *Am. J. Obstet. Gynecol.*, **134**, 431

Berger, S. A., Nagar, H. and Gordon, M. (1980). Antimicrobial prophylaxis in obstetric and gynecologic surgery. *J. Reprod. Med.*, **24**, 185

Berger, S. A., Nagar, H. and Weitzman, S. (1978). Prophylactic antibiotics in surgical procedures. *Surg. Gynecol. Obstet.*, **146**, 469

Breeden, J. T., Mayo, J. E. (1974). Low dose prophylactic antibiotics in vaginal hysterectomy. *Obstet. Gynecol.*, **43**, 379

Burke, J. F. (1967). The effective period of preventive antibiotic action in experimental incisions and dermal lesions. *Surgery*, **50**, 161

Chodak, G. W. and Plaut, M. E. (1977). Use of systemic antibiotics for prophylaxis in surgery. *Arch. Surg.*, **112**, 326

Chodak, G. W. and Plaut, M. E. (1978). Wound infections and systemic antibiotic prophylaxis in gynecologic surgery. *Obstet. Gynecol.*, **51**, 123

Chow, A. W., Marshall, J. R. and Guze, L. B. (1975). Anaerobic infections of the female genital tract: Prospects and perspectives. *Obstet. Gynecol. Surv.*, **30**, 477

Cruse, P. J. E. and Foord, R. (1973). A five-year prospective study of 23,649 surgical wounds. *Arch. Surg.*, **107**, 206

D'Angelo, L. J. and Sokol, R. J. (1980). Time-related peripartum determinants of postpartum morbidity. *Obstet. Gynecol.*, **55**, 319

Duff, P. (1982). Antibiotic prophylaxis for abdominal hysterectomy. *Obstet. Gynecol.*, **60**, 25

Gibbs, R. S., Hunt, J. E. and Schwarz, R. H. (1973). A follow-up study on prophylactic antibiotic in cesarean section. *Am. J. Obstet. Gynecol.*, **117**, 419

Gibbs, R. S., Jones, P. M. and Wilder, C. J. Y. (1978). Internal fetal monitoring and maternal infection following cesarean section. *Obstet. Gynecol.*, **52**, 193

Gilstrap III, L. C. and Cunningham, F. C. (1979). The bacterial pathogenesis of infection following cesarean section. *Obstet. Gynecol.*, **53**, 545

Goplerud, C. P., Ohm, M. J. and Galask, R. P. (1976). Aerobic and anaerobic flora of the cervix during pregnancy and the puerperium. *Am. J. Obstet. Gynecol.*, **126**, 858

Gordon, H. R., Phelps, D. and Blanchard, K. (1979). Prophylactic cesarean section antibiotics: Maternal and neonatal morbidity before or after cord clamping. *Obstet. Gynecol.*, **53**, 151

Grossman III, J. H. and Adams, R. L. (1979). Vaginal flora in women undergoing hysterectomy with antibiotic prophylaxis. *Obstet. Gynecol.*, **53**, 23

Grossman III, J. H., Greco, T. P., Minkin, M., Adams, R. L., Hierholzer, W. J. Jr., Andriole, V. T. (1979). Prophylactic antibiotics in gynecologic surgery. *Obstet. Gynecol.*, **53**, 537

Hamod, K. A., Spence, M. R. and King, T. M. (1982). Prophylactic antibiotics in vaginal hysterectomy: a review. *Obstet. Gynecol. Surv.*, **37**, 207

Hamod, K. A., Spence, M. R., Rosenshein, N. B. *et al.* (1980). Single-dose and multidose prophylaxis in vaginal hysterectomy: a comparison of sodium cephalothin and metronidazole. *Am. J. Obstet. Gynecol.*, **136**, 976

Hirschmann, J. V. and Inui, T. S. (1980). Antimicrobial prophylaxis: a critique of recent trials. *Rev. Infect. Dis.*, **2**, 1

Holman, J. F., McGowan, J. E. and Thompson, J. D. (1978). Perioperative antibiotics in major elective gynecologic surgery. *S. Med. J.*, **71**, 417

Jennings, R. H. (1978). Prophylactic antibiotics in vaginal and abdominal hysterectomy. *S. Med. J.*, **71**, 251

Larsen, B. and Galask, R. P. (1980). Vaginal microbial flora: practical and theoretical relevance. *Obstet. Gynecol. Suppl.*, **55**, 100S

Ledger, W. J., Sweet, R. L., Headington, J. T. (1973). Prophylactic cephaloridine in the prevention of postoperative pelvic infections in premenopausal women undergoing vaginal hysterectomy. *Am. J. Obstet. Gynecol.*, **115**, 766

Ledger, W. J., Gee, C. and Lewis, W. P. (1975). Guidelines for antibiotic prophylaxis in gynecology. *Am. J. Obstet. Gynecol.*, **121**, 1038

Lett, W. J., Ansbacher, R., Davison, B. L., Otterson, W. N. (1977). Prophylactic antibiotics for women undergoing vaginal hysterectomy. *J. Reprod. Med.*, **19**, 51

Mendelson, J., Portnoy, J., De Saint Victor, J. R., Gelfand, M. M. (1979). Effect of single and multidose cephradine prophylaxis on infectious morbidity of vaginal hysterectomy. *Obstet. Gynecol.*, **53**, 31

Mickal, A., Curole, D., Lewis, C. (1980). Cefoxitin sodium: double-blind vaginal hysterectomy prophylaxis in premenopausal patients. *Obstet. Gynecol.*, **56**, 222

Moellering Jr., P. C., Kung, K. J., Poitras, J. W. *et al.* (1977). Microbiologic basis for the rational use of prophylactic antibiotics. *S. Med. J. Suppl.*, **70**, 8

National Research Council, Division of Medical Sciences, Ad Hoc Committee of the Committee on Trauma. (1964). Post-operative wound infections: the influence of ultraviolet irradiation of the operation room and of various other factors. *Ann. Surg.*, **160** (Suppl. 2), 1

Neu, H. C. (1977). Clinical pharmacokinetics in preventive antimicrobial therapy. *S. Med. J. Suppl.*, **70**, 14

Ohm, M. J. and Galask, R. P. (1975). The effect of antibiotic prophylaxis on patients undergoing vaginal operations. *Am. J. Obstet. Gynecol.*, **123**, 590

Ohm, M. J., Galask, R. P. (1975). The effect of antibiotic prophylaxis on patients undergoing vaginal operations: II. alterations of microbial flora. *Am. J. Obstet. Gynecol.* **123**, 597

Ohm, M. J. and Galask, R. P. (1976). The effect of antibiotic prophylaxis on patients undergoing total abdominal hysterectomy. *Am. J. Obstet. Gynecol.*, **125**, 442

Ohm, M. J., Galask, R. P. (1976). The effect of antibiotic prophylaxis on patients undergoing total abdominal hysterectomy. *Am. J. Obstet. Gynecol.*, **125**, 448

Osborne, N. G., Wright, R. C. and Grubin, L. (1979). Genital bacteriology: A comparative study of premenopausal women with postmenopausal women. *Am. J. Obstet. Gynecol.*, **135**, 195

Phelan, J. P. and Pruyn, S. C. (1979). Prophylactic antibiotics in cesarean sections: A double-blind study of cefazolin. *Am. J. Obstet. Gynecol.*, **133**, 474

Polk, B. F., Shapiro, M., Goldstein, P. *et al.* (1980). Randomized clinical trial of perioperative cefazolin in preventing infection after hysterectomy. *Lancet*, **1**, 438

Roberts, J. M., Homesley, H. D. (1978). Low-dose carbenicillin prophylaxis for vaginal and abdominal hysterectomy. *Obstet. Gynecol.*, **52**, 83

Rudd, E. G., Cobey, E. A., Long, W. H. *et al.* (1982). Prevention of endomyometritis using antibiotic irrigation during cesarean section. *Obstet. Gynecol.*, **60**, 413

Shapiro, M., Munoz, A., Tager, I. B. *et al.* (1982). Risk factors for infection at the operative site after abdominal or vaginal hysterectomy. *N. Engl. J. Med.*, **307**, 1661

Shapiro, M., Schoenbaum, S. C., Tager, I. B. *et al.* (1983). Benefit–cost analysis of antimicrobial prophylaxis in abdominal and vaginal hysterectomy. *J. Am. Med. Assoc.*, **249**, 1290

Shapiro, M., Townsend, T. R., Rosner, B. *et al.* (1979). Use of antimicrobial drugs in general hospitals. *N. Engl. J. Med.*, **301**, 351

Sonne-Holm, S., Heisterberg, L., Hebjorn, S. *et al.* (1981). Prophylactic antibiotics in first-trimester abortions: A clinical, controlled trial. *Am. J. Obstet. Gynecol.*, **139**, 693

Stiver, H. G., Forward, K. R., Livingstone, R. A. *et al.* (1983). Multicenter comparison of cefoxitin versus cefazolin for prevention of infectious morbidity after nonelective cesarean section. *Am. J. Obstet. Gynecol.*, **145**, 158

Swartz, W. H. and Grolle, K. (1981). The use of prophylactic antibiotics in cesarean section. *J. Reprod. Med.*, **26**, 595

Vincelette, J., Finkelstein, F., Aoki, F. Y. *et al.* (1983). Double-blind trial of perioperative intravenous metronidazole prophylaxis for abdominal and vaginal hysterectomy. *Surgery*, **93**, 185

21
Pharmacokinetics and antimicrobial agents during pregnancy

P. J. JEWESSON and A. W. CHOW

PRINCIPLES OF ANTIMICROBIAL DRUG USAGE DURING PREGNANCY AND PUERPERIUM

Almost any infection that may be encountered in the nonpregnant individual can also occur during pregnancy. Pregnancy, however, influences both the frequency and nature of such infections. Some, such as bacteriuria and pyelonephritis, pose a particular threat to both mother and fetus. Others, such as syphilis and toxoplasmosis, may be relatively innocuous to the mother while resulting in high perinatal morbidity and mortality or congenital malformations. In contrast, certain infections such as cestodiasis (tapeworms) or giardiasis seldom pose any hazard either to the mother or fetus. In fact, the need for antimicrobial therapy in these latter instances is primarily determined by the safety and efficacy of available drugs.

Physicians managing infections during pregnancy must be equally cognizant of those circumstances under which antimicrobial therapy is urgent, and those for which antimicrobial therapy is best postponed until after delivery.

MATERNAL PHYSIOLOGIC AND PHARMACOKINETIC CONSIDERATIONS

The dynamic interactions of drug absorption, distribution, receptor activity, metabolism, and elimination are closely linked in at least three major functional compartments, those of the mother, placenta, and the fetus (Fig. 1). During pregnancy, a woman undergoes several physiologic changes that modify the pharmacokinetics of therapeutic agents. Important among these are maternal adaptations to increase the delivery of blood and nutrients to the fetus and to remove metabolic waste products from the mother and her fetus (Nation, 1980; Krauer and Krauer, 1977). These adaptations generally result

311

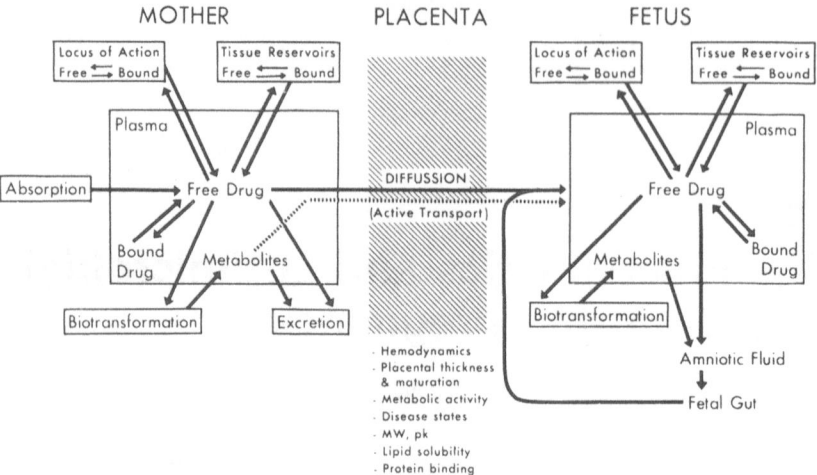

Fig. 1 Major pathways and interrelationships of drug pharmacokinetics in the mother, fetus, and placenta

in a marked increase in the intravascular and extravascular fluid volumes, the enhancement of cardiac output, renal blood flow, glomerular filtration rate, and augmentation of hepatic and other metabolic activities in the mother, fetus, and placenta (Ledger, 1977). As a consequence, the volume of distribution, as well as the metabolic degradation and renal clearance of a drug, can significantly alter in comparison with the nonpregnant state.

A decrease of plasma albumin concentration is also observed during pregnancy. This change may directly affect the ratio of bound versus free fractions of many antimicrobials and ultimately result in a lower total serum level of the drug, an increase in the tissue/plasma distribution ratio and an increase in the rate of drug clearance from the body.

Maternal gastrointestinal tone and motility may be diminished due to physical displacement by the enlarging uterus. This results in delayed gastric emptying and prolonged intestinal transit. Effects such as these may influence the bioavailability and effectiveness of drugs with acid-labile properties or site-specific absorption from the intestinal tract. Finally, the progressive thinning of the fetomaternal barrier as gestation advances results in increased transplacental diffusion and alternative routes of drug elimination from the mother (Krauer and Krauer, 1977; Landers et al., 1983).

The therapeutic implications of these pregnancy-associated physiologic changes are summarized in Table 1. Their net effect is that maternal antimicrobial concentrations tend to be lower than those reported for similar doses in nonpregnant patients. Overall, the percentage decrease ranges from 10% to 50% during late pregnancy (Landers et al., 1983), as was demonstrated for aminoglycosides (Good and Johnson, 1971; Weinstein et al., 1976), ampicillin (Philipson, 1977), and cefazolin (Bernard et al., 1977). Other antimicrobials for which decreased serum levels are likely in pregnancy include methicillin, cephalexin, cephalothin, the newer cephalosporins, erythromycin, and nitrofurantoin. Specific data, however, are lacking. Agents for which levels are probably unchanged in preg-

Table 1 Pregnancy associated physiologic alterations and their potential effect on antimicrobial pharmacokinetic parameters

Physiologic alteration during pregnancy	Pharmacokinetic effect	Therapeutic implications
Decreased gastrointestinal motility	Inhibit or enhance rate or extent of drug absorption	Unpredictable absorption of orally administered drugs
Expanded intravascular and extravascular volume	Increased volume of drug distribution Decreased plasma drug concentrations	Higher loading doses and more frequent dosing may be required
	Reduced plasma protein concentrations ↑ Drug clearance ↓ Total drug concentration ↑ Tissue/plasma drug distribution	Plasma concentrations of total drug will underestimate concentration of free drug and may lead to unnecessary increase in drug dosage
Thinning of fetomaternal barrier with advancing gestation	Increased transplacental diffusion Decreased maternal plasma concentration	Increase in drug dosage and adjustment of dosing interval may be required
Increased progesterone-activated hepatic drug metabolism	Increased rate of drug biotransformation to active or inactive metabolites Contribution by placenta and fetal liver possible	Increase in drug dosage and adjustment of dosing interval may be required
Increased renal blood flow and glomerular filtration rate	Increased drug clearance Decreased plasma drug concentrations	Increase in drug dosage and adjustment of dosing interval may be required

nancy include cephaloridine, clindamycin, chloramphenicol, metronidazole, and trimethoprim-sulfamethoxazole (Landers *et al.*, 1983).

The maternal adaptive changes likely to influence drug pharmacokinetics are most evident in the third trimester of pregnancy; however, the degree of change varies considerably from individual to individual.

FETAL EXPOSURE TO ANTIMICROBIAL DRUGS

Placental transfer and amniotic fluid

Antimicrobial drugs reach the fetus by placental transfer or by achieving sufficient concentrations in the amniotic fluid. Movement of compounds across the placenta is generally bidirectional, although net transfer occurs from mother to fetus for most substances. The transplacental passage of antimicrobials is regulated by many factors; the principal ones are the physiologic characteristics of the maternal–placental–fetal unit and the physiochemical properties of the drug (Mirkin, 1975). Physiologic factors include (1) hemodynamic changes in the maternal or fetal contribution to total placental blood flow, (2) the thickness and maturation of the placental membranes, and (3) the metabolic activity of placental tissues.

Although active and facilitated transport across the placenta has been demonstrated for some substances, transplacental passage of antimicrobials is primarily by simple diffusion (Hays, 1981). The rate-limiting factors in the placental transfer of antibiotics are identical to those which govern membrane diffusion by molecules. Therefore, diffusion across the placental barrier is directly proportional to the maternal–fetal concentration gradient and the surface area of the placenta; it is inversely proportional to the thickness of the placental membrane (Finster and Pederson, 1979). Early in pregnancy the placental membrane is relatively thick; this tends to reduce permeability. During the last trimester, however, the thickness of the trophoblastic epithelium diminishes markedly (from about $25\,\mu m$ early in gestation to about $2\,\mu m$ at birth), and passage of drugs is greatly facilitated (Hamod and Khouzami, 1982). Various disease states, including diabetes and toxemia of pregnancy, significantly alter the permeability characteristics of placental membrane (Hays, 1981). Drugs with molecular weights of less than 500 daltons, a high degree of lipid solubility, a low degree of ionization and low affinity for protein binding are able to traverse the placenta more readily. Since only the unbound (free) fraction of a drug is subject to placental transfer, the more a drug is bound to maternal plasma proteins, the less it is available for crossing to the fetus (Mirkin, 1975).

Although some variations exist in the placental transfer of antimicrobials, most follow a similar pattern. After a single intravenous infusion in the mother, peak antimicrobial concentrations in umbilical blood are usually attained within 30–60 minutes of attaining peak concentration in the maternal serum. Fetal-to-maternal peak serum level ratios range between 0.3 and 0.9 for ampicillin, cephalothin, clindamycin, carbenicillin and the aminoglycosides, while those for erythromycin and dicloxacillin are more limited (0.1 or less) (Nation, 1980). The relative concentrations in fetal and maternal circulation for ampicillin, methicillin, and dicloxacillin have been related to their respective capacities for protein binding. Ampicillin, which is bound to protein in the smallest proportion (20%), achieves high fetal and amniotic fluid levels, while methicillin (40% bound) and dicloxacillin (96% bound) achieve higher maternal levels and progressively lower levels in the fetus and amniotic fluid (Nation, 1980). On this basis, dicloxacillin may be suitable for treatment of a maternal infection but may not be useful for an intrauterine infection.

Fetal organs, especially the gastrointestinal tract, are in direct communication with the amniotic cavity and its fluid. Drugs present in the amniotic fluid are readily swallowed by the fetus and are therefore available for absorption from the fetal gut. A considerable time lag in antimicrobial penetration of amniotic fluid occurs after intravenous infusion in the mother. This delay, which may be as extensive as several hours, appears to stem from the fact that antimicrobial levels in amniotic fluid during the third trimester are largely dependent on antimicrobial excretion in fetal urine. The amount of drug excreted depends largely on the maturity and health of the fetus. Thus, amniotic levels in early pregnancy are much lower than those achieved at term, and negligible antimicrobial levels can be measured in the presence of intrauterine fetal death.

Drug disposition in the fetus

The fetal circulation and the flow pattern between various organs both play roles in determining the drug distribution to various fetal compartments. For example, because blood is shunted away from the lungs by way of the ductus of the foramen ovale, antimicrobial penetration at this anatomical site is particularly poor. Conversely, blood flow to the fetal kidneys is excellent, and antimicrobials are readily excreted in large amounts in the urine with subsequent delivery to the amniotic fluid. Since the fetal circulation varies greatly throughout different stages of pregnancy, significant variations in tissue distribution of different antimicrobials can be expected at various stages of gestation (Ledger, 1977; Schwartz, 1981).

The lipid solubility and protein-binding characteristics of antimicrobials are important determinants of their distribution in various fetal compartments and selective tissue uptake. Fetal serum levels tend to be considerably lower than maternal levels for antimicrobials that have good protein-binding characteristics, and approach maternal levels for those that are poor protein-binders. Occasionally drugs such as sulfisoxazole, which is more extensively bound in umbilical than maternal serum, may still achieve therapeutic concentrations in the fetus despite relatively high protein-binding in the mother (Hamar and Levy, 1980). As expected, higher fetal serum and amniotic fluid concentrations of antimicrobials can generally be attained by bolus rather than by continuous infusion of the drug in the mother and by multiple-dose therapy rather than single-dose (Philipson, 1982).

Until recently it was believed that the fetus lacked the necessary enzyme activity for biotransformation of drugs. It is now known, however, that fetal liver possesses many of the metabolic capabilities of the adult liver (Blake, 1982). Nevertheless, the fetus may not be capable of metabolizing certain drugs due to the immature metabolic activity of such enzymes as mono-oxygenases, epoxide hydrase, and glucuronyl transferase.

ANTIMICROBIALS IN BREAST MILK

Excretion of antimicrobials in breast milk is governed by the same principles that determine placental transfer. Most drugs enter the mammary alveolar cells in the nonionized, nonprotein-bound form (Anderson, 1977; Vorherr, 1974). Under normal conditions the pH of breast milk, which averages 6.8–7.0, is lower than that of plasma. Thus, weakly basic antimicrobials are less ionized in the maternal plasma, and more nonionized molecules are available to pass from plasma into milk (O'Brien, 1974). Such agents tend to have higher concentrations in breast milk and lower concentrations in maternal serum (Landers *et al.*, 1983). When the pH of plasma and human milk changes, the degree to which the drug is ionized and the amount that will be excreted into milk also changes. Drugs with higher volumes of distribution tend to result in lower maternal plasma levels and, therefore, lower drug concentrations in breast milk. Once inside the alveolar milk-secreting cells, antimicrobials readily enter milk, by diffusion primarily, although occasionally by active transport or by apocrine secretion. Lipid-soluble agents appear to reach peak levels in milk with a shorter lag interval and at higher concentrations than less lipid-soluble antimicrobials (Catz and Giaconia, 1972).

Although most antimicrobials administered to the nursing mother can be detected in her milk, deleterious effects on the neonate have only been occasionally encountered (Beeley, 1981c; Bowes, 1980). The drug concentration to which the infant is exposed is usually low and rarely reaches therapeutic or toxic levels. Moreover, drugs may be excreted in milk as inactive metabolites (e.g. 50% of chloramphenicol in breast milk is biologically inactive) and ingested by the infant, but remain unabsorbed or even be destroyed in the newborn gut (Stirrat, 1976). In spite of this, some antimicrobials that pass into breast milk are very potent, and it is important to be aware of possible dangers to the breast-fed infant when the mother is administered large doses of antibiotics, particularly when the nursling is premature or born with hereditary enzyme deficiencies and ineffective mechanisms for hepatic detoxification or renal clearance.

PROBLEMS IN TERATOGENICITY ASSESSMENT

Although the fetus is generally considered to be protected by the placental barrier, both dietary and therapeutic substances do in fact cross the placenta. The teratogenic potential of most therapeutic agents in humans remains largely unknown. Animal studies have been particularly unreliable in predicting human teratogenicity, and examples of false-positive and false-negative predictions based on these studies are well known. Thalidomide, the most potent human teratogen, produces little, if any, effect in the rat and mouse, while acetylsalicylic acid, which has a long history of safe use in human pregnancy, is responsible for a high incidence of malformations in the rat (Harbison, 1980). This variability in response to different substances remains the major shortcoming of preclinical safety assessments of pharmaceutic agents. It also accounts for much of the controversy regarding usage of many antimicrobial agents during pregnancy. The difficulty of separating potential adverse drug effects from an underlying disease process for which the drug was administered further complicates the issue and often renders it impossible to draw valid conclusions regarding drug toxicity (Hays, 1981). On the other hand, the condemnation of useful agents on the basis of unproven risks, particularly when therapy is clearly required, is unjustified and disconcerting. Clearly, more effective human data collection and carefully controlled, prospective epidemiologic and statistical investigations of drug safety during human pregnancy are urgently needed.

MATERNAL AND FETAL TOXICITY

There is no evidence that the overall incidence or severity of adverse reactions due to antimicrobial therapy in the mother is significantly influenced by pregnancy. Adverse reactions that are directly related to serum concentrations of the drug may, in fact, occur less frequently in pregnant women, since the attainable serum levels after a standard therapeutic dose are often lower in pregnancies. Nevertheless, one large prospective study demonstrated the risk of adverse reactions from all antimicrobials among medical and pediatric inpatients to be 4.4% (Caldwell and Cluff, 1974). These reactions were considered moderate to severe in over half of the patients and caused a prolongation of hospitalization in over 40% for cephalosporins, 5.7% for ampicillin, 7.7% for gentamicin, and 8.5% for methicillin. Skin rash and renal impairment were the most common clinical manifestations. Although these findings are not completely applicable to obstetric patients, the relative high rate of adverse reactions from antimicrobial therapy in general should alert the physician to a more careful analysis of the risk-versus-benefit considerations that attend each course of therapy in the pregnant mother.

Several agents are considered particularly dangerous to the mother and should be avoided during pregnancy. These include erythromycin estolate, tetracycline, and perhaps even isoniazid. Erythromycin estolate has been reported to cause subclinical but reversible hepatotoxicity in 10–15% of mothers administered the drug during late pregnancy (McCormack et al., 1977). This complication appears to be a hypersensitivity reaction, since it may rapidly return upon rechallenge. Similarly, tetracycline has been shown to cause a well-defined syndrome of fulminating hepatic decompensation associated with a high mortality rate in pregnant patients (Greene, 1976; Whalley et al., 1964). This syndrome appears to be specific to pregnant women who have reduced renal function. Finally, isoniazid also appears to possess greater potential for hepatotoxicity in pregnant women (Moellering, 1979).

The effects of drug exposure in the fetus are seldom an all-or-none phenomenon; only rarely do specific agents produce specific birth defects. The factors that determine the fetal reaction to intrauterine drug exposure are outlined in

Table 2 Factors influencing the risk of teratogenicity

Dosage, route of administration, and schedule of
  exposure to drug
Biologic and chemical half-life of the drug or
  metabolite
Transplacental diffusion and penetration into
  embryonic tissue by the drug
Detoxification ability of the maternal tissues
  (particularly the liver), placental membrane, and fetal
  or embryonic organs
Stage of embryonic or fetal development at time of
  exposure
Ability of damaged cells to repair or recover from drug
  insult
Genotype of the fetus and mother

Table 2. The complex interplay of these variables provides some explanation as to why a drug may be highly teratogenic under one set of experimental conditions and innocuous under another. There are five principal periods of concern for the use of drugs antenatally: (1) the preconception, or preimplantation period; (2) the postimplantation, or organogenesis period, which encompasses the first trimester; (3) the fetal development period, which encompasses the second and third trimesters; (4) the labor and delivery period; and (5) the breast-feeding period (Harbison, 1980). Animal studies suggest that preconception drug exposure in both the male and female may result in abnormal embryonic development or intrauterine death (Miller, 1981). During the first week after conception, prior to the actual implantation of the fertilized ovum within the uterus, it is probable that potential teratogens exert an all-or-none effect (i.e. the embryo either dies, or the damaged cells of the embryo are replaced by undifferentiated cells that develop in an entirely normal fashion). Differentiation of the embryo begins at 2 weeks, and it is during this period that most major morphological congenital abnormalities may be produced (Harbison, 1980). Drug exposure during the fetal development period in the second and third trimesters is associated with a much smaller risk of major birth defects since most major organ systems are already well developed and much less susceptible to teratogenic effects at this stage (Hays, 1981; Beeley, 1981a). It should be noted, however, that although the overall incidence of major congenital malformations is approximately 2–3% of all births, and minor defects may be evident in as many as 9%, the contribution of drug exposure to this problem is probably very small. It is estimated that only 10% of congenital malformations can be attributed any environmental causes, including drugs; 25% are due to genetic or chromosomal abnormalities. The remaining 65% of all reported congenital defects have no known identifiable cause (Beeley, 1981a).

The mechanisms by which exposure to a drug may exert a teratogenic effect are still poorly understood. Drugs may affect fetal development indirectly by their effects on maternal tissues; these effects include reduced blood oxygen-carrying capacity, hypo- or hyperglycemia, diminished vitamin availability, or alterations in the supply of hormones, amino acids, and trace elements (Harbison, 1980). Drugs may also exert a direct embryotoxic effect in the intrauterine environment. Alternatively, drugs may adversely affect the placenta by interfering with the normal passage of oxygen, glucose, or other nutrients (Yaffe, 1978). The placenta is an organ of major metabolic significance as it is capable of oxidation, reduction, conjugation and hydroxylation reactions (Hays, 1981). Changes in placental function are expected to adversely influence the disposition of many drugs and the subsequent development of the fetus (Yaffe, 1978).

THERAPEUTIC CONSIDERATIONS

The site and nature of an infection are critical considerations which influence the selection of therapy to ensure the optimal outcome. Although many antimicrobials cross the placenta and measurable concentrations can be detected in umbilical serum or amniotic fluid, the administration of antibiotics to the pregnant mother may not be the best way to treat a fetal infection *in utero* (Krauer and Krauer, 1977). Theoretically, antimicrobials that are intended for the fetus should have a high index of relative exposure; this is the ratio of the total area under the drug concentration time curve for the fetus to that of the mother. For certain infections (e.g. urinary tract), the lower serum antibiotic concentrations attained during pregnancy may be of little consequence, particularly if the site of infection is also the site of drug excretion and sufficient local drug concentrations are achieved to produce the desired therapeutic effect. In infections requiring high serum concentrations for therapeutic efficacy, however (e.g. infective endocarditis or pneumonias), much higher dosage schedules may be required than those recommended for nonpregnant patients. Such patients require close monitoring of serum drug levels to assure adequate dosage and avoid toxicity to the mother or the fetus.

The treatment of infections affecting the mother and the fetus requires special attention. In these cases the optimal antimicrobial should not only cure the infection promptly in the mother but should also be capable of readily crossing the placenta and achieving bactericidal levels in fetal tissues. Such an agent must be devoid of known teratogenic effects, have a wide margin of safety and readily possess the capacity to cure fetal infection at any stage of gestation (Schwarz, 1981). In the treatment of syphilis, penicillin achieves these desirable characteristics most closely. In the treatment of chorioamnionitis, however, ampicillin may be unsatisfactory, even though excellent maternal and fetal serum concentrations are achieved because peak amniotic fluid levels remain inadequate until 4–6 hours after initiation of therapy (Philipson, 1977). Moreover, the fetal lung which has been in contact with infected amniotic fluid would have low antibiotic concentrations because blood is shunted away from the lung by the fetal circulation. Therefore antimicrobial treatment of chorioamnionitis with intrauterine pneumonia is frequently suboptimal, and early delivery of the fetus is recommended. The efficacy of various antimicrobial regimens in the treatment of intrauterine fetal infection requires further study.

COMMONLY EMPLOYED ANTIMICROBIAL DRUGS

Antimicrobials considered safe for use in pregnancy

The penicillins are used most frequently and have proved the safest antimicrobials for use in pregnant women (Heinonen et al., 1977). Although allergic reactions to penicillins occur during pregnancy, there are no other known contraindications for their use. Maternal serum levels vary widely with the dosage and are usually lower than those in the nonpregnant individual as renal clearance is increased throughout pregnancy (Landers et al., 1983; Philipson, 1980). The apparent lack of toxicity with penicillins has led to a more extensive pharmacokinetic investigation than any other group of antibiotics. Accordingly, all penicillin derivatives cross the placenta and reach therapeutic levels in the fetus (Lewis, 1978; Pomerance and Yaffe, 1973). Amniotic fluid concentrations vary with the stage of gestation and the time elapsed since maternal ingestion. Fetal drug concentrations are almost nil during the first trimester and highest near term. All penicillin derivatives are excreted in small amounts in breast milk (Anderson, 1977; O'Brien, 1974).

Less information is available concerning the safety of cephalosporins during pregnancy, although the pharmacokinetics of this class of agents is similar to that of the penicillins. Maternal serum levels are lower and the half-life is shorter than in nonpregnant patients (Philipson, 1982; Yamada et al., 1980;

Bawdon *et al.*, 1982; Dubois *et al.*, 1981). The safety of second- and third-generation cephalosporins during pregnancy has not been thoroughly examined. They are, however, expected to retain the degree of safety provided by their predecessors.

Erythromycin and its salts are frequently administered to penicillin-allergic patients in the treatment of gonorrhea, syphilis, and chlamydial infections. Maternal serum levels of these agents are lower than in nonpregnant individuals, probably because they are inconsistently absorbed from the gastrointestinal tract during pregnancy (Philipson *et al.*, 1975). Although erythromycin crosses the placenta, its transplacental passage is unpredictable, and levels in fetal serum as well as amniotic fluid are typically low (Gribble and Chow, 1982). Erythromycin base has been widely used during pregnancy with no known deleterious effects to the mother or fetus. The estolate salt, however, is contraindicated during pregnancy.

Antimicrobials to be used with caution in pregnancy

Aminoglycosides are frequently used for serious infections during pregnancy, often in combination with penicillins or clindamycin in the treatment of pyelonephritis, septic abortion, or chorioamnionitis. Serum concentrations of gentamicin, kanamycin, and amikacin are consistently lower in pregnant patients who may require as much as twice the recommended dose of aminoglycosides to achieve therapeutic serum levels. Limited pharmacokinetic data indicate that there is a transplacental transfer of all aminoglycosides (Weinstein *et al.*, 1976; Pomerance and Yaffe, 1973; Yoshioka *et al.*, 1972). Only a small amount of active drug is detected in the amniotic fluid, though fetal serum concentrations may reach 30–50% of maternal serum levels (Landers *et al.*, 1983). Human studies have not demonstrated increased teratogenicity with these agents (Heinonen *et al.*, 1977). Ototoxicity in neonates has been reported in a number of fetuses whose mothers had received streptomycin and dihydrostreptomycin during their gestations for the treatment of tuberculosis (Snider *et al.*, 1980). Considering the widespread use of these agents, however, very few cases of ototoxicity in the neonate have been recorded following short-term maternal administration during late pregnancy (Assael *et al.*, 1982). With rare exceptions, only small groups of patients have been closely followed, and both cochleotoxicity and vestibulotoxicity are particularly difficult to monitor during early infancy.

The use of aminoglycosides during pregnancy is only indicated for severe infections and when suitable alternatives are unavailable. Extreme caution should be exercised, especially if preterm delivery is anticipated. Careful monitoring of maternal serum levels throughout therapy is strongly recommended, not only to minimize fetal exposure to excessive drug levels, but also to ensure optimal treatment outcome by avoiding subtherapeutic dosing in the mother.

Clindamycin has become more popular in the treatment of resistant anaerobic infections during the peripartal period, particularly for intra-amniotic and postpartum infections (Landers *et al.*, 1983). Serum levels of clindamycin in pregnant women are reported to be similar to those in nonpregnant patients, though its serum half-life is usually shorter. Transplacental transfer of clindamycin occurs rapidly, and therapeutic levels are achieved in fetal tissue (Philipson *et al.*, 1975; Weinstein *et al.*, 1976). Although no documentation of fetal toxicity due to clindamycin has been published to date, the potentially serious complication of pseudomembranous colitis in the mother must be considered.

Nitrofurantoin serum levels have been reported to decrease during pregnancy (Philipson, 1982). Nitrofurantoin has also been shown to cross the placenta and achieve a high fetal–maternal serum concentration ratio (Pomerance and Yaffe, 1973). Although the placenta is readily breached, therapeutic levels are not maintained in the cord serum, probably because of rapid renal excretion. Nitrofurantoin does not appear to attain significant concentrations in the amniotic fluid, and its excretion in breast milk is clinically insignificant (White and White, 1980). Nitrofurantoin is frequently chosen in the treatment of urinary infections in women during pregnancy; it appears to be safe both for mother and fetus. There is a theoretic risk of hemolysis in the fetus and neonate with relative glucose-6-phosphate dehydrogenase (G6PD) deficiency (Pomerance and Yaffe, 1973).

Nalidixic acid crosses the placenta with a high fetal–maternal serum concentration ratio. It is excreted in amniotic fluid and breast milk. Nalidixic acid has a low incidence of adverse side-effects, although it occasionally causes toxic psychosis and convulsions and should be avoided in patients with seizure disorders. It has been reported to cause increased intracranial pressure, papilledema, and bulging fontanelles in the newborn (Rao, 1974). Nalidixic acid should be used with caution during pregnancy and avoided altogether during the first trimester; its use is not recommended in nursing mothers and infants under 3 months of age.

Methanamine mandelate is absorbed rapidly following oral administration. Its distribution in maternal and fetal tissues and amniotic fluid has not been well studied. Nevertheless, it appears to be safe during pregnancy and can be used as a urinary antiseptic for treatment of bacteriuria. No increased risk to the fetus has been reported. Insignificant amounts of methanamine are excreted in breast milk (Anderson, 1977).

Metronidazole readily crosses the placenta (Pomerance and Yaffe, 1973). Metronidazole serum levels during pregnancy are comparable to those in nonpregnant women, and fetal serum concentrations approach maternal levels. Although metronidazole has been found to be carcinogenic in rodents and mutagenic for certain bacteria, there is no firm evidence that teratogenicity or an increased rate of congenital birth defects occurs in humans after maternal administration (Hamod and Khouzami, 1982). In spite of this, most obstetricians have refrained from using this drug during the first trimester and, when possible, during the last trimester and breastfeeding.

Sulfonamides are commonly employed for the treatment of asymptomatic bacteriuria or cystitis during pregnancy. All sulfonamide preparations readily cross the placenta and enter the fetal circulation and amniotic fluid (Pomerance and Yaffe, 1973). Passage into the breast milk also occurs (White and White, 1980). Direct toxic effects of sulfonamides to the fetus are not well documented. A theoretic risk of hemolysis from sulfonamides exists due to a relative deficiency of fetal G6PD and glutathione (Hamod and Khouzami, 1982).

Sulfonamides compete with bilirubin for albumin-binding sites (Hamar and Levy, 1980). In the fetus this competition is probably unimportant, as the placenta is fully capable of clearing unconjugated bilirubin. Once the fetus is born, however, the protection of the placenta is no longer available and the presence of long-acting sulfonamides then may predispose the fetus to hyperbilirubinemia with diffusion of free bilirubin into the central nervous system causing kernicterus (Stewart, 1981; Landers *et al.*, 1983). Therefore, long-acting sulfonamides, such as sulfamethoxydiazine, should not be administered during term pregnancy, since these drugs may remain at significant levels in the fetus for 4–6 days after maternal ingestion (Stirrat, 1976).

Antimicrobials contraindicated in pregnancy

Oxycycline, demeclocycline, and tetracycline all cross the placenta readily and appear in cord blood (Pomerance and Yaffe, 1973). These antimicrobials are specifically contraindicated during pregnancy because of adverse maternal and fetal effects. Pregnant women with underlying renal dysfunction or pyelonephritis appear to be particularly at risk for developing acute fatty necrosis of the liver and renal damage when administered high intravenous doses. These adverse effects are dose-related and associated with a high mortality (Moellering, 1979; Ledger, 1977). Adverse effects to the fetus occur particularly when these agents are administered during the second and third trimesters of pregnancy; discoloration and severe dysplasia of teeth and inhibition of bone growth have been documented (Landers *et al.*, 1983).

The fetal effects of tetracycline are mediated by two mechanisms: (1) interference with protein synthesis, and (2) chelation with calcium and other cationic substances. Congenital limb abnormalities and cataracts have also been observed in infants of mothers receiving large doses of the drug during the first 12 weeks of pregnancy (Pomerance and Yaffe, 1973). Tetracyclines chelate calcium in a dose-dependent manner and are deposited in developing long bones and teeth. These effects appear early in the second trimester when ossification centers begin to develop. Inhibition of bone growth and hypoplasia of the deciduous and permanent teeth may occur up to 6–8 years of age, if exposure is continued. The absorption of tetracycline by the infant via ingestion of breast milk is minimal due to chelation with milk calcium (Anderson, 1977).

Chloramphenicol is generally reserved for the treatment of severe infections when alternative agents are not available. Serum levels in pregnant women are comparable to nonpregnant individuals (Philipson, 1982) and transplacental passage of the drug occurs readily with fetal serum concentrations reaching 30–150% of simultaneous maternal levels (Scott and Warner, 1950). The use of chloramphenicol during late pregnancy is generally avoided because of the risk of development of blood dyscrasias and aplastic anemia. Serum levels in pregnant women are comparable to nonpregnant individuals (Philipson, 1982).

The well-described complications of gray syndrome have been reported primarily in premature infants who had received chloramphenicol postnatally. Gray syndrome is characterized by the rapid development of pallid cyanosis, abdominal distension, flaccidity, vomiting, irregular respiration, hypothermia, and acute respiratory failure (Leitman, 1979). It is caused by toxic accumulation of chloramphenicol, particularly in the preterm infant which lacks both the enzyme responsible for glucuronyl conjugation and mature renal function for effective tubular excretion of the free drug. The serum half-life for chloramphenicol is markedly prolonged in these neonates. The mortality associated with this syndrome may be as high as 40% (Schwarz, 1981). No characteristic pathologic features are noted postmortem. Although chloramphenicol is secreted in breast milk, the quantities are insufficient to induce the gray syndrome.

Trimethoprim-sulfamethoxazole (TMP-SMX) is best avoided during pregnancy, especially during the first and third trimesters. Folic acid antagonists are known teratogens and were formerly used as abortifacients. TMP-SMX has been reported to cause congenital anomalies such as cleft palates in rats (Landers *et al.*, 1983), although no cases of human birth abnormalities related to maternal ingestion have been recorded. Since both constituents of TMP-SMX readily cross the placenta and levels of fetal serum and amniotic fluid approach maternal serum levels, the risk of kernicterus and hemolysis from relative G6PD and glutathione deficiency in the fetus theoretically exists. TMP-SMX may cause megaloblastic anemia during pregnancy due to antifolate effects. This can be prevented by the concomitant administration of folinic acid which does not interfere with the antibacterial activity of TMP-SMX (Hamod and Khouzami, 1982).

LESS COMMONLY EMPLOYED ANTIMICROBIAL DRUGS

Antituberculous drugs

The outcome of pregnancy among women receiving antituberculosis therapy with the first-line agents such as isoniazid, ethambutol and rifampin does not differ significantly from other women and the use of these agents during pregnancy is not contraindicated (Snider *et al.*, 1980). The increased risk of ototoxicity in infants delivered by mothers who had received prolonged courses of streptomycin during pregnancy has been discussed previously. Streptomycin is no longer considered a first-line antituberculosis agent.

Antifungal drugs

Little data exists about the use of systemic antifungal drugs during pregnancy. The available evidence suggests that the adverse effects of amphotericin B are no worse in pregnant than among nonpregnant patients, and no increased incidence of teratogenesis or persistent toxic effects to the fetus has been reported (Ismail and Lerner, 1982). Flucytosine is teratogenic in rats; for this reason it is contraindicated during pregnancy (Bennett, 1977). Among the antifungal imidazoles, only miconazole and ketaconazole appear to be useful in systemic mycoses. Miconazole has thus far failed to fulfill a major role in antifungal chemotherapy, primarily because of its toxicity. Its safety during pregnancy is unknown. When used topically, miconazole is absorbed from the vagina in trace amounts, and its use in pregnancy should be carefully weighed against its potential risks. Ketoconazole is the first of the antifungal imidazoles to be well absorbed orally. It has unusual efficacy against diverse fungi,

323

including dermatophytes, as well as mucocutaneous candidiasis and deep mycosis. The pharmacokinetics of ketoconazole are incompletely defined; it has surprisingly few adverse effects when administered orally, although hepatitis and adrenal suppression have been reported (Graybull, 1983). The degree to which ketoconazole is absorbed by fetal tissues and amniotic fluid is unknown, and its safety in pregnancy has not been established. Griseofulvin is an antimicrobial with limited fungicidal activity that is used primarily for treatment of dermatophytic infections of the scalp and nails. It is inconsistently absorbed from the gastrointestinal tract and is extensively metabolized in the liver. Its ability to cross the placenta is poor and it is not detected in amniotic fluid (Rubin and Dvornik, 1965). Griseofulvin is embryotoxic and teratogenic in pregnant mice (Klein and Beall, 1972) and is not recommended for use in human pregnancy.

Antiviral drugs

Compared to the remarkable progress made in the treatment of bacterial infections in the past four decades, few major advances in antiviral chemotherapy have developed. These include the use of amantadine and derivatives for the prophylaxis and treatment of influenza, the use of vidarabine and acyclovir for the treatment of life-threatening herpes simplex and varicella-zoster infections, and use of acyclovir for genital herpes simplex infection. Idoxuridine and cytarabine are too toxic for systemic use and are primarily reserved for topical treatment of herpes keratitis.

Amantadine in large doses has been found to be embryotoxic and teratogenic for certain laboratory animals, and its use in pregnant women should be avoided. It is excreted in milk; other pharmacokinetic properties of this drug during pregnancy in humans are virtually unknown. Vidarabine is teratogenic in laboratory animals, and its use in pregnant women should be confined to life-threatening herpes infections. Acyclovir is only partially absorbed when administered orally. When infused intravenously, it is widely distributed in tissues and body fluids. Extensive studies have failed to demonstrate embryotoxicity or teratogenesis of acyclovir in laboratory animals (Tucker, 1982). Nevertheless, its safety in pregnancy has not yet been established. As a general rule, systemic antiviral agents should be avoided in pregnancy, particularly during the first trimester except in the presence of life-threatening infections in the mother. Whether treatment with antiviral agents near term is safe for the fetus and can prevent disseminated herpes simplex infection in the newborn remains to be determined.

Antiparasitic drugs

Since pregnancy complicated by malaria is of significant risk to the fetus and the mother (McGregor and Logie, 1970), treatment and prophylaxis are clearly indicated. Chloroquine is the drug of choice for chloroquine-sensitive malaria acquired during pregnancy. It is generally safe in pregnant women and poses little teratogenic risk. Chloroquine crosses the placenta and accumulates in fetal ocular tissue (Howard and Hill, 1979); it produces cochleovesticular damage after chronic administration at high doses (Matz and Naunton, 1968). It has not been found to have any harmful effect on the fetus when used in the dosages recommended for malaria prophylaxis.

Use of primaquine is not recommended during pregnancy. Since the fetal red blood cell is relatively deficient in G6PD and glutathione, the fetus is at increased risk for intravascular hemolysis and methemoglobinemia (Pomerance and Yaffe, 1973). Pregnant women for whom radical cure or terminal prophylaxis with primaquine is otherwise indicated should receive only chloroquine once weekly until delivery. Primaquine can then be administered after delivery. Women who are pregnant or are likely to become so should not travel to areas where the presence of chloroquine-resistant malaria requires prophylaxis with pyrimethamine-sulfadoxine (Fansidar). Pyrimethamine, a folic acid antagonist, is teratogenic in laboratory animals, and its safety in human pregnancy has not been established (Howard and Hill, 1979). It should be avoided, especially in the first trimester of pregnancy.

Dapsone in combination with pyrimethamine (Maloprim) has also been useful for treatment and prophylaxis of chloroquine-resistant falciparum malaria. However, this sulfone induces hemolytic anemia and methemoglobinemia, and several cases of agranulocytosis have been reported in association with its use as an antimalarial agent (Segal et al., 1973). Like pyrimethamine-sulfadoxine, its use during pregnancy is not recommended. Both tetracycline and quinine are contraindicated in pregnancy, unless they are required to treat life-threatening infections in the mother. Quinine in large doses was at one time widely used to induce abortion. Hypoplasia of the optic nerve and congenital deafness have both been reported after failure to terminate pregnancy (Beeley, 1981b). Quinine has also been reported to cause massive intravascular hemolysis followed by acute tubular necrosis and renal failure during pregnancy (Lang and Jones, 1964).

Amoebiasis may run a more fulminant course during pregnancy, and latent infections may be exacerbated (Trussel and Beeley, 1981). Treatment of amoebiasis during pregnancy is therefore generally warranted. Symptomatic infection should be treated with metronidazole plus diiodohydroxyquin; asymptomatic infection with diiodohydroxyquin alone. Subacute myelo-optic neuropathy has been reported with iodohydroxyquin, although only when administered in doses larger than recommended for amoebiasis; this complication is not as common as with iodochlorhydroxyquin. Diloxanide furoate is an alternative luminal amoebicide. Its safety during pregnancy has not been determined, and it should be avoided during pregnancy (Trussel and Beeley, 1981).

Toxoplasmosis acquired during pregnancy may lead to spontaneous abortion, premature birth, and, most importantly, congenital malformations (Desmonts and Couvreur, 1973). Women who acquire the disease during pregnancy, especially during the first 5 months, should be treated to prevent fetal and congenital complications. In nonpregnant patients, pyrimethamine plus sulfadiazine is the preferred therapy. Because of possible teratogenic effects of pyrimethamine and the potential adverse effects of sulfonamides to the fetus, however, this regimen cannot be advocated during pregnancy (Trussel and Beeley, 1981). Spiramycin, a macrolide antibiotic similar to erythromycin, is the drug of choice for treatment of toxoplasmosis during pregnancy (Scott, 1978).

Giardia lamblia seldom causes acute symptomatic infection except in compromised hosts. There are few studies of giardiasis during pregnancy. Symptomatic patients should be treated with metronidazole. Quinacrine is not recommended because it crosses the placenta and becomes a potential hazard to the fetus. Furazolidone, a nitrofuran effective in the treatment of giardiasis, is best avoided during pregnancy since it can cause agranulocytosis and acute hemolysis in individuals with G6PD deficiency.

Trichomonas vaginalis is a common protozoan. It can be identified in approximately 5% of infants born of untreated mothers, but very rarely causes symptomatic disease (Trussel and Beeley, 1981). In women with trichomonal vaginitis, metronidazole is highly effective, and the low risk of teratogenicity and carcinogenicity in humans suggests that it can be administered during pregnancy when therapy is clearly indicated (Roe, 1983).

Roundworm infestations, except for ascariasis and strongyloidiasis, are seldom significant during pregnancy, and treatment is usually unwarranted until after delivery. For enterobiasis, trichuriasis, and hookworm infections, the treatment of choice following delivery is mebendazole. Although it is poorly absorbed orally, mebendazole is teratogenic and embryotoxic in pregnant rats and is contraindicated during pregnancy (Keystone and Murdoch, 1979). Treatment of *Ascaris lumbricoides* during pregnancy should be limited to cases with heavy infestations or symptomatic disease. The treatment of choice for intestinal infection is piperazine, as there have been no reports of harmful effects to the fetus following maternal administration. Strongyloidiasis carries a serious potential risk and should always be treated, even in asymptomatic individuals. Thiabendazole is the drug of choice.

Since tapeworm infections generally are not life-threatening, it is recommended that treatment of pregnant women be postponed until after delivery. Niclosamide is the drug of choice. Cysticercosis due to *Taenia solium* larvae is best treated by surgical resection. Praziquantel, a new anticestodal drug, appears promising, particularly in neurocysticercosis. It is not known to have any teratogenic, embryotoxic, or mutagenic effects (Leopold *et al.*, 1978).

SUMMARY AND CONCLUSIONS

In this chapter we have examined the pharmacokinetic as well as therapeutic implications of antimicrobial therapy during pregnancy. While the need to evaluate critically the safety and potential teratogenicity of all therapeutic agents administered during pregnancy has been emphasized, the information currently available to assure the optimal usage of these drugs during the antenatal period is sparse. Precise pharmacokinetic data, particularly for the newer antifungal, antiviral, and antiparasitic agents, are lacking. While it is clear that all antimicrobial agents are potentially harmful to the fetus and that their administration during pregnancy must be limited to specific indications in both the mother and the fetus, more understanding of the nature and consequences of various infectious processes during pregnancy is needed. The potential risks and benefits of antimicrobial therapy must be individually assessed on the basis of relevant clinical and pharmacologic data that are appropriate to the specific clinical setting of both mother and fetus. Only in this manner can a more effective approach to antimicrobial therapy be developed for the pregnant patient.

References

Anderson, P. O. (1977). Drugs and breastfeeding: a review. *Drug Intel. Clin. Pharm.*, **11**, 208

Assael, B. M., Parini, R. and Rusconi, F. (1982). Ototoxicity of aminoglycoside antibiotics in infants and children. *Ped. Infect. Dis.*, **1**, 357

Bawdon, R. E., Cunningham, F. G., Quirk, J. G. *et al.* (1982). Maternal and fetal pharmacokinetics of moxalactam given intrapartum. *Am. J. Obstet. Gynecol.*, **144**, 546

Beeley, L. (1981a). Adverse effects of drugs in the first trimester of pregnancy. *Clin. Obstet. Gynecol.*, **8**, 261

Beeley, L. (1981b). Adverse effects of drugs in later pregnancy. *Clin. Obstet. Gynecol.*, **8**, 275

Beeley, L. (1981c). Drugs and breast feeding. *Clin. Obstet. Gynecol.*, **8**, 291

Bennett, J. E. (1977). Flucytosine. *Ann. Intern. Med.*, **86**, 319

Bernard, B., Barton, L., Abate, M. *et al.* (1977). Maternal-fetal transfer of cefazolin in the first twenty weeks of pregnancy. *J. Infect. Dis.*, **136**, 377

Blake, D. A. (1982). Requirements and limitations in reproductive and teratogenic risk assessment. In: Nietyl, J. R. (ed.) *Drug Use in Pregnancy*, p. 1. (Philadelphia: Lea & Febiger)

Bowes Jr., W. A. (1980). The effect of medications on the lactating mother and her infant. *Clin. Obstet. Gynecol.*, **23**, 1073

Caldwell, J. R. and Cluff, L. E. (1974). Adverse reactions to antimicrobial agents. *J. Am. Med. Assoc.*, **230**, 77

Catz, C. S. and Giaconia, G. P. (1972). Drugs in breast milk. *Ped. Clin. N. Am.*, **19**, 151

Desmonts, G. and Couvreur, J. (1974). Congenital toxoplasmosis: A prospective study of 378 pregnancies. *N. Engl. J. Med.*, **290**, 1110

Dubois, M., Delapierre, D., Chanteux, L. *et al.* (1981). A study of the transplacental transfer and the mammary excretion of cefoxitin in humans. *J. Clin Pharmacol.*, **21**, 477

Finster, M. and Pederson, H. (1979). Placental transfer and fetal uptake of drugs. *Br. J. Anaes.*, **51**, 25s

Good, R. G. and Johnson, G. N. (1971). The placental transfer of kanamycin during late pregnancy. *Obstet. Gynecol.*, **38**, 60

Graybull, J. R. (1983). Summary: potential and problems with ketoconazole. *Am. J. Med. Suppl.*, **74**, 86

Greene, G. (1976). Tetracycline in pregnancy. *N. Engl. J. Med.*, **295**, 512

Gribble, M. J. and Chow, A. W. (1982). Erythromycin. *Med. Clin. N. Am.*, **66**, 79

Hamar, C. and Levy, G. (1980). Serum protein binding of drugs and bilirubin in newborn infants and their mothers. *Clin. Pharmacol. Ther.*, **28**, 58

Hamod, K. A. and Khouzami, V. A. (1982). Antibiotics in pregnancy. In: Nietyl, J. R. (ed.) *Drug Use in Pregnancy*, p. 31. (Philadelphia: Lea & Febiger)

Harbison, R. D. (1980). Teratogens. In: Doull, J., Klaassen, C. D. and Amdur, M. O. (eds) *Caserett and Doull's Toxicology*, 2nd edn, p. 158. (New York: Macmillan)

Hays, D. P. (1981). Teratogenesis: A review of the basic principles with a discussion of selected agents: parts I-III. *Drug Intell. Clin. Pharm.*, **15**, 444

Heinonen, O. P., Slone, D. and Shapiro, S. (1977). *Antimicrobial and Antiparasitic Agents: Birth Defects and Drugs in Pregnancy*, p. 296. (Littleton, MA: Publishing Sciences Group)

Howard, F. M. and Hill, J. M. (1979). Drugs in pregnancy. *Obstet. Gynecol. Surv.*, **34**, 643

Ismail, M. A. and Lerner, S. A. (1982). Disseminated blastomycosis in a pregnant woman: Review of amphotericin B usage during pregnancy. *Am. Rev. Resp. Dis.*, **126**, 350

Keystone, J. S. and Murdoch, J. K. (1979). Mebendazole. *Ann. Intern. Med.*, **91**, 582

Klein, M. F. and Beall, J. R. (1972). Griseofulvin: A teratogenic study. *Science*, **175**, 1483

Krauer, B. and Krauer, F. (1977). Drug kinetics in pregnancy. *Clin. Pharmacol.*, **2**, 167

Landers, D. V., Green, J. R. and Sweet, R. L. (1983). Antibiotic use during pregnancy and the postpartum period. *Clin. Obstet. Gynecol.*, **26**, 391

Lang, P. A. and Jones, C. C. (1964). Acute renal failure precipitated by quinine sulfate in early pregnancy. *J. Am. Med. Assoc.*, **188**, 164

Ledger, W. J. (1977). Antibiotics in pregnancy. *Clin. Obstet. Gynecol.*, **20**, 411

Leitman, P. S. (1979). Chloramphenicol and the neonate: A 1979 review. *Clin. Perinatol.*, **6**, 151

Leopold, G., Ungethum, W., Groll, E. *et al.* (1978). Clinical pharmacology in normal volunteers of praziquantel, a new drug against schistosomes and cestodes. *Eur. J. Clin. Pharmacol.*, **14**, 281

Lewis, B. V., (1978). Drug therapy in pregnancy. *Practitioner*, **221**, 866

Logie, D. E. and McGregor, I. A. (1970). Acute malaria in newborn infants. *Br. Med. J.*, **3**, 404

Matz, G. J. and Naunton, R. F. (1968). Ototoxicity of chloroquine. *Arch. Otolaryngol.*, **88**, 50

McCormack, W. M., George, H., Donner, A. *et al.* (1977). Hepatotoxicity of erythromycin estolate during pregnancy. *Antimicrob. Agents Chemother.*, **12**, 630

Miller, R. K. (1981). Drugs during pregnancy: a therapeutic dilemma. *Rat Drug Ther.*, **15**, 1

Mirkin, B. L. (1975). Perinatal pharmacology, placental transfer, fetal localization and neonatal distribution of drugs. *Anaesthesiology*, **43**, 156

Moellering Jr., R. C. (1979). Special consideration of the use of antimicrobial agents during pregnancy, post partum, and in the newborn. *Clin. Obstet. Gynecol.*, **22**, 373

Nation, R. L. (1980). Drug kinetics in childbirth. *Clin. Pharmacol.*, **5**, 340

O'Brien, T. E. (1974). Excretion of drugs in human milk. *Am. J. Hosp. Pharm.*, **31**, 844

Philipson, A. (1977). Pharmacokinetics of ampicillin during pregnancy. *J. Infect. Dis.*, **136**, 370

Philipson, A. (1979). Pharmacokinetics of antibiotics in pregnancy and labor. *Clin. Pharmacol.*, **4**, 297

Philipson, A., Sabath, L. D. and Charles, D. (1975). Erythromycin and clindamycin absorption and elimination in pregnant women. *Clin. Pharmacol. Ther.*, **19**, 68

Philipson, A. E. L. (1982). Pharmacokinetics of antibiotics in the pregnant woman. In: Ledger, W. J. (ed.) *Antibiotics in Obstetrics and Gynecology*, p. 37. (The Hague: Martinus Nijhoff)

Pomerance, J. J. and Yaffe, S. J. (1973). Maternal medication and its effect on the fetus. *Curr. Prob. Ped.*, **4**, 1

Rao, K. G. (1974). Pseudotumor cerebri associated with nalidixic acid. *Urology*, **4**, 204

Roe, F. J. C. (1983). Toxicologic evaluation of metronidazole with particular reference to carcinogenic, mutagenic and teratogenic potential. *Surgery*, **93**, 158

Ross, S. M. (1982). Sexually transmitted disease in pregnancy. *Clin. Obstet. Gynecol.*, **9**, 565

Rubin, A. and Dvornik, D. (1965). Placental transfer of griseofulvin. *Am. J. Obstet. Gynecol.*, **92**, 882

Schwarz, R. H. (1981). Considerations of antibiotic therapy during pregnancy. *Obstet. Gynecol. Suppl.*, **58**, 95s

Scott, R. J. (1978). Toxoplasmosis. *Trop. Dis. Bull.*, **75**, 809

Scott, W. C. and Warner, R. F. (1950). Placental transfer of chloramphenicol (chloromycetin). *J. Am. Med. Assoc.*, **142**, 1331

Segal, H. E., Pearlman, E. J., Thiemann, W. *et al.* (1973). The suppression of plasmodium falciparum and plasmodium parasitemias by a dapsone-pyrimethamine combination. *J. Trop. Med. Hyg.*, **76**, 285

Snider Jr., D. E., Layde, P. M., Johnson, M. W. *et al.* (1980). Treatment of tuberculosis during pregnancy. *Am. Rev. Resp. Dis.*, **122**, 65

Stewart, K. S. (1981). Bacterial infections. *Clin. Obstet. Gynecol.*, **8**, 315

Stirrat, G. M. (1976). Prescribing problems in the second half of pregnancy and during lactation. *Obstet. Gynecol. Surv.*, **31**, 1

Trussel, R. R. and Beeley, L. (1981). Infestations. *Clin. Obstet. Gynecol.*, **8**, 333

Tucker, W. E. (1982). Pre-clinical toxicology profile of acyclovir: An overview. *Am. J. Med. Suppl.*, **73**, 27

Vorherr, H. (1974). Drug excretion in breast milk. *Postgrad. Med. J.*, **56,** 97

Weinstein, A. J., Gibbs, R. S. and Gailager, M. (1976). Placental transfer of clindamycin and gentamicin in term pregnancy. *Am. J. Obstet. Gynecol.*, **124,** 688

Whalley, J. P., Adams, R. H. and Combes, B. (1964). Tetracycline toxicity in pregnancy. *J. Am. Med. Assoc.*, **189,** 357

White, G. J. and White, M. K. (1980). Breastfeeding and drugs in human milk. *Vet. Human Toxicol.*, **22,** 1

Yaffe, S. J. (1978). Drugs and pregnancy. *Clin. Toxicol.*, **13,** 523

Yamada, N., Kido, K., Uchida, H. *et al.* (1980). Application of cephalosporins to obstetrics and gynecology: Transfer of cefazolin and cephalothin to uterine tissue. *Am. J. Obstet. Gynecol.*, **136,** 1036

Yoshioka, H., Morma, T. and Matsuda, S. (1972). Placental transfer of gentamicin. *J. Pediatr.*, **80,** 121

22
Culture diagnosis of genitourinary tract infections

M. P. SMELTZER

INTRODUCTION

In diagnosing a condition on the basis of culture one must consider when such a diagnosis is appropriate, how to collect the material necessary for analysis, and how to interpret the results. Accuracy parameters, i.e. sensitivity and specificity, are of importance, as is the role of culture diagnosis in comparison with other diagnostic techniques. The benefits of diagnosing by culture are that it can (1) define a specific cause and point to a specific treatment, (2) provide information that is relevant to the selection of therapy, such as antibiotic choice and dosage, (3) relate disease processes epidemiologically to specific causes, and (4) help prevent recurrence by implicating a source of infection.

The fact that a broad range of microflora reside in the genitourinary tract of men and women complicates culture diagnostic approaches. Infection with known pathogens is always a possibility; infection with an agent or agents from the indigenous flora also occurs, so commonly in fact, as not to raise an issue with clinicians.

Table 1 lists organisms most commonly found in the male and female genitourinary tract; Table 2 lists organisms associated with infections. Clearly, many organisms are found in both tables. In premenopausal women the organisms not usually associated with overt disease (avirulent organisms) include *Lactobacillus* species and diphtheroid bacilli, such as members of the genus *Cornynebacterium* (Ohm and Galask, 1975). In males, urethral cultures from normal individuals yield those two genera and *Staphylococcus epidermidis* as well (Bowie *et al.*, 1977a,b). Thus, the notation 'normal flora' is often returned to the clinician on a laboratory form when these organisms are found. Unfortunately, the clinician frequently fails to understand the implications of this finding. Infections arising from endogenous species are usually characterized by the predominance of the agent isolated in the laboratory. This is the case with *Escherichia coli* or the anaerobe *Bacteroides fragilis* (Larsen and

Table 1 Organisms common to the genitourinary area[a,b]

Organism	Location
Alpha-hemolytic streptococci	Urethra
Bacteroides spp.	Urethra
Candida albicans and other yeasts	Vagina
Corynebacteria spp.	Vagina, urethra
Enterobacteriaceae	Vagina, urethra
Enterococci	Vagina
Gardnerella vaginalis	Urethra
Group B Streptococci	Vagina
Lactobacilli	Vagina, urethra
Mycoplasma spp.	Vagina
Neisseria spp. (non-gonorrhea)	Vagina
Peptococcus spp.	Vagina, urethra
Peptostreptococcus spp.	Vagina, urethra
Staphylococcus aureus	Vagina
Staphylococcus epidermidis	Vagina, urethra
Trichomonas vaginalis	Vagina, urethra
Veridans streptococci	Vagina

[a] Bowie *et al.*, 1977a
[b] Isenberg and Painter, 1980

Galask, 1980) in vaginitis infections and with *Ureaplasma urealyticum* in male urethritis.

GENERAL CONCERNS

Culture techniques are often expensive, time-consuming, and sometimes fail to uncover an exact cause of infection. When infectious processes exist, however, cultural diagnostic techniques are the most specific methods available to define their causes. Cultural techniques are always appropriate when infections or symptoms cannot be categorized by faster and/or less expensive means, such as microscopic or serologic techniques. These latter methods are useful only when a specific etiology suggests itself; when this is not the case, then attempts to grow and identify the microbe are mandatory.

Collection of material for culture may involve the use of a swab, a loop, a syringe, or a scraping device, such as a scalpel. In general it is always better to collect a smaller sample free from contamination by adjacent surfaces than to collect a larger sample and risk exposing it to contamination. When a swab is used to collect the sample, the site of infection should be moist and the swab should be dry to assure absorption of microbe-containing material (Isenberg *et al.*, 1980). After sample collection, inoculation of adequate transport media and proper transport conditions are crucial to assure reliable results.

For genitourinary tract infections of unknown etiology, anaerobic cultures as well as a range of other cultures are required. Other cultures might include those for fungi, viruses, or parasites; generally, bacteria are ruled out first as causative microbes. An array of transport media or primary isolation media are needed to define comprehensively the bacterial flora. Several commercial collection and transport instruments are available. These usually consist of a swab (cotton, Dacron, or calcium alginate on a wooden, plastic, or metal shaft), which is placed into a tube containing maintenance media specially formulated to keep certain types of microbes alive during transport.

CULTURES IN REPRODUCTIVE HEALTH

Organisms that cause reproductive health problems are cultured from samples from the male urethra or prostate gland, or from the female vagina, cervix, various vulvar glands, urethra, rectum, and/or fallopian tubes via laparoscopy. Organisms found in these areas have already been listed (see Table 1). Problems in detecting these organisms by cultural techniques revolve around the time delay for obtaining results and the dependability of the results as a predictor of the cause of disease. Although automated and semi-automated bacterial identification systems have a high degree of accuracy, and effect considerable time savings, primary isolation is still necessary with specimens of high microbial heterogeneity as is the case in the female vagina (Woolfrey et al., 1983).

A few colorimetric tests are available for diagnosing specific diseases, such as gonorrhea and Group B streptococcal infections. Unfortunately, they are not used widely in clinical practice settings. These tests employ monoclonal antibodies that have been linked to an indicator enzyme that detects specific antigenic material. Their high specificity allows them to be effective even with contaminated samples. This technique is based upon ELISA (enzyme-linked immunosorbent assay) technology. ELISA has been adapted to detect many viral and bacterial diseases that might otherwise escape detection due to the small number and fastidious nature of the organism (Yolken, 1982).

ANAEROBES

Samples for anaerobic culturing should be taken only from active infection sites. Since most anaerobic infections are caused by endogenous species of microorganisms, contaminated specimens or screening samples may reveal anaerobes not involved in the disease process (Dowell and Allen, 1981).

Clinical samples should be placed in anaerobic transport containers and delivered to the laboratory as soon as possible; samples should be refrigerated only if there is a delay of 24 hours or longer. For swab samples, use anaerobic transport media, such as the Modified Cary-Blair or Port-A-Culmedia.[1] For tissue or fluid samples, use anaerobic tubes or containers; a commercially available container for tissues is the Anaerobic Culture Set.[2] The laboratory should examine the material microscopically and report these results immediately. Gram-stained smear results may confirm a suspicion so that treatment can be initiated or it may serve to narrow culture possibilities, thus reducing turnaround time.

[1] BBL, Cockeysville, MD
[2] Marion Scientific, Rockford, IL

Table 2 Pathogenic organisms of the genitourinary area[a,b]

Organism	Location	Disease
Acinetobacter spp.	Urethra, vagina	Urethritis
Candida albicans	Urethra, vagina	Candidiasis
Chlamydia trachomatis	Cervix, urethra, vagina	Cervicitis, nonspecific urethritis, various neonatal diseases; conjunctivitis, pneumonia, otitis media. Lymphogranuloma venereum
Cytomegalovirus	Cervix, urethra	Neonatal disease[c]
Enterobacteriaceae	Urethra, vagina	Pyelonephritis, cystitis, bacteriuria
Enterococcus	Urethra, vagina	Pyelonephritis, cystitis, bacteriuria
Gardnerella vaginalis	Urethra, vagina	Vaginitis[d]
Herpes simplex virus	Urethra, vagina, external genitalia	Herpetic lesions, neonatal herpes[e]
Moraxella spp.	Vagina	Postpartum complications
Mycoplasma spp.	Urethra, vagina	Nonspecific urethritis
Neisseria gonorrhoeae	Cervix, urethra, vagina, glands	Cervicitis, PID, urethritis
Peptococcus spp.	Vagina	Postpartum or postoperative complications
Peptostreptococcus spp.	Vagina	Puerperal fever
Staphylococcus aureus	Urethra, vagina	Urethritis, furunculosis
Streptococcus agalactiae	Vagina	Various diseases of the neonate; endocarditis, abscess, meningitis, myocarditis, osteomyelitis, septicemia[f]
Treponema pallidum	External genitalia	Syphilis
Trichomonas vaginalis	Urethra, vagina	Vaginitis, nonspecific urethritis

[a] Bowie *et al.*, 1977a
[b] Isenberg and Painter, 1980
[c] Starr and Friedman, 1980
[d] Pheifer *et al.*, 1978
[e] Rawls, 1980
[f] Wilkinson, 1978

Primary isolation of anaerobes involves the following: (1) the use of nonselective, selective, and enriched media; (2) the use of reduced media; (3) the use of an anaerobic holding jar for uninoculated plates; (4) incubation in an anaerobic system; and (5) anaerobic conditions during inspection of colonies and subculture (Dowell and Allen, 1981). Nonselective media for isolation of anaerobes in the genitourinary tract should include CDC anaerobe blood agar (Dowell *et al.*, 1977), enriched thioglycollate broth, blood agar incubated in a candle extinction jar or a CO_2 incubator, and cooked meat–glucose medium (CMG) (Dowell, 1975). All plated media should be held in an anaerobic system for 4–18 hours before use; liquid media can be heated for 10 minutes in a boiling water bath. Selective media for isolation of *Bacteroides* and *Fusobacterium* species is kanamycin–vancomycin blood agar (KVA). For isolation of *Peptococcus* and *Peptostreptococcus* species and other anaerobes of interest, phenylethylalcohol agar (PEA) is used. Plated cultures should be incubated at 35–37 °C for a minimum of 48 hours; incubation for 72–96 hours is preferred; broth cultures should be incubated at least 1 week unless growth is noted earlier. For colonial observation and subculture, an anaerobic glove box or a VPI roll-streak system is useful. To a great degree, sensitivity of anaerobic cultures depends on collection and transport. Samples contaminated with other material yield meaningless results. However, if meaningful primary isolation is accomplished, very few tests are necessary to identify the genus designation of a urogenital isolate. For a Gram-negative bacillus, gas–liquid chromatography distinguishes between *Bacteroides* and *Fusobacterium* organisms (Finegold and Citron, 1980). For speciation and differentiation of Gram-positive cocci (*Peptococcus* and *Peptostreptococcus*), as well as further characterization of *Bacteroides* and *Fusobacterium*, biochemical and antimicrobic testing are necessary. These tests include the use of anaerobic blood agar for determining resistance to penicillin, rifampin, and kanamycin, as well as for demonstrating the ability to reduce nitrites. A *presumpto* plate is inoculated to test for indole production, lipase production esculin hydrolysis, catalase production, and bile susceptibility (Dowell and Hawkins, 1974). Fermentation studies are also necessary for complete speciation (Dowell and Allen, 1981).

SEXUALLY TRANSMITTED ORGANISMS

Among the organisms to be considered here are *Neisseria gonorrhoeae*, *Trichomonas vaginalis*, herpes simplex virus, *Chlamydia trachomatis*, and *Ureaplasma urealyticum*. These are the most common sexually transmitted pathogens, those which are responsible for the most severe clinical complications and devastating impacts on reproductive health. The health consequences of pelvic inflammatory disease (PID) are discussed elsewhere in this volume (see Chapter 17). Each organism presents different challenges to *in vitro* cultivation.

Neisseria gonorrhoeae

The gonococcus is a fastidious organism with stringent transport requirements. The type of transport system depends on the distance and time between collection and primary culturing. Selective transport systems that have been recommended over others include Transgrow and JEMBEC. However, a recommended system that involves direct inoculation onto selective media, such as the Improved Thayer–Martin (ITM) medium (Martin and Lewis, 1977) or New York City (NYC) medium (Faur *et al.*, 1973) is the most sensitive isolation procedure. Specimen collection remains critical to culture accuracy; because of the organism's sensitivity to physical and chemical factors, no lubricants other than water should be used (Kellogg, 1977). The specimen should be obtained from a specific site with little or no contamination from adjacent material and should be taken with a low toxicity swab (cotton, wool, calcium alginate).

Following collection, cultures are placed in a CO_2 environment (3–8%) as soon as possible. This environment can be created with a CO_2 incubator, a candle-extinction jar, or a plastic bag with a CO_2 tablet. Selective transport systems sometimes provide adequate CO_2 for growth initiation. Cultures should be delivered to the laboratory within 48 hours for incubation at 36–37°C and subsequent identification. *N. gonorrhoeae* is generally identified presumptively, using colonial morphology, oxidase reaction, cellular morphology, and Gram-stain reaction. Experience in gonococcal identification is necessary for accurate laboratory diagnosis, especially when only presumptive criteria are used. Some indigenous *Neisseria* species exhibit colonial morphology that has only subtle differences, and even some *Moraxella* organisms appear as *N. gonorrhoeae* except for slight morphologic differences.

Although presumptive identification is 98–99.99% specific (Kellogg, 1977; Smeltzer *et al.*, 1980), confirmatory testing is necessary for medicolegal cases and useful for quality control purposes. Confirmation can be accomplished by carbohydrate degradation, FA procedures, or coagglutination with prepared antibody complexes (Kellogg, 1977). Culture diagnosis of gonorrhea has been greatly aided by the development of antibiotic-containing selective media. As with diagnosis of other anogenital infections, contamination is a major problem in gonorrhea diagnosis. Other problems include the following: (1) the need for a CO_2 environment and (2) the need for prompt incubation, because the organism cannot survive in a holding medium.

A new technique for diagnosis of gonorrhea is an ELISA procedure called Gonozyme.[3] Because this technique does not require viable organisms, transport is much less critical; culture is still recommended, however, to support a positive ELISA result and to provide colonies for B-lactamase testing.

B-lactamase is an enzyme that is produced by *N. gonorrhoeae* and other organisms, that inactivates penicillin and makes these organisms completely resistant to treatment with this medication. Penicillinase-producing *N. gonorrhoeae* (PPNG) organisms frequently spread in urban areas from prostitutes to their consorts. To stem the spread of this strain, the Centers for Disease Control (CDC) recommend that all gonococcal isolates be tested for B-lactamase production. At the present time, however, only viable organisms can be analyzed. The most efficient method is the chromogenic cephalosporin reaction, which is available commercially as Cefanase.[4]

The specificity of the culture technique, which may be defined as the frequency with which a test is negative when the disease is not present, is, in the diagnosis of gonorrhea, approximately the same for both male urethral infections and cervical infections. The sensitivity of the culture procedure (the frequency with which a test is positive when disease is present) varies according to the site of infection. For male urethral cultures and cervical cultures, the sensitivity can approach about 98% and 95%, respectively under optimal conditions (Smeltzer *et al.*, 1979). As certain negative factors are introduced, however, the sensitivity is reduced appreciably. Negative factors and their effects include delayed incubation and absence of carbon dioxide. If CO_2 is present, holding a specimen on selective media at 24–30°C for 24 hours has

[3] Abbott Laboratories, North Chicago, IL
[4] BBL, Cockeysville, MD

little effect on recovery (immediate incubation = 79/79; delayed incubation = 74/79) (Sng et al., 1982). Approximately 38% of clinical isolates will not produce viable colonies without CO_2 (Morse et al., 1977). If viable organisms are present, colonies with prompt incubation develop in 24 hours 65% of the time in a CO_2 environment, and in 48 hours 95% of the time (Smeltzer et al., 1979). Dependable gonorrhea culture results are now the rule for health facilities with an easily accessible laboratory.

Trichomonas vaginalis

Culture diagnosis of this infection is not widely practiced, and as a result, countless individuals are undiagnosed and untreated. Dehydrated culture media are available (Trichose 1[5]) as are several formulations for laboratory prepared media (Diamond, 1957). All of these media require supplementation with animal serum to support growth of T. vaginalis and antibiotics to inhibit contaminants. When laboratory facilities are accessible daily, culture techniques prove valuable. Even when kept at room temperature for up to 8 hours prior to incubation, cultures are 50% more sensitive than 0.85% NaCl wet mounts (Spence et al., 1980). Incubation time can vary from 3 to 7 days; however, daily examination is useful for detection of motile organisms. Examination consists of microscopic observation of culture broth under a coverslip. It is not productive to examine culture sediment, but rather an interface approximately 15 mm from the bottom of a 13×75 mm test tube containing 5 ml of Diamond's media yields better results quantitatively. Cultures for T. vaginalis can be inoculated with the same swab used to prepare NaCl wet preps. Processing can be dependent on negative wet prep. results. Cultures are especially valuable when small numbers of organisms are present, such as with asymptomatic disease or with treatment failures.

Herpes simplex virus (HSV)

The culturing of this pathogen, which can be grown readily in a number of cell culture systems, is a routine diagnostic procedure. Primary rabbit kidney cells are the easiest to prepare, and the most sensitive (Rawls, 1979). Specimen collection involves scraping material from the base of lesions, swabbing vaginal or urethral secretions, or swabbing vesicular lesions. Dry swabs should be used for collection, and the specimen should be placed in transport broth as soon as possible. The most common transport system is 'virocult' which contains a modified Liebovitz medium. This system keeps isolates viable for 1–19 days at ambient temperatures (Rawls, 1979).

Following primary inoculation, cell cultures are incubated at 33–34 °C, and the cell surface is examined for changes indicating cell destruction (cytopathic effects (CEP)) daily for up to 7 days. HSV cytopathic effects are quite distinct and may occur in 12–24 hours depending on the number of 'virus' particles present in the sample. Often this is sufficient for tentative diagnosis; however, serologic testing to identify and type the virus as 1 or 2 is indicated in some

[5] BBL, Cockeysville, MD

instances. Neutralization tests or immunofluorescence are the most common confirmatory and typing procedures (Rawls, 1980).

Chlamydia trachomatis

Although sometimes erroneously classified as a bacterium, *C. trachomatis* is an obligate intracellular parasite that must be cultured in living cells. As in the case with other organisms, collection and transport systems critically affect culture results. The most productive collection sites are the cervix and the urethra. Collection swabs must have a cotton or calcium-alginate tip and a plastic or wire shaft. The swab for urethral sampling must be small enough to reach 3–4 cm up the urethra, such as Calgi-swabs I and IV[6] or ENT Sterile Applicator No. 1054.[7] The swab for cervical sampling should be sturdy enough to allow for a scraping action. All of these considerations are critical to the culture process (Mårdh and Zeeberg, 1981).

The collection swabs are placed in sucrose-phosphate buffer (2-SP) for transporting. Samples should be refrigerated (4 °C) immediately for cell culture inoculation within 24 hours. If inoculation is delayed beyond 24 hours, samples must be frozen at −70 °C. The culture methods available for detecting *Chlamydia* require the expertise and equipment found in tissue culture labs since this organism is fragile and does not survive normal transport conditions.

Antibody levels (microimmunofluorescence) range from 25% to 40% in a normal population, and as high as 70% in sexually active women without active chlamydial infection (Schachter and Dawson, 1977), which makes serologic testing an unlikely diagnostic tool. Other methods, including ELISA and direct FA, are being developed, but culture is currently the best diagnostic approach.

If the specimen has reached the laboratory in a condition amenable to growth, culture problems center around cell monolayer sensitivity and identification procedures. The most sensitive cells and the ones used in most laboratories are McCoy cells. These cells are grown in monolayers on glass coverslips, then inoculated with an aliquot from a 2-SP transport broth tube. It appears that different McCoy cell lines perform differently (Smith *et al.*, 1982), making quality control and willingness to use new cell lines important to the culture system. McCoy cells can be passed up to 100 times and can be frozen at −70 °C for future use; therefore, when a line is found that is sensitive with the method being used, it can be used indefinitely. To support *Chlamydia*, McCoy cells need to be nonreplicating. There are a number of ways to halt cell division; the use of cycloheximide is easy and produces good results (Ripa and Mårdh, 1977).

Inoculated cell culture vials are centrifuged to increase the number of chlamydial bodies taken into the cells; this increases the isolation rate significantly. These vials are then seeded with maintenance media (Eagles' MEM) containing cycloheximide and incubated at 35 °C for 2–3 days. Incubation for 2 days is sufficient time for inclusion bodies to develop. Inclusion bodies can be detected by several methods, any one of which constitutes identification. Staining of monolayers to reveal chlamydial inclusions can be accomplished

[6] Indox Corp., Glenwood, IL
[7] Medical Wire & Equipment Co., England

with iodine, Giemsa stain, or fluorescent antibodies. Iodine is the fastest and least expensive method. It is as sensitive as Giemsa but, unlike Giemsa, iodine is a transient stain, making immediate examination necessary and slide retention impractical. Fluorescent staining using monoclonal antibodies significantly decreases slide examination time and increases slide sensitivity (Stephens *et al.*, 1982). Overall the sensitivity of culture diagnosis has not been determined (Wentworth, 1977). Specificity is probably very good (95–99%), especially when experienced personnel are involved.

Other sexually transmitted pathogens

Other sexually transmitted pathogens that can compromise reproductive health are *Ureaplasma urealyticum*, *Candida albicans*, and *Gardnerella vaginalis*. *U. urealyticum*, although clearly implicated in disease processes of the genital tract, is a questionable pathogen (Schwartz *et al.*, 1978) and may represent an opportunistic infection. *U. urealyticum* is easily transported and cultured in selective medium. Problems revolve around its designation as the causative agent when isolated. *C. albicans* and *G. vaginalis* are often diagnosed microscopically. Transport and culture of either organism is not difficult. *C. albicans* is part of the indigenous vaginal flora, making culture for this organism nonproductive. *G. vaginalis*, previously named *Haemophilus vaginalis* and *Corynebacterium vaginalis*, is associated with nonspecific vaginitis. Problems with culture diagnosis are usually associated with the small colony size (0.5 mm diameter). These colonies may be overlooked unless there is strong interest in searching for their presence. Use of a magnifying lens is helpful for observation of the agar surface.

Group-B streptococci, *Staphylococcus aureus*, and enteric pathogens

The diagnosis and treatment of these organisms offer different challenges. Group-B streptococci and *S. aureus* are usually isolated on blood agar and differentiated by Gram's stain or by the catalase reaction. Identification is generally possible within 24 hours, and culture diagnosis presents few problems.

Enteric organisms found in the genitourinary tract play a role in postoperative opportunistic infections (Larsen and Galask, 1980). These agents can be cultured using differential media and selective broths or transport media. The problem of selecting the primary culturing media is usually solved by inoculating several different types, including blood agar, MacConkeys agar, and XLD agar. Important concerns with enterics are species identification and sensitivity testing. There are a number of commercially available species identification kits, including the Mini-tek,[8] Micro ID,[9] and API 20-E[10] systems. These products rely on large numbers of isolates to arrive at computer-based identification guidelines. Antibiotic sensitivity testing is discussed in another chapter of this volume.

[8] BBL, Cockeysville, MD
[9] General Diagnostics, Morris Plains, NJ
[10] Anylab Products, Plainview, NY

CONCLUSION

Culture diagnosis is an essential tool in the characterization of infectious processes. Results of a culture test, however, are subject to interpretation, especially results that are inconsistent with other findings.

Many factors influence the value of a culture test. Due to the dynamic nature of microorganisms, the sensitivity of culture diagnosis may sometimes be called into question. In addition to microbial characteristics, lack of sensitivity could result from the culture process itself, i.e. the collection technique, transport medium, transport conditions, or primary culturing. The use of an inappropriate protocol may also contribute to sensitivity problems. The causative agent may be inhibited by something inherent in the technique. There may be an indigenous agent present that inhibits the growth of the infectious agent *in vitro* but not *in vivo*.

The goal is to create a system sensitive enough to detect disease only when it is present. Until such a system is available for all of the possible disease entities, interpretive guidelines need to be developed. Clinical presentation is important, as is history, and other nonlaboratory parameters. A culture result is only another parameter to be assessed and utilized intelligently to arrive at a final decision.

References

Bowie, W. R., Pollock, H. M., Forsyth, P. S. *et al.* (1977). Bacteriology of the urethra of normal men and men with nongonococcal urethritis. *J. Clin Microbiol.*, **6**, 482

Bowie, W. R., Wang, S. P. and Alexander, E. R. *et al.* (1977). Etiology of nongonococcal urethritis: evidence for *Chlamydia trachomatis* and *Ureaplasma urealyticum*. *J. Clin. Invest.*, **59**, 735

Diamond, L. S. (1957). Media for isolation of *Trichomonas vaginalis*. *J. Parasitol.*, **43**, 488

Dowell, V. R. (1975). Methods for isolation of anaerobes in the clinical laboratory. *Am. J. Med. Technol.*, **41**, 32

Dowell, V. R. and Allen, S. D. (1981). Anaerobic bacterial infections. In Ballows, A. and Hausler Jr., W. J. (eds.) *Diagnostic Procedures for Bacterial, Mycotic, and Parasitic Infections*, 6th edn. (Washington: American Public Health Association)

Dowell, V. R., Lombard, G. L., Thompson, F. S. *et al.* (1977). *Media for Isolation, Characterization and Identification of Obligatory Anaerobic Bacteria*. (Atlanta: Center for Disease Control)

Dowell, Jr., V. R. and Hawkins, T. M. (1974). *Laboratory Methods in Anaerobic Bacteriology, DHEW No. 74-8272*. (Atlanta: Center for Disease Control)

Faur, Y. C., Weisburd, M. H. and Wilson, M. E. (1973). A new medium for the isolation of pathogenic *Neisseria* (NYC medium) II. *Health Lab. Sci.*, **10**, 55

Finegold, S. E. and Citron, D. M. (1980). Gram-negative nonsporeforming anaerobic bacilli. In Lennette, E. H., Balows, A., Hausler Jr., W. J. (eds.) *Manual of Clinical Microbiology*, 3rd edn. (Washington: American Society of Microbiology)

Isenberg, H. D. and Painter, B. G. (1980). Indigenous and pathogenic microorganisms of humans. In Lennette, E. H., Balows, A., Hausler Jr., W. J. *et al.* (eds.) *Manual of Clinical Microbiology*, 3rd edn. (Washington: American Society of Microbiology)

Isenberg, H. D., Washington II, J. A., Balows, A. *et al.* (1980). Collection, handling, and processing of specimens. In Lennette, E. H., Balows, A. and Hausler Jr., W. J. *et al.* (eds.) *Manual of Clinical Microbiology*, 3rd edn. (Washington: American Society of Microbiology)

Kellogg Jr., D. S. (1977). Current methods for laboratory diagnosis of gonococcal infections. In Roberts, R. B. (ed.) *The Gonococcus*. (New York: Wiley & Sons)

Larsen, B. and Galask, R. P. (1980). Vaginal microbial flora: practical and theoretic relevance. *Obstet. Gynecol.*, **55**, 1005

Mårdh, P.-A. and Zeeberg, B. (1981). Toxic effect of sampling swabs and transportation test tubes on the formation of intracytoplasmic inclusions of *Chlamydia trachomatis* in McCoy cell cultures. *Br. J. Vener. Dis.*, **57**, 268

Martin Jr., J. E. and Lewis, J. (1977). Anisomycin: improved antimicotic activity in Modified Thayer-Martin medium. *Pub. Hlth. Lab.*, **35**, 53

Morse, S. A., Miller, R. D. and Hebler, B. H. (1977). Physiology and metabolism of *Neisseria gonorrhoeae*. In Roberts, R. B. (ed.) *The Gonococcus*. (New York: Wiley & Sons)

Ohm, M. J. and Galask, R. P. (1975). Bacterial flora of the cervix from 100 prehysterectomy patients. *Am. J. Obstet. Gynecol.*, **122**, 683

Pheifer, T. A., Forsyth, P. S., Durfee, M. A. *et al.* (1978). Nonspecific vaginitis. *N. Engl. J. Med.*, **298**, 1429

Rawls, W. E. (1979). Herpes simplex virus types 1 and 2 and herpes virus semiae. In Lennette, E. H. and Schmidt, N. J. (eds.) *Diagnostic Procedures for Viral, Rickettsial and Chlamydial Infections*, 5th edn. (Washington: American Public Health Association)

Rawls, W. E. (1980). Herpes simplex viruses. In Lennette, E. H., Ballows, A., Hausler Jr., W. J. *et al.* (eds.) *Manual of Clinical Microbiology*, 3rd edn. (Washington: American Society of Microbiology)

Ripa, K. T. and Mårdh, P.-A. (1977). New simplified culture technique for *Chlamydia trachomatis*. In Hobson, D. and Holmes, K. K. (eds.) *Nongonococcal Urethritis and Related Infections*, p. 323. (Washington: American Society for Microbiology)

Schachter, J. and Dawson, C. R. (1977). Comparative efficacy of various diagnostic methods for chlamydial infection. In Hobson, D. and Holmes, K. K. (eds.) *Nongonococcal Urethritis and Related Infections*. (Washington: American Society for Microbiology)

Smeltzer, M. P., Curran, J. W. and Lossick, J. G. (1979). A comparative evaluation of media used to culture *N. gonorrhoeae*. *Pub. Hlth. Lab.*, **37**, 43

Smeltzer, M. P., Curran, J. W. and Stuart, S. T. *et al.* (1980). Accuracy of presumptive criteria for culture diagnosis of *Neisseria gonorrhoeae* in low-prevalence populations of women. *J. Clin. Microbiol.*, **11**, 485

Smith, T. F., Brown, S. D. and Weed, L. A. (1982). Diagnosis of *Chlamydia trachomatis* by cell cultures and serology. *Lab. Med.*, **13**, 92

Sng, E. H., Rajan, V. S., Yea, K. L. *et al.* (1982). The recovery of *Neisseria gonorrhoeae* from clinical specimens: effects of different temperatures, transport, times, and media. *Sex. Transm. Dis.*, **9**, 74

Spence, M. R., Hollender, D. H., Smith, J. *et al.* (1980). The clinical and laboratory diagnosis of *Trichomonas vaginalis* infection. *Sex. Transm. Dis.*, **7**, 168

Starr, S. E. and Friedman, H. M. (1980). Human cytomegalovirus. In Lennette, E. H., Balows, A., Hausler, Jr., W. J. *et al.* (eds.) *Manual of Clinical Microbiology*, 3rd edn. (Washington: American Society of Microbiology)

Stephens, R. S., Kuo, C. and Tam, M. R. (1982). Sensitivity of immunofluorescence with monoclonal antibodies for detection of *Chlamydia trachomatis* inclusions in cell culture. *J. Clin. Microbiol.*, **16**, 4

Swartz, S. L., Kraus, S. J. and Herrmann, K. L. *et al.* (1978). Diagnosis and etiology of nongonococcal urethritis. *J. Infect. Dis.*, **138**, 445

Wentworth, B. B. (1977). Sensitivity of cell culture for isolation of *Chlamydia trachomatis* from genital sources. In Hobson, D. and Holmes, K. K., (eds.) *Nongonococcal Urethritis and Related Infections*. (Washington: American Society for Microbiology)

Wilkinson, H. W. (1978). Group B streptococcal infections. *Ann. Rev. Microbiol.*, **32**, 41

Woolfrey, B. F., Lally, R. T. and Quall, C. O. (1983). Evaluation of auto scan-3 and sceptor systems for enterobacteriaceae identification. *J. Clin. Microbiol.*, **17**, 807

Yolken, R. H. (1982). Enzyme immunoassays for the detection of infectious antigens in body fluids: current limitations and future prospects. *Rev. Infect. Dis.*, **4**, 35

23
Local immune response to bacterial infection of the male urinary tract

J. E. FOWLER, Jr.

INTRODUCTION

The precise role of the immune response in the defense against urinary tract infection has not been clearly defined. Several observations, however, suggest that local antibody secretions may contribute to the prevention or containment of such infections, at least in the male.

Urinary pathogens are rarely isolated from the urethras of normal men despite the proximity of the urinary meatus to the Gram-negative bacteria of the anus and perineum. The incidence of urinary tract infection among males with no underlying urologic disorders is remarkably low, and clinically apparent infections of the prostate, seminal vesicles, and epididymis, which communicate directly with the urethra, are uncommon complications of documented bacteriuria. Finally, and perhaps most important, antibody against infecting bacteria can be detected in the urine, prostatic fluid, and seminal fluid of men with urinary tract infection.

This chapter will review our own recent observations, as well as those of others, concerning the concentrations of immunoglobulin (Ig) in male genital secretions and the local immune response of the male genital tract to bacteriuria and bacterial prostatitis. Because of frequent misconceptions about the microbiology of the normal male genitourinary system and because the significance of the local immune response to infection is based in part upon the degree of antigenic stimulation in normal health, the chapter will also examine the microbiology of this organ complex and the techniques that may be applied for the localization of bacterial infections. Since the primary concern of this volume is reproductive physiology and health, secretion of Ig by the bladder and the kidneys, which is quantitatively less than that of the male reproductive organs, will not be addressed in detail.

LOCAL IMMUNITY

Mucosal surfaces exposed to the external environment, as well as the mucosa of the bowel, are continually colonized by bacteria of varying pathogenicity. The containment of commensural, and the elimination of pathogenic, bacteria are critical to the prevention of superficial and invasive infections. A variety of nonspecific humoral, cellular, and physical host defense mechanisms contribute to this process. There is evidence that antibody secretion is also an important component of the mucosal defenses (Tomasi, 1976; Hanson and Brandtzaeg, 1979).

Local immunity, which is generated primarily by the secretory immune system, is characterized by the secretion of Ig classes in proportions different from those found in the serum, and by a regulation of antibody secretion that is largely independent of the systemic antibody response. The synthesis of antigen-specific Ig is induced by stimulation of lymphoid cells in the lamina propria of the mucous membrane and adjacent secretory glands. By mechanisms that are not completely understood, plasma cells committed primarily to the synthesis of immunoglobulin A (IgA) with specificity for the stimulating antigen subsequently populate the lamina propria at the site of antigenic challenge. The IgA released by these cells is thought to be in the dimeric form, and each dimer is complexed with a polypeptide (secretory component) during passage through the mucosal epithelium. Secretory component confers resistance to proteolysis, a biologically advantageous property for antibody in the external secretions. Immunoglobulin M (IgM) in mucosal secretions may also be synthesized in part by plasma cells in the lamina propria and may complex with secretory component. The major proportion of immunoglobulin G (IgG) is derived from serum transudate.

Most of our knowledge concerning the secretory immune system has stemmed from studies of the easily accessible ocular, oral, mammary, and respiratory secretions and from studies of gastrointestinal immunology. Advances in the understanding of infectious disorders of the genitourinary tract have also stimulated interest in the local immune processes of this organ complex. The relative concentrations of Ig classes and the presence of secretory IgA (S-IgA) in both female and male genital secretions suggest secretory immunity. Gonococcal urethritis in the male is accompanied by the local secretion of antigen-specific S-IgA (Tramont, 1977), while IgA directed against *Candida albicans* (Waldman *et al.*, 1972) and the polio vaccine (Ogra and Ogra, 1973) can be detected in vaginal fluid after topical application. These observations are also consistent with a secretory immune response. Finally, there is now convincing evidence of a profound local immune response by the prostate to Gram-negative bacterial infection of the genitourinary tract.

MICROBIOLOGY OF THE MALE GENITOURINARY TRACT

Investigations into the normal microbiology of the secretory organs and mucosal surfaces of the male genitourinary system have been complicated by the difficulty of selectively isolating fluids from specific anatomic sites. Urine, urethral washings, ejaculate, and fluid obtained by digital massage of the prostate all can be cultured. The ejaculate, however, is a complex fluid derived from the glands of Cowper and Littré, the prostate, the ampulla of the vas deferens, the epididymis, and the seminal vesicles (Polakaski *et al.*, 1976). Similarly, fluid obtained by massage of the prostate (expressed prostatic secretion, EPS) is derived primarily from the prostate but may also contain fluids from the seminal vesicles and ampulla of the vas deferens (Fair and Cordonnier, 1978). Furthermore, the voided urine, ejaculate, and EPS all are subject to contamination by the urethral flora.

 Gram-positive bacteria of limited pathogenicity, usually staphylococci, streptococci, and diphtheroids, can be isolated from urethral cultures of approximately 90% of men who have no clinical evidence of genitourinary infection (Stamey, 1980; Anderson and Weller, 1979; Klousia *et al.*, 1978; Holmes *et al.*, 1975). *Mycoplasma hominis* and *Ureaplasma urealyticum* colonize the distal urethra of approximately 30–50% of normal men (Klousia *et al.*, 1978; Holmes *et al.*, 1975; Ulstein *et al.*, 1976). These same organisms are frequently isolated from the voided urine, ejaculate, and EPS of normal men (Stamey, 1980; Ulstein *et al.*, 1976; Berger *et al.*, 1982).

There is considerable evidence that bladder urine and the components of genital secretions are normally sterile before micturition, emission, or expression, but are contaminated during transit through the urethra. For example, urine aspirated directly from the bladders of normal men is invariably sterile. Similarly, fluid obtained from the vas deferens during elective vasectomy was cultured for *M. hominis* and *U. urealyticum* (Taub *et al.*, 1973) in a group of 98 males. Each specimen was culture negative despite prior isolation of at least one of these organisms from the urethra in 25% of cases. In addition, among men with acute epididymitis, the cultures of epididymal aspirates uniformly contain only one identifiable infecting microorganism or no identifiable microorganisms (Berger *et al.*, 1978).

A noninvasive method for estimating urethral contamination of male genital secretions enhances our understanding of the microbiology of the male genitourinary tract in addition to providing a practical means for localizing bacterial infection within the male reproductive organs (Meares and Stamey, 1968). In this technique a quantitative culture of the first 10 ml of voided urine (the VB_1) identifies the urethral flora and provides an estimate of the anticipated contribution of urethral bacteria to subsequent specimens; this is then compared to quantitative cultures of the midstream urine (the VB_2), the EPS, and the first 10 ml of urine voided after prostatic massage (the VB).

In the normal male the concentration of a bacterium in the VB_1 specimen generally exceeds that in the VB_2 specimen and a bacterium isolated from the VB_2 is almost always present in the VB_1. If this be the case, the site of colonization is localized to the urethra rather than the bladder urine. Moreover, the concentration of an isolate in the EPS specimen is usually equivalent to or less than 5 times greater than the concentration of the same isolate in the VB_1. Among men with bacterial infections of the prostate who do not have coexisting bacteriuria or who are receiving an antibiotic that suppresses the growth of bacteria in the bladder urine and urethra, the concentration of the infecting

345

organism in the EPS characteristically exceeds that in the VB_1 by more than tenfold. The concentration of the infecting organism in the VB_3, which contains residual intraurethral prostatic fluid, may also exceed that of the VB_1. If the urine is infected with high concentrations of bacteria (10^5/ml in the VB_2), quantitative differences between the VB_1, EPS, and VB_3 isolates are difficult to detect and the infection cannot be localized. A comparison of the quantitative culture of the VB_1 to that of an ejaculate specimen obtained shortly after voiding may also localize bacterial infection to the prostate or to other reproductive glands contributing to the ejaculate (Mobley, 1975).

The value of this widely used technique is due largely to the fact that bacteria in the urine and the urethra generally are more susceptible to antimicrobial therapy than bacteria within the internal, secretory organs. Therefore, contamination of EPS or the ejaculate by coexisting pathogenic bacteria within the urethra can be minimized and the infection localized to the prostate. If the urethral flora is not suppressed or eliminated, however, or if strict criteria are not used in the interpretation of culture data, quantitative culture results may be misleading.

To demonstrate this concept we performed bacterial localization cultures in six male volunteers of proven fertility who were not receiving antibiotics and who had no histories of genitourinary disorders (Table 1). The EPS was

Table 1 Genitourinary bacteriology of five volunteer men with no histories of genitourinary disorders

	Colonies per ml					
Patient no.	VB_1	VB_2	EPS	VB_3	Seminal fluid	Organism
1	7500	2200	1000	1700	6000	Staphylococcus
	2500	700	0	100	1500	Enterococcus
2	2000	100	15,000	600	1000	Staphylococcus[a]
	2000	1000	15,000	600	1000	Diphtheroids[a]
3	1000	40	4000	900	6000	Staphylococcus[a,b]
	0	0	4000	0	6000	Diphtheroids[a,b]
4	200	0	100	100	140	Staphylococcus
	400	0	2700	1600	1800	Streptococcus[a,b]
	0	0	0	0	700	Diphtheroids[b]
5	100	200	0	60	800	Staphylococcus[b]
	0	0	0	0	3000	Diphtheroids[b]
6	100	80	550	80	340	Stapylococcus
	0	0	550	0	0	Diphtheroids[a]

[a] Culture results suggest prostatic infection
[b] Culture results suggest infection of glands contributing secretions to the ejaculate

obtained after collection of the VB_2, and the seminal fluid was obtained by masturbation approximately 1 hour before the urine and EPS specimens. None of the patients had increased numbers of leukocytes in the urine, EPS, or seminal fluid. In each case the concentration of an isolate in the VB_1 exceeded that in the VB_2. However, the concentration of 7 of the 9 EPS isolates and of 7 of the 12 seminal fluid isolates exceeded the concentration of the same isolate in the corresponding VB_1 specimen. Indeed, 2 of the EPS isolates and 3 of the seminal fluid isolates were not recovered from the corresponding VB_1. This finding undoubtedly results from an increased susceptibility to urethral contamination due to: (1) the greater viscosity of these secretions compared to urine, and (2) the slow movement of prostatic fluid and the initial portions of the ejaculate along the urethra. Extraurethral contamination also may have been introduced during masturbation. Were it not for the knowledge that: (1) these bacterial isolates rarely cause genitourinary infection, (2) these patients had no clinical evidence of genitourinary infection, and (3) specific organisms were often isolated from one genital secretion but not the other, 4 of the 6 culture studies would have suggested infection of the secretory reproductive glands by at least one organism. Two additional bacterial localization studies were performed in each volunteer over the ensuing 2 months. In many cases organisms that differed from the initial genital fluid isolates were cultured from the second and third EPS and seminal fluid specimens. Since spontaneous resolution of bacterial infection of the male reproductive organs is unlikely, the possibility that the EPS or seminal fluid isolates actually infected the secretory reproductive glands seems extremely remote.

URINARY TRACT INFECTION IN THE MALE

In the absence of urologic instrumentation or anatomical abnormalities of the genitourinary tract, urinary tract infection in the male is remarkably infrequent (Stamey, 1980). The vast majority of infections are caused by Enterobacteriaceae, *Pseudomonas*, or enterococcus. Concurrent infection of the male reproductive organs, and the prostate in particular, may occur because of their direct linkage to the urinary tract. Acute prostatic infections, which are always accompanied by infected urine and manifested by symptoms of bacteriuria and severe prostatic tenderness, are not difficult to diagnose or eradicate. In contrast, chronic bacterial prostatitis may be associated with sterile urine, is frequently manifested only by vague pelvic discomforts, and is often refractory to antimicrobial therapy.

Increased numbers of leukocytes in the EPS (>10–20 per HPF) are invariably observed in cases of chronic bacterial prostatitis. This finding, however, is nonspecific, and quantitative culture of the urine, EPS or seminal fluid in the manner described above is necessary to establish the diagnosis.

A series of bacterial localization cultures in a man with chronic bacterial prostatitis due to an 01 *Escherichia coli* are shown in Table 2. The Gram-negative bacterium isolated from the urine and EPS was always an 01 *E. coli* and the urine and EPS cultures often were negative during treatment but invariably became positive when antibiotics were withheld. Moreover, the concentration of leukocytes in the EPS was persistently increased. When isolated, the concentration of the infecting *E. coli* was usually more than 10 times greater in the EPS than in the VB_1. Despite unequivocal evidence of persistent prostatic infection, the patient was entirely asymptomatic during antimicrobial therapy. This phenomenon is characteristic of chronic bacterial prostatitis.

Table 2 Case 1: Genitourinary bacteriology of J.G., a 44-year-old male with chronic *E. coli* bacterial prostatitis

Date	Days on (+) or off (−) drug	Colonies per ml				Organism	EPS leukocytes per HPF
		VB_1	VB_2	EPS	VB_3		
1979-1981	3 episodes of symptomatic culture documented *E coli* bacteriuria						
27 Aug. 1981	First visit	1000	1000	100,000	–	*E. coli* (01)	40
8 Sept. 1981	+10 TMP-SMX	0	0	0	0	–	15
8 Oct. 1981	+ 30 TMP-SMX	0	0	0	0	–	40
3 Nov. 1981	+55 TMP-SMX (s)	0	0	0	0	–	15
9 Feb. 1982	−36 TMP-SMX (s)	100,000	85,000	25,000	85,000	*E. coli* (01)	30
9 Mar. 1982	+28 TMP-SMX (s)	0	0	0	0	–	20
6 Apr. 1982	+56 TMP-SMX (s)	0	0	0	0	–	20
15 June 1982	+70 Nitrofurantoin (s)	0	0	0	0	–	25
10 Aug. 1982	+126 Nitrofurantoin (s)	0	0	180	200	*E. coli* (01)	25
14 Oct. 1982	−7 Nitrofurantoin (s)	100	0	20,000	40	*E. coli* (01)	40
9 Dec. 1982	+56 Nitrofurantoin (s)	100	20	500	40	*E. coli* (01)	40
17 Feb. 1983	+70 TMP-SMX	60	80	2100	120	*E. coli* (01)	40
9 Apr. 1983	+122 TMP-SMX	0	0	0	0	–	25
9 June 1983	+183 TMP-SMX	0	0	0	20	*E. coli* (01)	20
5 July 1983	+26 Nitrofurantoin (s)	20	0	0	20	*P. aeruginosa*	15

From Fowler, J. E., Jr. and Mariano, M. (1983b). Bacterial infection and male infertility: Absence of IgA with specificity for *E. coli* in seminal fluid of infertile men. *J. Urol.*, **130**, 171

TMP-SMX = Trimethoprim-sulfamethoxazole in full dosage (160–800 mg b.i.d.);
TMP-SMX (s) = Trimethoprim-sulfamethoxazole in suppressive dosage (40–200 mg q.h.s.);
Nitrofurantoin (s) = Nitrofurantoin in suppressive dosage (100 mg q.h.s.)

The positive localization cultures in this case are not dissimilar to some of the localization cultures in normal volunteer men (see Table 1). However, the persistence of increased numbers of EPS leukocytes and the intermittent isolation of a single pathogenic bacterium from the EPS despite prolonged antimicrobial therapy indicate chronic prostatic infection. On the other hand, among the untreated volunteers the microscopic appearance of the EPS was normal and the bacterial isolates from serial EPS and seminal fluid specimens were variable, indicating urethral contamination of the EPS rather than infection of the prostate.

IMMUNOGLOBULIN IN MALE GENITAL SECRETIONS

Investigations of Ig concentrations in male genital secretions have been necessarily limited to assays of the EPS and seminal fluid. Among men with no clinical evidence of prostatic inflammation, the average concentrations of EPS IgG and IgA are reported to range from 15 to 49 mg/dl and from 5 to 131 mg/dl, respectively (Gray et al., 1973; Grayhack et al., 1979; Wishnow et al., 1982). A portion of EPS IgA appears to be in the form of S-IgA (Gray et al., 1973; Shortliffe et al., 1981a). IgM is often undetectable with assays of low sensitivity (Gray et al., 1973).

The concentrations of seminal fluid Ig in apparently normal men are substantially less than those of EPS. IgG is usually present in concentrations of 5–14 mg/dl, while IgA, when detectable, is in concentrations of 0.5–3 mg/dl. IgM has generally not been measurable (Sullivan and Quinlivan, 1980; Azim et al., 1978; Uehling, 1971; Tauber et al., 1975; Friberg, 1980). A portion of seminal fluid IgA is also present in the secretory form (Soliman and Olesen, 1976; Sullivan and Quinlivan, 1980). These data are consistent with observations that the concentrations of IgG and IgA are greater in the initial portions of the ejaculate, which are derived largely from prostatic secretions, than in the terminal portions, which are composed primarily of fluid from the seminal vesicles (Rumke, 1974; Tauber et al., 1975). IgE in extremely low concentrations (1–2 ng/ml), but not IgD, has also been detected in seminal fluid (Friberg, 1980). The concentrations of IgD and IgE in prostatic fluid have not been reported.

Our own studies of EPS and seminal fluid Ig parallel these data. We employ an indirect solid-phase radioimmunoassay (SPRIA) to quantitate class-specific Ig in biologic fluids (Fowler et al., 1982). The sensitivity of the assay is 0.01 mg/dl. Among men who have no histories of genitourinary infection, sterile or contaminated EPS, and normal EPS leukocyte concentrations, the mean concentrations of EPS IgG, IgA, and IgM were 18.4, 7.9, and 0.29 mg/dl, respectively (Table 3).

We are unaware of any substantive data concerning intrasubject variability of EPS Ig concentrations in healthy men. Among men with well-suppressed or recently eradicated bacterial infections of the prostate, however, the variability in serial specimens is not great (see below).

Our investigations of Ig in the seminal fluid (Fowler and Mariano, 1983a), as well as those described previously, have explored the possible relationships between Ig concentrations and male infertility and are limited to the study of men between the ages of approximately 20 and 40 years. The mean concentrations of seminal fluid IgG and IgA among men of proven fertility with no histories of genitourinary disorders were significantly lower than those in the EPS of the normal men that we have studied (see Table 3). Seminal fluid IgM was usually not measurable (<0.04 mg/dl). Nonetheless, IgM was undoubtedly present since a portion of the ejaculate is derived from prostatic secretions and

Table 3 Immunoglobulin concentrations in seminal fluid of normal men and in prostatic fluid (EPS) of normal men and men with bacteriuria and bacterial prostatitis

Patient group (no.)	Mean age (years)	Mean Ig (mg/dl)±1 S.D. (number specimens assayed)			
		IgG	IgA	IgM	IgG/IgA
Seminal fluid					
Normal men (16)	29.4	2.7±1.8 (16)	0.5±0.2 (16)	–	5.5±3.5 (16)
EPS					
Normal men (37)	51.1	18.4±18.7[a]	7.9±7.7[a]	0.29±0.30	4.0±3.3
Bacteriuric patients (10)	49.0	20.5±19.5 (8)	45.3±66.8[b] (9)	0.97±0.70[b] (8)	1.4±1.0[c] (8)
Bacterial prostatitis patients (9)	59.1	48.9±77.2 (8)	67.1±54.6[b] (9)	2.40±3.10[b] (8)	1.1±1.1[c] (8)

[a] Significantly greater ($p<0.01$) than corresponding mean Ig concentration in seminal fluid
[b] Significantly greater ($p<0.01$) than corresponding mean Ig concentration in EPS of normal men
[c] Significantly less ($p<0.01$) than corresponding mean ratio in EPS of normal men

IgM is almost always detected in the EPS when highly sensitive assays are employed. Seminal fluid Ig concentrations appear to remain relatively stable for a given individual over the course of time (Uehling, 1971; Fowler and Mariano, 1983a).

On the basis of these collective observations it appears that the prostate gland and the male reproductive tract should be considered as part of the secretory immune system. This concept is further supported by investigations of the local immune response of the reproductive organs to urinary tract infection.

LOCAL IMMUNE RESPONSE TO URINARY TRACT INFECTION

Increased Ig concentrations and antibody against infecting bacteria have been detected in the urine of men and women with urinary tract infection (Thomas and Forland, 1982). The magnitude of this immune response, primarily of the IgG and IgA classes, depends in part on the duration and extent of the infection. In men, the titer of antibacterial Ig in urine is greater when there is coexisting bacterial prostatitis than when there is no evidence of prostatic infection.

The presence of antibody in the EPS against bacteria infecting the prostate has been demonstrated with indirect immunofluorescent techniques (Jones, 1974). Using indirect SPRIA methodology, Shortliffe et al. (1981a,b) quantitated total and antigen-specific Ig in the serum and the EPS of two men with bacterial prostatitis. In both cases infection was accompanied by increases in the concentrations of EPS IgA, but the serum IgG and IgA concentrations remained relatively constant. Serum antibody directed against the infecting organisms was primarily of the IgG class, whereas the EPS antibody was predominantly IgA.

We have also assessed the nonspecific and specific local immune response of the genital tract to both bacteriuria and bacterial prostatitis (Fowler *et al.*, 1982; Fowler and Mariano, 1982, 1983b, 1984). The mean concentrations of EPS IgA and IgM among men with bacteriuria and bacterial prostatitis were significantly greater than among men with no histories of genitourinary infection (Table 3). The mean ratios of EPS IgG to IgA were significantly less for these two groups of infected patients than for the uninfected group. This suggests that bacterial infection of the urine or of the urine and the prostate is associated with a relatively greater increase in IgA secretion than IgG secretion.

Class-specific antibacterial Ig was quantitated with indirect SPRIA methodologies (Shortliffe *et al.*, 1981a). In these assays formalinized whole bacteria were used as the antigen, serial twofold dilutions of EPS, seminal fluid, or serum were the primary antibody, and ^{125}I-labeled antihuman IgG, IgA, or IgM were the secondary antibody (Fig. 1). Nonspecific binding of primary and

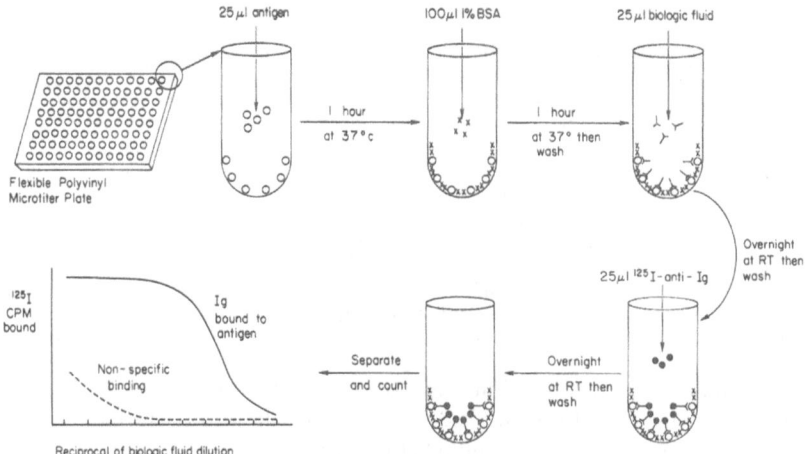

Fig. 1 Methods of indirect SPRIA for quantitating class-specific antibacterial Ig in EPS, seminal fluid, and serum. Formalinized whole bacteria (the antigen in the assay system) coat the wells of the microtiter plate; 1% bovine serum albumin (BSA) coats the remaining surface of the wells to reduce nonspecific binding of primary and secondary antibody. Serial 2-fold dilutions of the biologic fluid of interest (the primary antibody in the assay system) are added to each well and the antibody with specificity for bacterial antigen binds to the bacteria. ^{125}I-labeled antihuman IgG, A, or M (the secondary antibody in the assay system) binds to Ig of the corresponding class that is fixed to the bacteria. The CPM of the bound secondary antibody in each well is measured in a gamma counter and the resultant SPRIA curve (CPM of bound secondary antibody vs. the reciprocal of the primary antibody dilution) is compared to a standard curve (Fig. 2) to quantitate antibacterial class-specific Ig in the biologic fluid

secondary antibody in each assay was assessed using wells with no antigen. The configurations of the binding curves generated with immune specimens are identical to those generated in the indirect SPRIA for total class-specific Ig where antihuman IgG, IgA, or IgM is used as the antigen (Fig. 2). Further, the plateau regions of the binding curves, which reflect saturation binding of primary antibody to antigen, are in general quantitatively similar in the two assay systems. For these reasons, total Ig and antibacterial Ig of a given class are quantitated by reference to the same standard curve (Fig. 2). Our methods

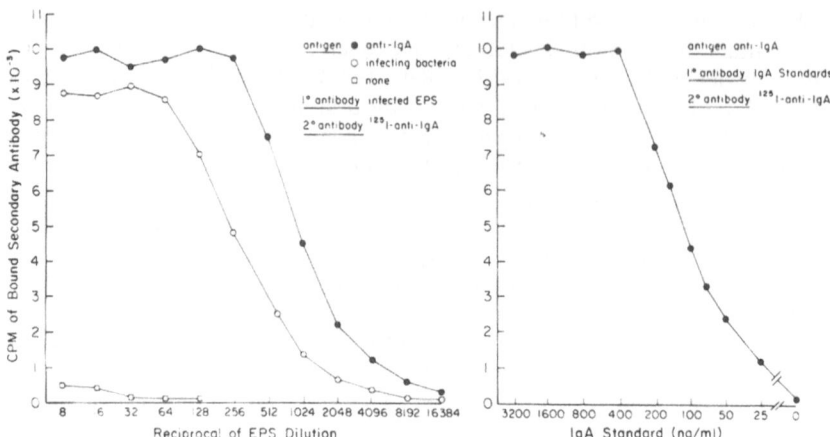

Fig. 2 Comparison of standard SPRIA curve with SPRIA curves for quantitation of total Ig and antibacterial Ig in EPS. (Right) ●——● standard SPRIA curve (CPM of bound secondary antibody vs. concentration of IgA standard) is generated with antihuman IgA as antigen, IgA standards as primary antibody, and ^{125}I-labeled antihuman IgA as secondary antibody. (Left) ●——● SPRIA curve to quantitate total IgA in EPS (CPM of bound secondary antibody vs. reciprocal of EPS dilution) is generated with antihuman IgA as antigen, serial 2-fold dilutions of EPS from chronic bacterial prostatitis patient as primary antibody, and ^{125}I-labeled antihuman IgA as secondary antibody. O——O SPRIA curve to quantitate antibacterial IgA in EPS is generated with infecting *E. coli* from patient with chronic bacterial prostatitis as antigen, serial 2-fold dilutions of EPS as primary antibody, and ^{125}I-labeled antihuman IgA as secondary antibody. Note that the configuration and the height of the plateau region of the three curves are roughly equivalent. Both total and antibacterial IgA in the EPS are therefore quantitated by reference to the same standard curve

for calculating Ig concentrations have been reported previously (Fowler *et al.*, 1982). The concentrations of class-specific Ig binding to bacterial antigen are expressed as mg units/dl (Wishnow *et al.*, 1982).

Class-specific antibody against the infecting bacterium, or bacterium of the same species as that which caused the infection, has been quantitated in the EPS of 12 bacteriuric and 10 bacterial prostatitis patients. Measurable antibacterial EPS IgA was detected in specimens from each of the bacterial prostatitis patients and from all but one of the bacteriuric patients (Table 4). Measurable antibacterial EPS IgG was detected less frequently and was quantitatively smaller, while measurable antibacterial EPS IgM was never observed. When only those patients with measurable antibacterial Ig were considered, the mean amounts of antibacterial IgG and IgA expressed alone or as a function of total EPS Ig were not significantly different in the bacteriuric and bacterial prostatitis groups ($p > 0.05$).

We then assessed the specificity of measurable EPS antibacterial IgG and IgA as an indicator of past or ongoing bacterial infection of the genitourinary tract. The EPS of men without histories suggestive of past infection and with normal EPS leukocyte concentrations and sterile or contaminated EPS was assayed. A mixture of *Proteus mirabilis*, *Klebsiella pneumoniae*, and *Pseudomonas aeruginosa*, or a mixture of eight *E. coli* 0-serotypes that commonly cause urinary infection, was used as the antigen in the assay system. In only

Table 4   Antibacterial immunoglobulin in prostatic fluid (EPS)

	Patient group		
	Control	Bacteriuric	Bacterial prostatitis
Number specimens with measurable antibacterial Ig (%)			
IgG	1/17 (6%)	4/8 (50%)	7/8 (88%)[b]
IgA	0/23 (0%)	11/12 (92%)	10/10 (100%)
IgM	0/10 (0%)	0/5 (0%)	0/3 (0%)
Mean antibacterial Ig (mg units/dl) $\pm$ 1 SD[a]			
IgG	0.5	0.96 $\pm$ 1.2	0.78 $\pm$ 1.0
IgA	–	3.0 $\pm$ 5.4	5.5 $\pm$ 7.6
Mean $\dfrac{\text{antibacterial Ig}}{\text{total Ig}}$ ($\times$100) $\pm$ 1 SD			
IgG	0.9	4.8 $\pm$ 2.7	3.0 $\pm$ 3.3
IgA	–	5.6 $\pm$ 6.3	12.8 $\pm$ 17.1

[a] Includes only those specimens with measurable antibacterial Ig
[b] Includes patient with IgG multiple myeloma and no antibacterial IgG

one case was there measurable EPS Ig directed against bacterial antigen (IgG, 0.5 mg units/ml binding to *E. coli*) (see Table 4). Composites of the curves generated with these control specimens contrast sharply with composites of the curves generated with EPS from the bacteriuric and bacterial prostatitis patients (Fig. 3).

Antibody directed against bacterial antigen may also be detectable in the seminal fluid of men with urinary tract infection. We assayed the seminal fluid of the patient with an 01 *E. coli* chronic bacterial prostatitis (see Table 2), and the seminal fluid of 86 fertile and infertile men with no histories of genitourinary infection, for IgA directed against antigen in the mixture of eight common *E. coli* 0-serotypes (Fowler and Mariano, 1983b). Antibacterial IgA was easily measured in the specimen from the bacterial prostatitis patient but was not detectable in specimens from the uninfected men (Fig. 4). The latter observation provides further evidence that Ig directed against Gram-negative enteric bacteria is not usually present in the reproductive secretions of men with no histories of genitourinary infection. This finding also indirectly supports the concept that this organ system is rarely infected by Gram-negative bacteria.

The precise antigen or antigens to which EPS or seminal fluid antibacterial Ig bind could not be determined from these studies since whole bacteria are used in the assays. However, we (Fowler and Mariano, 1982) and others (Wishnow *et al.*, 1982) have demonstrated that EPS antibody directed against *E. coli* has minimal cross-reactivity with other enterobacteria, and vice-versa, and that antibody directed against *E. coli* is relatively specific for the 0-antigen (Fowler and Mariano, 1983b).

As is characteristic of the secretory immune system, the secretion of antigen-specific IgA by the prostate appears to be largely independent of the systemic immune response. Class-specific antibacterial Ig was measured in both the serum and the EPS of ten men with bacteriuria or bacterial prostatitis

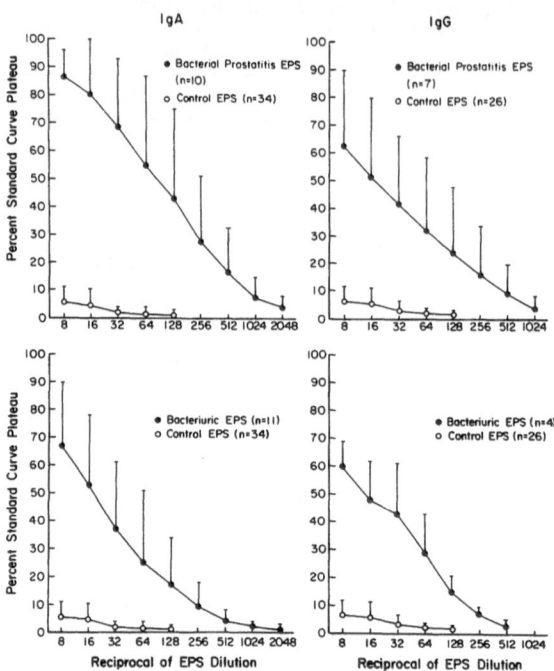

Figure 3 SPRIA curves for quantitation of antibacterial IgG and IgA in EPS of men with and without histories of urinary infection. (Left top) ●——● A composite of 10 SPRIA curves each generated with infecting bacteria (or bacteria of same species) as antigen serial 2-fold dilutions of EPS from patient with bacterial prostatitis (and measurable antibacterial EPS IgA) as primary antibody and ¹²⁵I-labeled antihuman IgA as secondary antibody. ○——○ A composite of 36 SPRIA curves generated with mix of eight common *E. coli* 0-serotypes (22 curves) or mix of *P. mirabilis*, *P. aeruginosa* and *K. pneumoniae* (14 curves) as antigen serial 2-fold dilutions of EPS from one of 23 men with no histories of genitourinary infection as primary antibody and ¹²⁵I-labeled antihuman IgA as secondary antibody. CPM of the bound secondary antibody is expressed as percentage of the plateau region of a standard SPRIA curve generated on the same day. Bars indicate +1 standard deviation of binding at each dilution. (Left bottom) ●——● A composite of 11 SPRIA curves each generated with the same antigen and secondary antibody as above, but with serial 2-fold dilutions of EPS from a patient with history of bacteriuria (and measurable antibacterial EPS IGA). ○——○ Same as above. (Right top) ●——● A composite of 7 SPRIA curves each generated with infecting bacteria (or bacteria of same species) as antigen serial 2-fold dilutions of EPS from patient with bacterial prostatitis (and measurable antibacterial EPS IgG) as primary antibody and ¹²⁵I-labeled antihuman IgG as secondary antibody. ○——○ A composite of 26 SPRIA curves generated with a mix of eight common *E. coli* 0-serotypes (16 curves), or a mix of *P. mirabilis*, *P. aeruginosa* and *K. pneumoniae* (10 curves) as antigen; serial 2-fold dilutions of EPS from one of 17 men with no histories of genitourinary infection as primary antibody; ¹²⁵I-labeled antihuman IgG as secondary antibody. CPM of bound secondary antibody is expressed as percent of plateau region of standard SPRIA curve generated on the same day. Bars indicate +1 standard deviation of binding at each dilution. (Right bottom) ●——● A composite of four SPRIA curves generated with same antigen and secondary antibody as above but with serial 2-fold dilutions of EPS from patient with history of bacteriuria (and measurable antibacterial EPS IgG) as primary antibody. ○——○ Same as above

IMMUNE RESPONSE TO INFECTION OF THE MALE URINARY TRACT

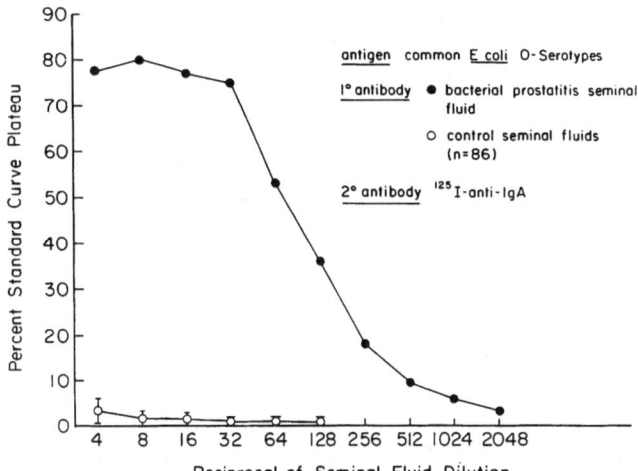

Fig. 4 ●———● SPRIA curve generated with a mix of eight common *E. coli* 0-serotypes as antigen, serial 2-fold dilutions of seminal fluid from patient with *E. coli* chronic bacterial prostatitis as primary antibody, and ^{125}I-labeled antihuman IgA as secondary antibody. ○———○ A composite of 86 SPRIA curves each generated with the same antigen and secondary antibody as above, but with serial 2-fold dilutions of seminal fluid from fertile and infertile men with no history of genitourinary infection as primary antibody. Bars indicate ±3 standard deviations of binding at each dilution. None of the fertile or infertile controls had measurable antibacterial seminal fluid IgA

Table 5 Antibacterial immunoglobulin in prostatic fluid (EPS) and serum of bacteriuric and bacterial prostatitis patients

	Mean $\dfrac{Antibacterial\ Ig}{Total\ Ig}$ $(\times 100) \pm 1\ SD$		Mean ratio $\dfrac{EPS}{Serum} \pm 1\ SD$
	EPS	Serum	
IgG (n = 8)	3.5 ± 2.6	1.2 ± 1.5	4.0 ± 4.4
IgA (n = 10)	10.6 ± 9.6[a]	0.5 ± 0.3	38.7 ± 42.2[b]
IgM (n = 6)	0.0 ± 0.0	1.8 ± 1.9	–

[a] Significantly greater than corresponding serum value, $p<0.01$
[b] Significantly greater than corresponding ratio for IgG, $p = 0.02$

(Table 5). The mean concentration of EPS antibacterial IgA expressed as a function of the corresponding total EPS IgA concentration was significantly greater than that of concurrent serum samples ($p<0.01$). On the other hand, the mean fraction of EPS IgG with specificity for bacterial antigen was similar to that of serum ($p>0.05$). The mean ratio of EPS to serum antibacterial Ig when expressed as a function of total Ig of the corresponding specimen was 4.0 for IgG and 38.7 for IgA ($p = 0.02$). These data suggest that EPS antibacterial IgA is locally synthesized and secreted but that EPS antibacterial IgG is largely a transudate from serum.

Absorption of immune EPS with antihuman secretory component removed 70–100% of the IgA with specificity for bacterial antigen (Fowler and Mariano, 1982). This finding indicates that antibacterial EPS IgA is primarily in the secretory form and is also consistent with a secretory immune response of the prostate to infection of the genitourinary tract.

The apparent secretory immunity of the prostate can be further characterized by longitudinal studies of EPS from men with urinary infection. Other investigators (Shortliffe *et al.*, 1980b) have shown that antibacterial EPS IgA may be detectable for more than 1 year following eradication of a prostatic infection. Our studies of bacteriuric men indicate that antibacterial IgA may also be detected in EPS as long as 1 year following curative treatment of infection confined to the bladder (Fowler and Mariano, 1982). We have now assayed in a longitudinal fashion EPS from three men with conclusive bacteriologic documentation of prostatic infection. Their cases are discussed below.

J.G., a 44-year-old man, had experienced three episodes of culture-proved *E. coli* bacteriuria before visiting our clinic with acute symptomatic bacteriuria in September of 1981. The culture data obtained during 19 months of treatment have been described above (see Table 2). We do not know if his previous infections were caused by the 01 *E. coli*, but the recurrent nature of these three uncharacterized infections and the subsequent inability to sterilize the prostate suggest that this is the case. Serial assays of this patient's EPS and serum for total Ig and for Ig directed against the infecting 01 *E. coli* (Fig. 5) demonstrated the following: (1) the anticipated relationship between total EPS IgG and IgA concentrations had reversed; (2) there was minimal variation in the concentration of EPS IgM; (3) antibacterial EPS IgG and IgA were generally measurable despite culture-negative EPS on six occasions; (4) antibacterial EPS IgA levels were substantially greater than IgG; (5) there was no measurable antibacterial EPS IgM; (6) there were no clear correlations between total and antibacterial EPS Ig concentrations and treatment; (7) the fraction of EPS IgA directed against the infecting bacterium greatly exceeded that of serum IgA; (8) the fraction of EPS IgG directed against the infecting bacterium approximated that of serum IgG; and (9) antibacterial IgM was measurable in the serum but not the EPS.

The second patient, W.L., a 64-year-old man, had experienced intermittent symptoms suggestive of bacteriuria for 3 years prior to evaluation in our clinics (Table 6). When first evaluated he had symptoms of acute bacteriuria but no signs or symptoms of acute bacterial prostatitis. The EPS was purulent and *Proteus mirabilis* was localized to the prostate. Despite treatment with full and then suppressive doses of trimethoprim, the infection could not be eradicated. Serial assays of the EPS for total Ig and for Ig directed against the infecting *P. mirabilis* (Fig. 6) demonstrated the following: (1) the concentrations of IgG and IgA decreased dramatically after administration of full-dose trimethoprim, but subsequently increased after 3 months of treatment with suppressive doses of trimethoprim; (2) the concentrations of IgM varied minimally; (3) antibacterial IgA and IgG were consistently measurable with the exception of the first specimen; (4)

IMMUNE RESPONSE TO INFECTION OF THE MALE URINARY TRACT

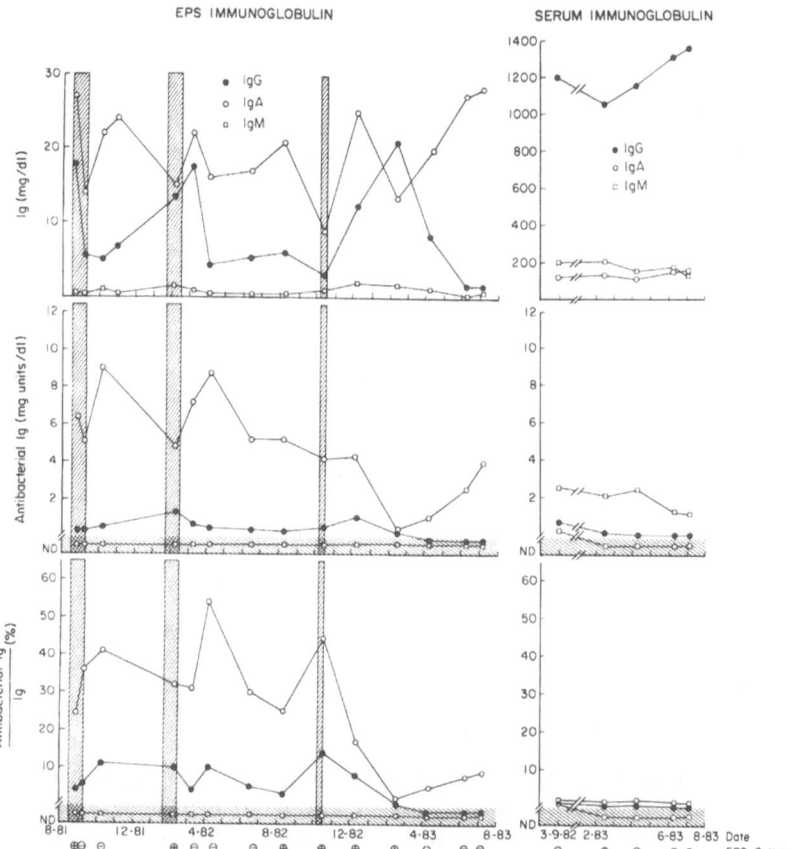

Fig. 5 Total and antibacterial IgG, A, and M in EPS and serum of J.G. (Case 1), a 44-year-old man with an *E. coli* chronic bacterial prostatitis (see text and Table 2). Vertical shaded areas indicate periods when symptomatic. Horizontal shaded areas labeled ND indicate that antibacterial Ig was not detectable. (From Fowler, J. E., Jr. and Mariano, M. (1984). Longitudinal studies of prostatic fluid immunoglobulin in bacterial prostatitis. *J. Urol.*, **131**, 363)

antibacterial IgA levels were substantially greater than those of IgG; (5) the alterations observed in total IgG and IgA levels during the initial months of therapy were not associated with comparable changes in antibacterial IgG and IgA levels; and (6) antibacterial IgM was unmeasurable.

The third case, that of a 79-year-old man (W.G.), was particularly enlightening because of co-existing multiple myeloma of the monoclonal IgG lambda chain variety. This patient had suffered two episodes of bacteriuria during the 3 years prior to study, but neither had been caused by the *Pseudomonas* that acutely infected his prostate in September 1982 (Table 7). Treatment with tobramycin and then with suppressive doses of trimethoprim-sulfamethoxazole eradicated this patient's infection. Serial assays of his EPS and serum for total Ig and for Ig directed against the infecting *Pseudomonas* (Fig. 7) demonstrated the following: (1) the concentration of EPS IgG underwent a dramatic and sustained decrease after initiation of antimicrobial therapy and eradication of the infection; (2) the concentrations of EPS IgA and IgM, and serum IgG, IgA, and IgM varied minimally; (3) EPS

357

IgA concentrations were lower than expected for a man with bacterial prostatitis; (4) antibacterial EPS IgG and IgM levels were undetectable, but a gradual increase in antibacterial EPS IgA concentrations were observed; and (5) antibacterial serum IgM levels were measurable, but antibacterial serum IgG and IgA could not be detected.

Table 6 Case 2: Genitourinary bacteriology of W.L., a 64-year-old male with chronic *Proteus mirabilis* bacterial prostatitis[a]

Date	Days on (+) or off (−) drug[b]	Colonies per ml				Organism	EPS Leukocytes per HPF
		VB_1	VB_2	EPS	VB_3		
1979-1982	Intermittent dysuria and frequency						
12 Aug. 1982	First visit	1000	200	7000	240	P. mirabilis	50
17 Aug. 1982	+5 TMP	320	140	3000	600	P. mirabilis	50
14 Sept. 1982	+33 TMP	200	70	60,000	360	P. mirabilis	50
12 Oct. 1982	+28 TMP (s)	100	100	2300	300	P. mirabilis	30
2 Dec. 1982	+80 TMP (s)	1100	100	2000	200	P. mirabilis	30
13 Jan. 1983	+122 TMP (s)	800	60	10,000	60	P. mirabilis	30

[a] From Fowler, J. E., Jr. and Mariano, M. (1984). Longitudinal studies of prostatic fluid immunoglobulin in bacterial prostatitis. *J. Urol.*, **131**, 363
[b] TMP = Trimethoprim in full dosage (100 mg b.i.d.)
TMP (s) = Trimethoprim in suppressive dosage (50 mg q.h.s.)

These longitudinal data all support the observations that bacterial infection of the genitourinary tract results in a relatively greater increase of EPS IgA than EPS IgG concentrations, that EPS antibody directed against bacterial antigen is primarily of the IgA class, and that secretion of antibacterial IgA is largely independent of the systemic antibody response. In addition, the impact of acute prostatic inflammation on total EPS Ig concentrations is clearly demonstrated in Cases 2 and 3. In both cases there were notable dissociations between the elevated total EPS Ig levels that accompanied the symptomatic prostatic inflammation and the corresponding levels of antibacterial EPS Ig of the same class. Moreover, in Cases 1 and 3 the fluctuations of total EPS Ig were not accompanied by similar changes in total serum Ig. These considerations indicate that increased total EPS Ig concentrations associated with acute prostatic inflammation result from enhanced nonspecific transudate of serum Ig into the prostatic fluid. As demonstrated previously, there is wide variability of total EPS Ig concentrations among men with bacteriuria and bacterial prostatitis. The relationship between prostatic inflammation and total EPS Ig levels may account for these observations since the intervals beween the initiation of treatment and EPS procurement were not standardized.

Unique insights into the relationship between serum and EPS Ig concentrations are provided by Case 3. Due to the IgG multiple myeloma the serum concentrations of IgG were consistently elevated and serum concentrations of IgA and IgM were consistently decreased. During acute infection of the prostate

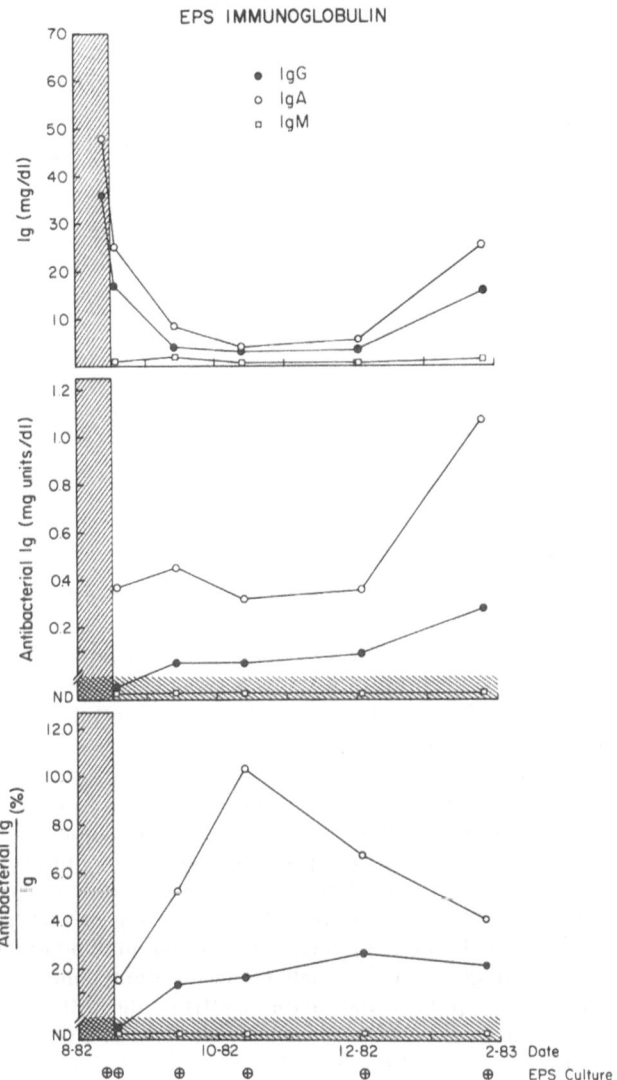

Fig. 6 Total and antibacterial IgG, A, and M in EPS of W.L. (Case 2), a 64-year-old man with a *P. mirabilis* chronic bacterial prostatitis (see text and Table 6). Vertical shaded area indicates period when symptomatic. Horizontal shaded areas labelled ND indicate that antibacterial Ig was not detectable. (From Fowler, J. E., Jr. and Mariano, M. (1984). Longitudinal studies of prostatic fluid immunoglobulin in bacterial prostatitis. *J. Urol.*, **131**, 363)

Table 7 Case 3: Genitourinary bacteriology of W.G., a 79-year-old man with multiple myeloma and non-aeruginosa *Pseudomonas* acute bacterial prostatitis[a]

Date	Days on (+) or off (−) drug[b]	Colonies per ml				Organism	EPS leukocytes per HPF
		VB_1	VB_2	EPS	VB_3		
1980-1982	Two episodes of culture-documented bacteriuria (non-Pseudomonas)						
12 Aug. 1982	First visit	—	100,000	—	—	*Pseudomonas*	—
16 Aug. 1982	+4 Tobramycin	300	0	7800	200	*Pseudomonas*	50
19 Aug. 1982	+7 Tobramycin	0	0	330	400	*Pseudomonas*	50
1 Sept. 1982	+13 TMP-SMX (s)	0	0	0	0	—	30
14 Oct. 1982	+56 TMP-SMX (s)	0	0	0	0	—	5
1 Dec. 1982	+101 TMP-SMX (s)	0	0	0	0	—	5
29 Dec. 1982	−28 TMP-SMX (s)	0	0	0	0	—	5
7 Mar. 1983	−96 TMP-SMX (s)	0	0	0	0	—	5

[a] From Fowler, J. E., Jr. and Mariano, M. (1984). Longitudinal studies of prostatic fluid immunoglobulin in bacterial prostatitis. *J. Urol.*, **131**, 363
[b] TMP-SMX (s) = Trimethoprim-sulfamethoxazole in suppressive dosage (40–200 mg q.h.s.)

the total EPS IgG concentrations were markedly elevated, but there was little change in the concentrations of total EPS IgA. This observation supports the notion that elevated total EPS IgG and IgA concentrations during prostatic inflammation result primarily from nonspecific increases in the diffusion of Ig from the serum.

The prostatic infections in Cases 1 and 2 appeared to be longstanding and both were resistant to antimicrobial therapy. The infection in Case 3 appeared to have developed shortly before presentation and was promptly eradicated. We have not had the opportunity to characterize in a longitudinal fashion the systemic and local immune responses following eradication of bacterial infection of the prostate among men with normal immune functions. Further, the number of patients studied is small. Generalizations concerning the duration of these immune responses and factors contributing to the magnitude of the responses, are therefore difficult to make. Nonetheless, during the periods of observation the concentration of antibacterial EPS IgA in Case 3 approached that in Case 2. Conversely, the concentration of antibacterial EPS IgA in Case 1 exceeded that in Case 2 by as much as 10-fold. These preliminary observations raise the possibility that the magnitude of the secretory immune response may be unrelated to the duration of infection or the response of the infection to antimicrobial therapy. Such findings may account in part for the observation that the concentrations of antibacterial EPS IgA among men with bacteriuria but no clinical or bacteriologic evidence of prostatic infection and among men with documented bacterial prostatitis are quantitatively similar.

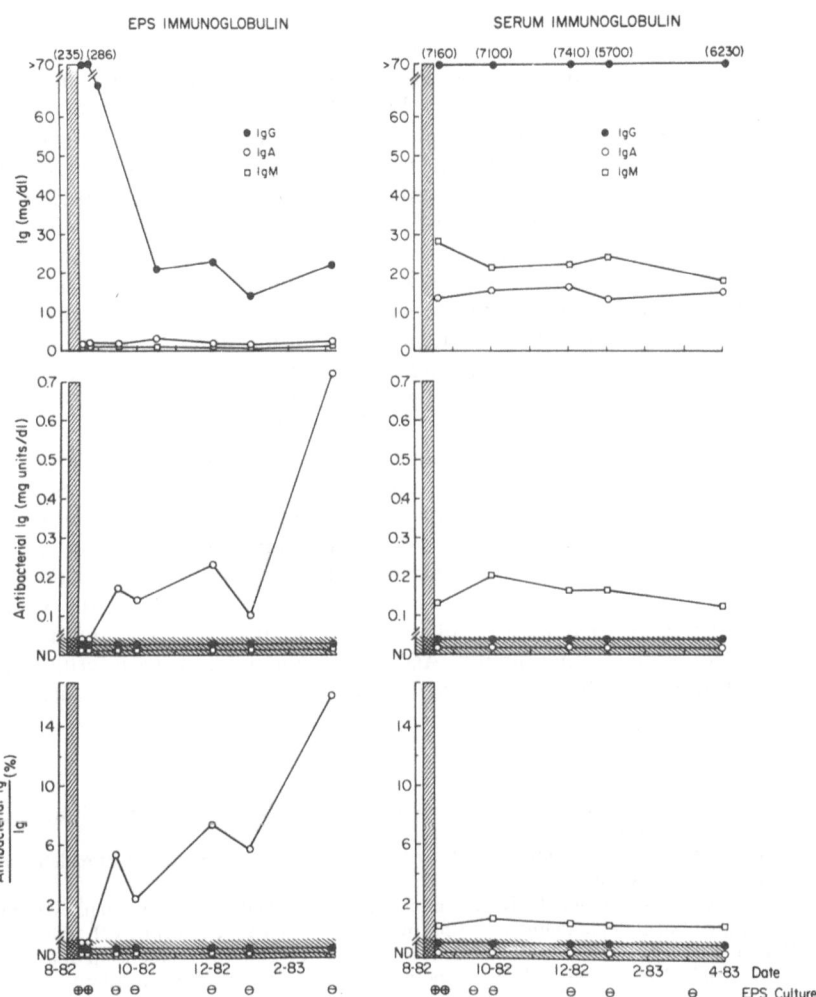

Fig. 7 Total and antibacterial IgG, A, and M in EPS and serum of W.G. (Case 3), a 79-year-old male with acute *Pseudomonas* bacterial prostatitis and IgG monoclonal multiple myeloma (see text and Table 7). Vertical shaded area indicates period when symptomatic. Horizontal shaded areas labelled ND indicate that antibacterial Ig was not detectable. (From Fowler, J. E., Jr. and Mariano, M. (1984). Longitudinal studies of prostatic fluid immunoglobulin in bacterial prostatitis. *J. Urol.*, **131**, 363)

POTENTIAL APPLICATIONS OF ASSAYS FOR ANTIMICROBIAL IMMUNOGLOBULIN IN THE STUDY OF GENITOURINARY DISORDERS

Bacteriuria and bacterial prostatitis are uncommon infectious disorders in the male. Diagnosis is not difficult with routine culture techniques and cure or symptomatic control is usually achievable with antimicrobial therapy. An understanding of the local secretory immune response to such infections, however, may enhance the investigations of more common infectious or inflammatory disorders of the genitourinary tract. It has already been shown, for example, that inflammatory disorders of the prostate that are accompanied by purulent but sterile EPS are not associated with detectable antibacterial EPS Ig (Wishnow *et al.*, 1982). This important observation argues against the possibility that this common but poorly understood syndrome is due to bacterial infection. The possibility that viruses, anaerobic bacteria, *Chlamydia trachomatis* or *Ureaplasma urealyticum* might be etiologic factors in these infections may be illuminated by the assay of genital secretions for antibody against these microorganisms.

Subclinical infection of the male reproductive tract is considered by many as a major cause of impaired fertility. IgA directed against *E. coli* is never detectable in the seminal fluid of infertile men with no histories of urinary infection (Fowler and Mariano, 1983b). Circumstantial evidence exists that persistent asymptomatic colonization of the urethra by *U. urealyticum* may impair fertility in the male (Toth *et al.*, 1983). Infection of the secretory reproductive organs might explain the postulated adverse impact of such colonization on seminal quality. Assays of seminal fluid from infertile men for Ig with specificity for *U. urealyticum* may help to clarify these issues.

References

Anderson, R. U. and Weller, C. (1979). Prostatic secretion leukocyte studies in nonbacterial prostatitis (prostatosis). *J. Urol.*, **121**, 292

Azim, A. A., Fayad, S., Fattah, A. A. *et al.* (1978). Immunologic studies of male infertility. *Fertil. Steril.*, **30**, 426

Berger, R. E., Alexander, E. R., Harnisch, J. P. *et al.* (1978). Etiology, manifestations and therapy of acute epididymitis: prospective study of 50 cases. *J. Urol.*, **121**, 750

Berger, R. E., Karp, L. E., Williamson, R. A. *et al.* (1982). The relationship of pyospermia and seminal fluid bacteriology to sperm function as reflected in the sperm penetration assay. *Fertil. Steril.*, **37**, 557

Fair, W. R., Jr. and Cordonnier, J. J. (1978). The pH of prostatic fluid: a reappraisal of therapeutic implications. *J. Urol.*, **120**, 695

Fowler, J. E., Jr., Kaiser, D. L. and Mariano, M. (1982). Immunologic response of the prostate to bacteriuria and bacterial prostatitis: Part I. Immunoglobulin concentrations in prostatic fluid. *J. Urol.*, **128**, 158

Fowler, J. E., Jr. and Mariano, M. (1982). Immunologic response of the prostate to bacteriuria and bacterial prostatitis: Part II. Antigen specific immunoglobulin in prostatic fluid. *J. Urol.*, **128**, 165

Fowler, J. E., Jr. and Mariano, M. (1983a). Immunoglobulin in seminal fluid of fertile, infertile, vasectomy and vasectomy reversal patients. *J. Urol.*, **129**, 869

Fowler, J. E., Jr. and Mariano, M. (1983b). Bacterial infection and male infertility: Absence of IgA with specificity for E. coli in seminal fluid of infertile men. *J. Urol.*, **130**, 171

IMMUNE RESPONSE TO INFECTION OF THE MALE URINARY TRACT

Fowler, J. E., Jr. and Mariano, M. (1984). Longitudinal studies of prostatic fluid immuno-globulin in bacterial prostatitis. *J. Urol.*, **131**, 363

Friberg, J. (1980). Immunoglobulin concentration in serum and seminal fluid from men with and without sperm-agglutinating antibodies. *Am. J. Obstet. Gynecol.*, **136**, 671

Gray, S. P., Billings, J. and Blacklock, N. J. (1973). Prostatic fluid immunoglobulin levels in prostatitis. *Urol. Nephrol.*, **73**, 20

Grayhack, J. T., Wendel, E. F., Oliver, L. *et al.* (1979). Analysis of specific proteins in prostatic fluid for detecting prostatic malignancy. *J. Urol.*, **121**, 295

Hanson, L. A. and Brandtzaeg, P. (1979). The mucosal defense system. In Stiehm, E. R. and Fulginiti, V. A. (eds) *Immunologic Disorders in Infants and Children*, 2nd edn (Philadelphia: W. B. Saunders)

Holmes, K. K., Handsfield, H. H., Wang, S. P. *et al.* (1975). Etiology of nongonococcal urethritis. *N. Engl. J. Med.*, **292**, 1999

Jones, T. C. (1974). Prostatitis as cause of antibody-coated bacteria in urine. Letter to the Editor, *N. Engl. J. Med.*, **291**, 365

Klousia, J. W., Madden, R. L., Fucillo, D. A. *et al.* (1978). The etiology of nonspecific urethritis in active duty marines. *J. Urol.*, **120**, 67

Meares, E. M. and Stamey, T. A. (1968). Bacterial localization patterns in bacterial prostatitis and urethritis. *Invest. Urol.*, **5**, 492

Mobley, D. F. (1975). Semen cultures in the diagnosis of bacterial prostatitis. *J. Urol.*, **114**, 83

Ogra, P. L. and Ogra, S. S. (1973). Local antibody response to polio vaccine in the human female genital tract. *J. Immunol.*, **110**, 1307

Polakaski, K. L., Syner, F. N. and Zaneveld, L. J. D. (1976). Biochemistry of human seminal plasma. In; E. S. E. Hafez, (ed.) *Human Semen and Fertility Regulation in Men*, p. 355. (St. Louis: C. V. Mosby)

Rumke, P. (1974). The origin of immunoglobulins in semen. *Clin. Exp. Immunol.*, **17**, 287

Shortliffe, L. M. D., Wehner, N. and Stamey, T. A. (1981a). Use of a solid-phase radioimmu-noassay and formalin-fixed whole bacterial antigen in the detection of antigen-specific immunoglobulin in prostatic fluid. *J. Clin. Invest.*, **67**, 790

Shortliffe, L. M. D., Wehner, N. and Stamey, T. A. (1981b). The detection of a local prostatic immunologic response to bacterial prostatitis. *J. Urol.*, **125**, 509

Soliman, H. A. and Olesen, H. (1976). Concentration of the secretory IgA of seminal fluid in normal subjects in decreased fertility and in aspermia. *Clin. Chim. Acta*, **69**, 543

Stamey, T. A. (1980). *Pathogenesis and Treatment of Urinary Tract Infections*. (Baltimore: Williams & Wilkins)

Sullivan, H. and Quinlivan, W. L. G. (1980). Immunoglobulins in the semen of men with azoospermia, oligospermia, or self-agglutination of spermatozoa. *Fertil. Steril.*, **34**, 465

Taub, R. G., Madden, D. L., Fuccillo, D. A. *et al.* (1973). The male as a reservoir of infection with cytomegalovirus, herpes, and mycoplasma. *N. Engl. J. Med.*, **289**, 697

Tauber, P. F., Zaneveld, L. J. D., Propping, D. *et al.* (1975). Components of human split ejaculates. I. Spermatozoa, fructose, immunoglobulins, albumin, lactoferrin, transferrin, and other plasma proteins. *J. Reprod. Fertil.*, **43**, 249

Thomas, V. L. and Forland, M. (1982). Antibody-coated bacteria in urinary tract infections. *Kid. Intern.*, **21**, 1

Tomasi, T. B., Jr. (1976). *The Immune System of Secretions*. (Englewood Cliffs: Prentice-Hall)

Toth, A., Lesser, M. L., Brooks, C. *et al.* (1983). Subsequent pregnancies among 161 couples treated for T-mycoplasma genital-tract infection. *N. Engl. J. Med.*, **308**, 505

Tramont, E. C. (1977). Inhibition of adherence of Neisseria gonorrhoeae by human genital secretions. *J. Clin. Invest.*, **59**, 117

Uehling, D. (1971). Secretory IgA in seminal fluid. *Fertil. Steril.*, **22**, 769

Ulstein, M., Capell, P., Holmes, K. K. *et al.* (1976). Nonsymptomatic genital tract infection and male infertility. In Hafez, E. S. E., (ed.) *Human Semen and Fertility Regulation in Men*, p. 355. (St. Louis: C. V. Mosby)

Waldman, R. H., Cruz, J. M. and Rowe, D. S. (1972). Intravaginal immunization of humans with *Candida albicans*. *J. Immunol.*, **109**, 662

Wishnow, K. I., Wehner, N. and Stamey, T. A. (1982). The diagnostic value of the immunologic response in bacterial and non-bacterial prostatitis. *J. Urol.*, **127**, 689

24
Genital infection and neoplastic changes of the cervix

LUIS IGLESIAS-CORTIT and JAVIER IGLESIAS-GUIU

INTRODUCTION

In this chapter we will discuss cervical intraepithelial neoplasia (CIN), a disease entity first proposed by Richart in 1967, together with atypical changes that take place in the cervix. These changes include the evolutionary stages of mild dysplasia (Reagan and Hicks, 1953) and the development of carcinoma *in situ* (Ferenczy, 1977).

Dysplasia can arise from a squamous metaplasia or from normal squamous epithelium and then evolve into carcinoma *in situ*; it is believed that this process may go on to develop into invasive carcinoma. Several factors thought to influence this process have been studied from an epidemiologic standpoint; some of these are considered below.

EPIDEMIOLOGY OF CERVICAL NEOPLASIA

Factors which may affect the incidence of cervical neoplasia include the number of births, marital status, sexual activity, socioeconomic status, race, contraceptive method, inherited factors, and prior incidence of venereal infection.

Number of births

A relationship has been established between the number of children a woman has borne and the incidence of cervical neoplasia. It has been observed that the probabilities of incurring this disease are doubled among women with five or more children (Maliphant, 1978). In one study of 213 CIN patients, a high correlation between the incidence of CIN and the number of term pregnancies, preterm pregnancies, and abortions was found; on the other hand, correlation with the age of first child was observed (Iglesias-Cortit *et al.*, 1982). According to Boyd and Doll (1964), the number of births is significant.

Marriage status

CIN occurs more frequently among married women than among unmarried women who do not engage in sexual intercourse (Boyd and Doll, 1964). It is hardly ever observed among nuns (Gagnon, 1950). There also appears to be some connection between the age of marriage and the occurrence of CIN (Rotkin, 1967). It is more common among those women whose husbands had formerly been married to women with cancer of the uterine cervix (Kessler, 1976). It is therefore believed that certain men are themselves 'high-risk factors', for reasons that are not entirely clear, and that the wives of these men are at greater risk for developing cervical neoplasia (Singer *et al.*, 1976).

Sexual activity

The association between marriage and the appearance of cervical neoplasia is believed to be related to the act of coitus. Carcinoma of the uterine cervix is more common among women who begin their sexual activity at a relatively younger age (Wynder *et al.*, 1954; Martin, 1967; Iglesias-Cortit *et al.*, 1982). CIN is more frequent in women who have had several partners, as is the case with women who have been married several times, or among prostitutes (Martin, 1967; Rotkin, 1967).

Although not universally agreed upon, there is some evidence that cervical cancer occurs less frequently among women whose husbands have been circumcised (Wynder *et al.*, 1954). In addition, there is a higher risk of the disease among women whose husbands had suffered from venereal infection and there is some evidence that this finding is related to the herpesvirus type 2 (Kessler, 1981).

Socioeconomic status

A higher incidence of neoplasia has been found in women from the lower socioeconomic classes (Terris *et al.*, 1967). In our population, however, this correlation is not present (Iglesias-Cortit *et al.*, 1982).

Race

Certain races appear at greater risk for developing cervical neoplasia. For example, Jewish women have a lower incidence of carcinoma of the uterine cervix (Vineberg, 1919; Clemmesen, 1965); the same is true for some communities in India (Wynder *et al.*, 1954). In the United States (Wynder *et al.*, 1954), there is higher incidence of cervical carcinoma among black women.

Contraceptive method

Some workers have raised the possibility of a connection between the use of hormonal contraceptives and the appearance of cervical neoplasia. It was found that there were more women with carcinoma *in situ* among those taking hormonal oral contraceptives than among those who used the diaphragm (Melamed *et al.*, 1969). A higher incidence of dysplasia and carcinoma *in situ* have been found in women who have taken hormonal contraceptives for more than 6 years (Stern *et al.*, 1977). On the other hand, no correlation between the use of hormonal contraceptives and the incidence of CIN was observed in our population (Iglesias-Cortit *et al.*, 1982).

Heredity

Although Stern *et al.* (1967) believe that heredity may play a role in the onset of CIN, we were unable to find a connection between heredity and CIN (Iglesias-Cortit *et al.*, 1982).

Venereal infections

The possibility that the incidence of cervical neoplasia is somehow related to the incidence of genital infection has been under investigation for several years. Several agents may be related to the appearance and progression of the disease.

We studied the aspect of genital infection in a group of patients with diagnosed CIN and compared it with the findings in a control group of the same age and marital status. A higher incidence of nonspecific, mixed flora, including *Trichomonas* and *Gardnerella* infections, was found in the neoplasia group than in the control group. This difference was statistically significant (Fig. 1) and this finding further supports the idea of a relationship between cervical neoplasia and genital infection.

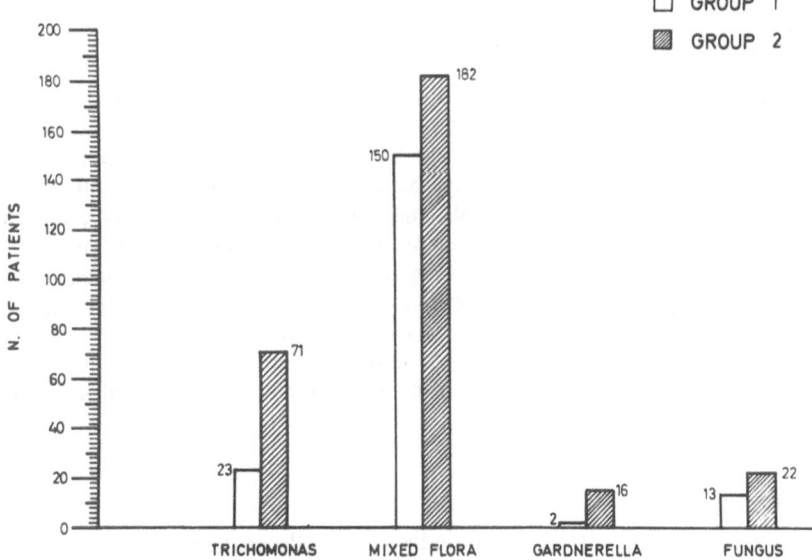

Fig. 1 Degree of vaginal infection found in the two groups of patients studied. Group 1 is the control group and Group 2 is the neoplasia group. Infection is clearly higher in the neoplasia group

We did not find, however, any similar influence on the later evolution of the neoplasia. It would seem, therefore, that these infections influence the onset of neoplastic disease, but that, once established, they have no further effect on it (Iglesias-Cortit *et al.*, 1982). Such influences have already been described, mainly in connection with *Trichomonas* infections (Meisels, 1969; Szell *et al.*, 1967), syphilis (Rojel, 1953), and gonorrhea (Ferenczy, 1977).

A great deal of evidence points to a relationship between viral infections, including the herpes simplex type 2 virus (HSV-2) on which most studies have been done, and cervical neoplasia. The papillomavirus, which is responsible for cervical and vulvar condylomas, is another of the viruses associated with cervical neoplasia. Some relationship with the cytomegaloviruses, which some researchers have implicated in neoplastic transformations, has also been observed. Another agent that may be associated with cervical neoplasia is *Chlamydia trachomatis*, which has frequently been thought to have a role in some neoplastic transformations. Although it has not been shown conclusively that these agents cause CIN, they are now considered to be the most likely factors responsible for the cellular transformations that lead to cervical carcinoma.

ETIOLOGY OF CERVICAL INTRAEPITHELIAL NEOPLASIA

We have already noted that cervical dysplasia arises from squamous metaplasia. Among the factors which may alter the normal processes of metaplastic differentiation and maturation and lead to carcinoma *in situ*, are viral infections, spermatozoa, and smegma.

Viral infections

It has long been thought that viruses may be etiologic agents in the dysplastic change that eventually leads to CIN. It is now known that viruses are obligate intracellular parasites and that when the cells of the host organism are attacked by them, there is frequently no adverse effect in the host cells. Viruses, however, can also destroy cells and kill them or, more rarely, initiate an adaptation process. When this adaptation occurs, cellular functions, as well as the morphology and growth capacity, undergo changes. An oncogenic capacity is then acquired (Stoker and McPherson, 1961; Strohl *et al.*, 1967). These cells are called transformed cells, and it is accepted that this transformation is associated with the presence of genetic viral material inside the cells. The relationship between viral infections and cervical neoplasia will be discussed in greater detail below.

Spermatozoa

Spermatozoa may also have some bearing on the incidence of cervical neoplasia. Smegma or some substance present in the seminal fluid have been implicated in the genesis of uterine cervical cancer (Doll *et al.*, 1966). Apparently, there is a lower cervical cancer rate among women whose husbands have been vasectomized (Swan and Brown, 1979) than among women whose husband's foreskins remain intact.

The idea that spermatozoa can give rise to cervical neoplasia is based on the fact that the nucleic acid in the sperm head can become integrated into the host cell in the same way as the viruses (Coppleson and Reid, 1967). Spermatozoa or other carcinogenic substances may be able to penetrate the cells in the metaplasic phase (Reid and Coppleson, 1978). Current knowledge indicates that there are two basic proteins, protamines and histones, capable of dissolving the mucoid coat of the cell.

The protamine–histone ratio in the sperm head fluctuates among individuals and this ratio has been shown to vary linearly in social groups where women show a greater frequency of cervical neoplasia (Reid and Coppleson, 1978). The idea that the protamine–histone ratio in the sperm of certain epidemiologic groups may affect neoplastic mechanisms would also justify the finding that the wives of husbands of blue-collar workers have a higher cancer rate, as already mentioned.

Smegma

A higher incidence of carcinoma of the penis has been demonstrated in uncircumcised males. There also appears to be a correlation between the occurrence of carcinoma of the penis and cervical cancer (Doll *et al.*, 1966). Tumors have been produced in certain animals by administering or applying smegma (Wynder and Hoffman, 1967).

VIRAL INFECTION AND CERVICAL NEOPLASIA

Virus and cancer

Viral genital tract infections, both in the female and in the male, have been linked to the onset of CIN (Rawls *et al.*, 1968). This association was first suggested when it was discovered that atypical results were obtained from cervical biopsies performed on women with cytologically diagnosed herpes infection. It was later observed that the genital herpes infectious process frequently preceded the appearance of cervical neoplasia by about 10 years (Naib *et al.*, 1969).

Another connection between viral infection and cervical neoplasia was shown in the early seroepidemiologic studies of 1968; these studies examined the possibility of neutralizing antibodies acting against HSV-2 virus in groups of women with or without neoplasia (Nahmias and Dowdle, 1968; Rawls *et al.*, 1968). For such studies to be of any value, however, case comparisons must be properly controlled for the complicating factors of age, sexual activity, social status, and age at first coitus. In those studies where these factors have been taken into account, a close association between HSV-2 and cervical cancer was found.

The next sections will examine the various viral infections and the roles they play in the onset of cervical neoplasia.

Herpesvirus

The herpesviruses have been found to infect man and all animal species studied to date. The HSV-2 virus is a member of the human herpes-viridae family, which also includes herpes simplex type 1 (HSV-1), cytomegalovirus, the varicella-zoster virus, and the Epstein-Barr virus (EBV).

The herpesviruses are relatively large (150 nm) in size, they have complex morphology and are enveloped in a capsid. The capsid has cubic or icosahedral symmetry and contains double-stranded DNA. It has 162 capsomers and is surrounded by a lipid-containing cover. The virions are found in the nucleus of the infected cells and acquire their cover by budding through the nuclear membrane.

The HSV-2 virus shares 50% of its DNA base sequence with HSV-1. Although these viruses are different antigenically, they contain at least one glycoprotein with a crossed reaction. The HSV-2 is very cytopathic for the majority of host cells and brings about lysis in 18–24 hours. It can cause keratoconjunctivitis, encephalitis, and genital infections. Once the primary infection has taken place the viruses enter the latent phase in which there is no clinical or cytopathologic evidence of the infection. Several different factors can reactivate the virus, with a subsequent recurrence of the lesions and other symptoms. It has been shown that herpesviruses reside in some ganglia during the latent phase (Baringer and Swoveland, 1973; Bestian et al., 1972; Stevens et al., 1972; Baringer, 1975).

Serologic reaction of the herpesviruses

Several workers have found positive serologic reactions against HSV-2 in patients with dysplastic changes, varying degrees of dysplasia, and carcinoma of the uterine cervix. The results are shown in Table 1. The most conclusive finding was that dysplasia and carcinoma in situ appear more frequently in those women who have suffered HSV-2 infections. It can therefore be said that HSV-2 infection increases the likelihood of neoplasia (Nahmias et al., 1970).

Antigens have been found in biopsies performed on cervical tumors. One of

Table 1 Positive serologic reactions found against HSV-2 antibody in different stages of cervical neoplasia (Nahmias et al., 1970)

| Author | Type of neoplasia | Positive cases | | | |
| | | Patients | | Controls | |
		N	%	N	%
Nahmias	In situ carcinoma	57	65	82	15
Aurelian	Invasive cancer	—	100	—	68
Rawls and Adam	In situ carcinoma	—	42	—	17
	Invasive cancer	—	45	—	17
Thiry	Cervical atypia	—	20	—	8
	Dysplasia	—	40	—	8
	Carcinoma	—	75	—	8

these antigens, AG-4, was found in 90% of the biopsies performed on patients with cervical carcinoma compared to only 10% of the control group. AG-4 antibodies were found in higher proportions in patients with invasive carcinoma than in those with carcinoma *in situ*; furthermore, AG-4 antibody levels were higher in carcinoma *in situ* than in patients with dysplasia (Aurelian *et al.*, 1973, 1975). In those women in whom the tumors had been successfully excised, no antibodies against the AG-4 antigen were found, but a very high proportion was found in patients with recurrent neoplasia (Aurelian *et al.*, 1973, 1975; Hollinshead *et al.*, 1976). The HSV-TAA (HSV-tumor-associated antigen) has also been studied and antibodies against it were found in 80% of patients with carcinoma of the cervix (Notter and Docherty, 1976). UP-134, another HSV-2-specific antigen, has also been studied, and antibodies against it were found in 90% of patients with cervical carcinoma.

HSV-2 and mRNA have also been studied using molecular hybridization techniques; their presence was detected in varying proportions in neoplastic cells. These molecular and seroepidemiologic studies show a clear relationship between HSV-2 and cervical carcinoma, although a cause-and-effect relationship has not been definitively established.

Oncogenic potential of HSV

It was possible to induce neoplastic growth by inoculating newborn hamsters with HSV-2-transformed cells that had been inactivated. The viral genome persists in the transformed cells, and only a portion of it is necessary to maintain the transformations (Galloway *et al.*, 1980). It appears obvious, therefore, that HSV-2 has the potential to produce neoplastic disease in animals. The ability of these viruses to transform cells *in vitro* and the ability of the transformed cells to produce tumors *in vivo* is currently the most convincing evidence of their oncogenic potential. While viral infections are very common among humans, the incidence of cervical neoplasia is relatively rare, which leads to the conclusion that other factors, in addition to the viruses, must be responsible for the disease.

Papillomavirus

Condyloma acuminatum was described in detail by the ancient Greeks and Romans, although it was not until the late 17th and early 18th centuries that it was shown to be different from syphilis, and not until 1900, when the gonococcus was isolated, that it was distinguished from gonorrhea. For a long time it was widely believed that these warts were caused by the irritation of genital secretions. Although some misinformed individuals still hold this opinion, the viral etiology of condylomas was finally established by Ciuffo in 1907. Later studies using electron microscopy identified the virus with certainty (Strauss *et al.*, 1949; Almeida *et al.*, 1962).

The usual sites of condylomas are the penis, anus, vulva, vagina, and sometimes the cervix. They appear less frequently in extragenital areas, such as the scrotum, nipple, urethra, bladder, or mouth, and changes identical to those of condylomata acuminatum have recently been described in the bronchial tree. The viral agents found in condylomas are members of the Papovaviri-dae family and are of the same morphology and size as the papillomavirus (55 nm). The virus has a naked icosahedral capsid with 72 capsomers. Its genome consists of a covalent DNA molecule with a molecular weight of 5×10^6.

Biologic and serologic studies have shown that there are at least five serotypes and six subtypes of the papillomavirus.

Condylomata of the cervix and carcinoma

Carcinoma of the cervix often clinically resembles a venereal disease, as does cervical dysplasia. As many as 70% of cases of cervical condylomas have been confused with mild dysplasia (Meisels *et al.*, 1977).

Histologic studies have recently shown that 90% of papillomavirus infections in women who have undergone surgery for pre-invasive or invasive neoplasia are subclinical. In hysterectomized patients in a matched-control group this figure was 12%. Therefore, subclinical infection by papillomavirus is closely related to cervical malignancy (Reid *et al.*, 1982). It would be necessary, however, to carry out a longitudinal epidemiologic study to establish that infection by papillomavirus is related to a high incidence of neoplasia or that the viral genetic information persists in the tumor cells.

Carcinogenesis of the papillomavirus

What evidence is there linking papillomaviruses to carcinogenesis? Reid (1982) points to the following clinical observations:

(1) The prevalence of subclinical infection by papillomavirus, which was established by Meisels and Fortin (1976), who observed that in 70% of mild dysplasias, viral infections were present. Reid found them in 25% of biopsies exhibiting atypical epithelium.

(2) The persistent nature of subclinical infection by papillomavirus. Condyloma lesions regress after a time, as a result of the immunologic processes of the organism, but a latent stage lasting several years follows, and later reactivation has frequently been observed.

(3) The strong similarities between the epidemiologic profiles of infection by papillomavirus and those of cervical neoplasia. Both disease entities are related to sexual activity, and there exist male vectors that are of importance in the appearance of each.

(4) The evidence suggesting an association between infection by papillomavirus and cervical neoplasia. Both entities, for example, have been observed in histologic studies.

(5) The evidence suggesting that infection by papillomavirus precedes any neoplastic change. Some studies have shown that vulvar carcinoma can appear after several years of the presence of condylomas (zur Hausen, 1977; Orth *et al.*, 1977).

(6) The oncogenicity of the papillomaviruses, which was established conclusively by Noonan and Butel in 1978. The viral genome has been found in spontaneous tumors in animals (Lancaster *et al.*, 1977) and in experimentally induced tumors (Stevens and Wettstein, 1979).

(7) The detection of persistent viral genetic information in tumor cells. It would appear to be possible to study the tumor cells to prove this point (zur Hausen *et al.*, 1981).
(8) Morphologic evidence of the possible progression of subclinical infection by papillomavirus. Subclinical papillomatose infection frequently coexists at the site of cervical intraepithelial neoplasia, and there are examples of an apparent transition (Reid *et al.*, 1980).

All of this evidence suggests the likelihood of a causal relationship between the incidence of papillomavirus infection and the onset of cervical neoplasia. Although papillomavirus infection is transmitted sexually and cervical neoplasia is also believed to be contracted in the same way, epidemiologic evidence must be accumulated to establish that infection by papillomavirus always precedes cervical neoplasia.

Nevertheless, our current knowledge of these phenomena leads us to consider patients with papillomavirus infections as being at higher risk for undergoing the changes associated with CIN compared to women who have not been exposed to the virus.

Cytomegalovirus

Cytomegalovirus infection is due to a DNA-containing virus of the herpes group. The virus was identified by Smith in 1956. Although it is associated with the appearance of giant cells in the tissues of the host, infection by cytomegalovirus in adults is not associated with any apparent clinical manifestation.

Cytomegalovirus infection occurs on a worldwide basis. The incidence of antibodies against the cytomegalovirus increases with age and 50% of all adults show evidence of having been infected. Fifty percent of Western women, however, reach reproductive age with no antibodies. Seroconversion, therefore, usually takes place between 15 and 35 years, coinciding with the period at which sexual activity and pregnancy are most likely.

The possible significance of this observation lies in the fact that congenital malformations such as cataracts and congenital heart diseases have been reported in connection with the disease (Charles, 1980). Cytomegalovirus infection occurs at the reproductive age and, for that reason, has been thought to play a part in the genesis of cervical neoplasia.

Although the conclusive studies to support this belief have not been conducted, there are some indications that it may be true. In a recent study involving 33 women the infection rate for cytomegalovirus was found to be 28%. When these patients had a Papanicolaou test and colposcopic examination, it was found that cytomegalovirus was present in 18% of normal cells, while the figure for atypical or metaplastic cells was 36%. The prevalence of cytomegaloviruses, therefore, appears to increase in abnormal cytologic situations and, in fact, exceeds 33% when severe dysplasia or carcinoma *in situ* are present (Chiang *et al.*, 1981). Thus, although there is little evidence at present regarding the genesis of cervical neoplasia by cytomegalovirus, investigations on the subject have begun to appear.

Chlamydia trachomatis

Epidemiologically, *C. trachomatis* is similar to HSV-2 virus in terms of the frequency of infection and the effect on cells. In the light of this similarity it has been suggested that the TRIC agent may be associated with the incidence of cervical neoplasia. For example, high serologic reactivity titers against *Chlamydia* antigens have been found in patients with cervical dysplasia. Since these titers were also found in high proportions in women without dysplasia, this finding may indicate that these women have been exposed to sexually transmitted diseases (Schachter *et al.*, 1975).

Immunoassay techniques have been used to study the presence of antibodies against *C. trachomatis* and HSV-2 virus in cervical secretions. Using this method a higher incidence of *Chlamydia* antibodies was observed in women with malignant or premalignant cervical changes. The incidence was lower in women suffering from cervicitis and almost nonexistent in the control group (Kalimo *et al.*, 1981). Therefore it would appear that chlamydial IgA antibodies are produced in women with atypical cervical lesions. What remains to be seen is whether this phenomenon is coincidental or etiologic.

There are indications, therefore, that chlamydiae may also be considered as potential etiologic agents in the appearance of cervical dysplasia. The evidence available at the present time, however, is only suggestive, since no consistent facts have been brought to light, although epidemiologically this infectious agent is now believed to be the cause of genital infections more frequently than a few years ago.

INFECTION BY PROTOZOA AND CARCINOMA

Trichomonas vaginalis

T. vaginalis infection is usually asymptomatic in men, although the male is the carrier; it is found in the female sexual partners of all carriers.

Trichomonas infection is considered the most widely sexually transmitted disease. It is estimated that 2.5 million people are affected annually in the USA. The incidence among sexually active women is 50–75% (Charles, 1980). The fact that this infection has epidemiologically been found to be more common in women with dysplasia and carcinoma of the cervix than in control groups leads us to consider whether it may be an etiologic factor in neoplastic changes (Meisels, 1969; Szell *et al.*, 1967).

Among 213 patients with cervical intraepithelial neoplasia we found that infection by *Trichomonas* and its pathogenic persistence were found very common. Both the incidence and the persistence of the infection were significantly higher in patients with neoplasia than in the control group (Fig. 2). This finding has led us to hypothesize that the presence of *Trichomonas* and other infectious agents may play an important role in the appearance of neoplasia (Iglesias-Cortit *et al.*, 1982).

No difference in the incidence or persistence of this infection was found, however, among the varying degrees of severity of cervical intraepithelial

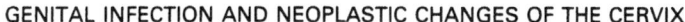

GENITAL INFECTION AND NEOPLASTIC CHANGES OF THE CERVIX

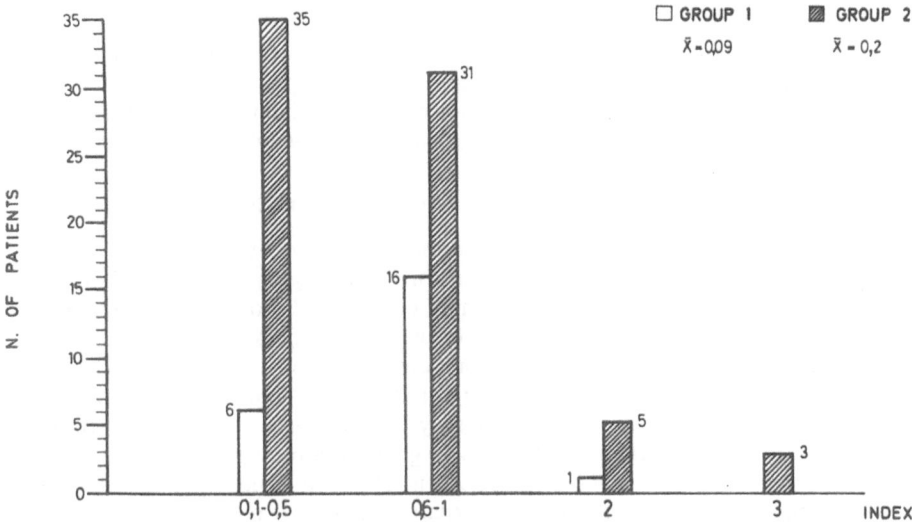

Fig. 2 Incidence and prevalence of *Trichomonas* infection. The number of infections per year was significantly higher in the neoplasia group (Group 2)

☐ TRICHOMONAS
▥ MIXED FLORA
▨ GARDNERELLA

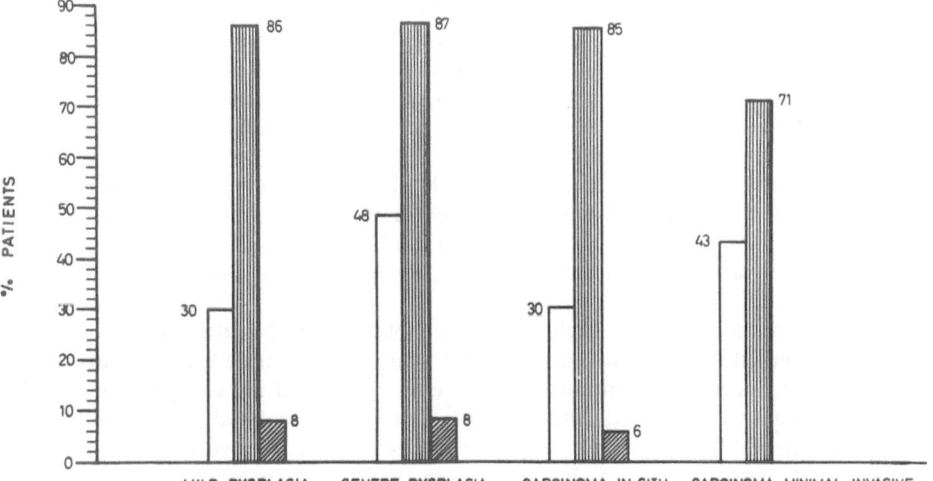

Fig. 3 The frequency of infection in various types of neoplasia. The incidence of infection is similar among the different grades of severity of neoplasia

neoplasia (Fig. 3). We can therefore state that, after the onset of the disease, *Trichomonas* infections do not appear to influence the speed of growth.

OTHER INFECTIONS

According to some authors these sexually transmitted diseases may have some relation to the appearance of cervical dysplasia. This aspect of these diseases, however, has not been studied in depth. In our series we found that nonspecific mixed flora infections were the most common type of infections, both in the neoplasia group and in the control group. The frequency and persistence of nonspecific mixed flora infection, however, was significantly higher in the neoplasia group than in the control group (Iglesias-Cortit *et al.*, 1982).

Control of genital infections as a prophylaxis to CIN

Since carcinoma of the uterine cervix may be a sexually transmitted disease, prophylaxis should be directed towards protection against this type of disease. It is of utmost importance to implement educational programs on this subject in schools, and doctors should be made aware of the possible increased hazards of STDs. Information designed to prevent infection by STDs should also be provided for the general public. High-risk groups should be identified and special efforts applied so that people may be aware of the standards of hygiene necessary to reduce the risk of STDs. In general, however, it is from the high-risk groups that the poorest response is obtained. The condom should be recommended for use among the sexually active as it provides an extremely efficient barrier against STDs.

Screening strategies for the detection of cervical neoplasia should be directed towards incorporating such examinations into the services that people use voluntarily. Since family planning services screen large, apparently healthy, population groups, such centers can provide great support in the discovery and control of cancer of the uterine cervix. In our own population, cervical intraepithelial neoplasia was diagnosed earlier and at less serious stages in patients using oral contraceptives than in those not using the pill (Iglesias-Cortit *et al.*, 1982).

Chemical vaginal contraceptives should also be recommended because they help prevent vaginal infection and disease. It has been shown that some of these preparations prevent the growth of the HSV-2 virus and could, therefore, become of paramount importance in the prevention of the spread of this disease (Singh *et al.*, 1976).

The frequency with which the Papanicolaou test should be conducted is controversial at this point in time. The Walton Committee recommends that it is only necessary to conduct the test every 3 years if the two previous tests were negative. Obviously this is insufficient for the high-risk group, and it is recommended that patients engaging in sexual activity have this test once a year (Richart and Barron, 1981). In those patients where atypical cell changes have been detected the Papanicolaou test should be performed as often as every 3 months (Barber, 1981).

References

Almeida, J. D., Howatson, A. F. and Williams, M. G. (1962). Electron microscopic study of human warts: site of virus production and nature of the inclusion bodies. *J. Inv. Dermatol.*, **38**, 337

Aurelian, L., Cornisti, J. D. and Smith, M. F. (1975). Herpes-virus type 2-induced tumor specific antigen (AG-4) and specific antibodies in patients with cervical cancer and controls. In The, G., Epstein, M. A. and zur Hausen, H. (eds) *Oncogenesis and Herpes viruses*, vol. 2, p. 79. (Lyon: International Agency for Research on Cancer)

GENITAL INFECTION AND NEOPLASTIC CHANGES OF THE CERVIX

Aurelian, L., Davis, H. J. and Julian, C. G. (1973). Herpes virus type 2 induced tumor specific antigen in cervical carcinoma. *Am. J. Epidemiol.*, **98**, 1

Barber, H. R. K. (1981). Uterine cancer (prevention). *Cancer*, **47**, 1126

Baringer, J. R. (1975). Herpes simplex virus in human sensory ganglia. In The, G., Epstein, M. A. and zur Hausen, H. (eds) *Oncogenesis and Herpesviruses*, vol. 2, p. 73. (Lyon: International Agency for Research on Cancer)

Baringer, J. R. and Swoveland, D. (1973). Recovery of herpes simplex virus from human trigeminal ganglia. *N. Engl. J. Med.*, **288**, 648

Bestian, F. O., Rabson, A. S., Lee, C. L. *et al.* (1972). Herpes virus hominis: isolation from human trigeminal ganglion. *Science*, **178**, 306

Boyd, J. T. and Doll, R. (1964). A study of the aetiology of carcinoma of the cervix uteri. *Br. J. Cancer*, **18**, 419

Charles, D. (1980). *Infections in Obstetrics and Gynecology: Viral Infections.* (Philadelphia: W. B. Saunders)

Chiang, W. T., Chen, H. M. and Hsieh, C. V. (1981). Cytomegalovirus infection of the uterine cervix: Local cervical infection and antibody response. *Int. J. Gynecol. Obstet.*, **3**, 19

Ciuffo, G. (1907). Innesto positivo con filtrato di verruca volgare. *G. Ital. Mal. Ven. Pelle*, **48**, 12

Clemmesen, J. (1965). *Statistical Studies in the Etiology of Malignant Neoplasms.* (Kovenhaun: Munksgaard)

Coppleson, M. and Reid, B. (1967). *Preclinical Carcinoma of the Cervix Uteri.* (Oxford: Pergamon Press)

Coppleson, M. and Reid, B. (1968). The etiology of squamous carcinoma of the cervix. *Obstet. Gynecol.*, **32**, 432

Doll, R., Payne, O. and Waterhouse, J. (1966). *Cancer Incidence in Five Continents.* (Berlin: Springer)

Ferenczy, A. (1977). Cervical intraepithelial neoplasia. In Blaustein, A. (ed.) *Pathology of the Female Genital Tract.* (Berlin: Springer)

Gagnon, F. (1950). Contribution to the study of etiology and prevention of cancer of the cervix of the uterus. *Am. J. Obstet. Gynecol.*, **60**, 516

Galloway, D. A., Copple, C. D. and McDougall, J. K. (1980). Analysis of viral DNA sequences in hamster cells transformed by herpes simplex virus type 2. *Proc. Natl. Acad. Sci. USA*, **77**, 2279

Hollinshead, A. C., Chretien, P. B., Lee, O. *et al.* (1976). In vivo and in vitro measurements of the relationship of human squamous carcinomas to herpes simplex virus tumor-associated antigens. *Cancer Res.*, **36**, 821

Iglesias-Cortit, L., Domenech, J. M., Cobo, E. *et al.* (1982). Oral contraceptives and risk of developing cervical dysplasia and carcinoma in situ. *Contr. Deliv. Syst.*, **3**, 115

Kalimo, K., Terho, P., Honkonen, E. *et al.* (1981). Chlamydia trachomatis and herpes simplex virus IgA antibodies in cervical atypia. *Br. J. Obstet. Gynecol.*, **88**, 1130

Kessler, I. I. (1976). Human cervical cancer as a venereal disease. *Cancer Res.*, **36**, 783

Kessler, I. I. (1981). Etiological concepts in cervical carcinogenesis. *Gynecol. Oncol.*, **12**, 57

Lancaster, W. D., Olsen, C., Mein, C. *et al.* (1977). Bovine papilloma virus: Presence of viral specific DNA in naturally occurring equine tumors. *Proc. Natl. Acad. Sci. USA*, **74**, 524

Maliphant, R. G. (1978). Incidence of cancer of uterine cervix. *Br. Med. J.*, **1**, 949

Martin, C. E. (1967). Marital and coital factors in cervical cancer. *Am. J. Publ. Health*, **5**, 803

Meisels, A. (1969). Microbiology of the female reproductive tract as determined in the cytologic specimen. III. In presence of cellular atypias. *Acta Cytol.*, **13**, 64

Meisels, A. and Fortin, R. (1976). Condylomatous lesions of the cervix and vagina. I. Cytologic patterns. *Acta Cytol.*, **20**, 505

Meisels, A., Fortin, R. and Roy, M. (1977). Condylomatous lesions of the cervix. II. Cytologic, colposcopic and histopathologic study. *Acta Cytol.*, **21**, 379

Melamed, M. R., Ross, L. G., Flehinger, B. J. *et al.* (1969). Prevalence rates of uterine cervical carcinoma in situ for women using diaphragm or contraceptive oral steroids. *Br. Med. J.*, **3**, 195

Nahmias, A. J. and Dowdle, W. R. (1968). Antigenic and biologic differences in herpes virus hominis. *Prog. Med. Virol.*, **10**, 110

Nahmias, A. J., Josey, W. E., Naib, Z. M. *et al.* (1970). Antibodies to herpes virus hominis types 1 and 2. II. Women with cervical cancer. *Am. J. Epidemiol.*, **91**, 547

Naib, Z. M., Nahmias, A. J., Josey, W. E. *et al.* (1969). Genital herpetic infection: Association with cervical dysplasia and carcinoma. *Cancer*, **23**, 940

Noonan, C. A. and Butel, J. S. (1978). Transformation by viruses: Simian virus 40 as a model system. *Natl. Cancer. Inst. Monogr.*, **48**, 227

Notter, M. F. D. and Docherty, J. J. (1976). Comparative diagnostic aspects of herpes simplex virus tumor-associated antigens. *J. Natl. Cancer Inst.*, **57**, 438

Orth, G., Breitburd, F., Favre, M. *et al.* (1977). Papillomaviruses: Possible role in human cancer. In Watson, J. (ed.) *Origins of Human Cancer*, p. 1043. (Cold Spring Harbor NY)

Rawls, W. E., Laurel, D., Melnick, J. L. *et al.* (1968). A search for viruses in smegma, premalignant and early malignant cervical tissues: The isolation of herpes viruses with distinct antigenic properties. *Am. J. Epidemiol.*, **87**, 647

Reagan, J. W. and Hicks, D. J. (1953). A study of in situ and squamous cell cancer of the uterine cervix. *Cancer*, **6**, 224

Reid, B. L. and Coppleson, M. (1978). The natural history of the origin of cervical cancer. In MacDonald, R. R. (ed.) *Scientific Basis of Obstetrics and Gynecology*, 2nd edn, p. 427. (London: Butterworth)

Reid, R., Laverty, C. R., Coppleson, M. *et al.* (1980). Noncondylomatous cervical wart virus infection. *Obstet. Gynecol.*, **55**, 476

Reid, R., Stanhope, C. R., Herschman, B. R. *et al.* (1982). Genital warts and cervical cancer. I. Evidence of an association between subclinical papillomavirus infection and cervical malignancy. *Cancer*, **50**, 377

Richart, R. M. (1967). The natural history of the cervical intraepithelial neoplasia. *Clin. Obstet. Gynecol.*, **10**, 747

Richart, R. M. and Barron, B. A. (1981). Screening strategies for cervical cancer and cervical intraepithelial neoplasia. *Cancer*, **47**, 1176

Rojel, J. (1953). Interrelation between uterine cancer and syphilis. *Acta Pathol. Microbiol. Scand.*, **97**, Suppl. 8

Rotkin, I. D. (1967). Sexual characteristic of a cervical cancer population. *Am. J. Publ. Health*, **57**, 815

Schachter, J., Hill, E. C., King, E. B. *et al.* (1975). Chlamydial infection in women with cervical dysplasia. *Am. J. Obstet. Gynecol.*, **123**, 753

Singer, A., Reid, B. L. and Coppleson, M. (1976). A hypothesis: The role of a high-risk male in the etiology of cervical carcinoma. *Am. J. Obstet. Gynecol.*, **126**, 110

Singh, B., Postic, B. and Cutler, J. (1976). Viricidal effect of certain chemical contraceptives on type 2 herpesvirus. *Am. J. Obstet. Gynecol.*, **126**, 422

Smith (1956). Propagation in tissue cult of a cytopathogenic virus from human salivary gland disease. *Proc. Soc. Exp. Biol. Med.*, **92**, 424.

Stern, E., Forsythe, A. B. and Coffelt, C. F. (1977). Steroid contraceptive use and cervical dysplasia: Increased risk of progression. *Science*, **196**, 1462

Stern, E., Lachembruch, P. A. and Dixon, W. J. (1967). Cancer of the uterine cervix. II. A biometric approach to etiology. *Cancer*, **20**, 190

Stevens, J. G. and Wettstein, F. O. (1979). Multiple copies of shope virus DNA are present in cells of benign and malignant non-virus-producing neoplasms. *J. Virol.*, **30**, 891

Stevens, J. G., Nesburn, A. B. and Cook, M. L. (1972). Latent herpes simplex virus from trigeminal ganglia of rabbits with recurrent eye infection. *Nat. New Biol.*, **235**, 216

Stoker, M. and McPherson, I. (1961). Studies on transformation of hamster cells by papillomavirus in vitro. *Virology*, **14**, 359

Strauss, M. J., Shaw, E. W., Bunting, H. *et al.* (1949). Crystalline virus-like particles from skin papillomas characterized by intranuclear inclusion bodies. *Proc. Soc. Exp. Biol. Med.*, **72**, 46

Strohl, W. A., Rabson, A. L. and Rouse, H. (1967). Adenovirus tumorogenesis: a role of viral genome in determining tumour morphology. *Science*, **156**, 1631

Swan, S. H. and Brown, W. L. (1979). Vasectomy and cancer of cervix. *N. Engl. J. Med.*, **301**, 46

Szell, L., Traub, A., Ember, M. *et al.* (1967). Die rolle der trichomoniasis in der Entsteung der Prablastomatosen de portio uteri. *Z. Gynak.*, **89**, 312

Terris, M., Wilson, F., Smith, H. *et al.* (1967). The relationship of coitus to carcinoma of the cervix. *Am. J. Publ. Health*, **57**, 840

Vineberg, H. N. (1919). The relative infrequency of cancer of the uterus in women of the Hebrew race. In *Contributions to Medical and Biological Research*, vol. 2, p. 1223. (New York: Paul B. Hodber)

Wynder, E. I., Cornfield, J., Schroff, P. D. *et al.* (1954). Study of environmental factors in carcinoma of the cervix. *Am. J. Obstet. Gynecol.*, **68**, 1016

Wynder, E. I. and Hoffmann, D. (1967). Relaciones entre la epidemiologia y la carcinogenesis experimental. *Muench. Med. Wochenschr.* (Spanish edition), **5**, 432

zur Hausen, H. (1977). Human papillomaviruses and their possible role in squamous cell carcinoma. *Cur. Topics Microbiol. Immunol.*, **79**, 225

zur Hausen, H., deVilliers, E. M. and Gissman, L. (1981). Papillomavirus: Infections and human genital cancer. *Gynecol. Oncol.*, **12**, 5124

Index